Facial Aesthetic Surgery

"The desire to look young and attractive is no preogative to any one class. The world is made up of a penn' worth of all sorts, and it is not everybody's good fortune to grow more graceful and beautiful in advancing age. The operations for removal of eyelid wrinkles, cheek folds, and fat in the neck are justifiable if the patients are chosen with honest discrimination."

Sir Harold Gillies

Facial Aesthetic Surgery

M. Eugene Tardy Jr., M.D., F.A.C.S.
Professor of Clinical Otolaryngology
Director of the Division of
Facial Plastic and Reconstructive Surgery
University of Illinois Medical Center
Chicago, Illinois
Professor of Clinical Otolaryngology
Indiana University School of Medicine
Indianapolis, Indiana

J. Regan Thomas, M.D., F.A.C.S.
Assistant Clinical Professor
Division of Facial Plastic and Reconstructive Surgery
Department of Otolaryngology-Head and Neck Surgery
Washington University School of Medicine
St. Louis, Missouri
Director
The Facial Plastic Surgery Center
St. Louis, Missouri

Robert J. Brown, B.A.

With Approximately 900 Illustrations

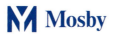

St. Louis Baltimore Boston Chicago London Philadelphia Sydney Toronto

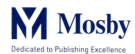
Dedicated to Publishing Excellence

Editor: Robert Hurley
Editorial Asitant: Mia Carino
Project Manager: Nancy C. Baker

Copyright © 1995 by Mosby–Year Book, Inc.

All rights reserved. No part of this publication may be reproduced, stored in a retrieval system, or transmitted, in any form or by any means, electronic, mechanical, photocopying, recording, or otherwise, without prior written permission from the publisher.

Permission to photocopy or reproduce solely for internal or personal use is permitted for libraries or other users registered with the Copyright Clearance Center, provided that the base fee of $4.00 per chapter plus $.10 per page is paid directly to the Copyright Clearance Center, 27 Congress Street, Salem, MA 01970. This consent does not extend to other kinds of copying, such as copying for general distribution, for advertising or promotional purposes, for creating new collected works, or for resale.

Printed in the United States of America
Composition by Clarinda
Color Separator: Clarinda Color
Printing/binding by Walsworth

Mosby–Year Book, Inc.
11830 Westline Industrial Drive
St. Louis, Missouri 63146

Library of Congress Cataloging-in-Publication Data

Tardy, M. Eugene, 1934-
　　Facial aesthetic surgery / M. Eugene Tardy, Jr., J. Regan Thomas,
　Robert J. Brown
　　　　p.　　cm.
　　Includes bibliographical references and index.
　　ISBN 0-8016-6090-4
　　1. Face—Surgery.　2. Surgeery, Plastic,　I. Thomas, J. Regan.
　II. Brown, Robert J. (Robert James), 1960-　　. III. Title.
　　[DNLM: 1. Surgery, Plastic, 2. Face—surgery. 3. Neck—Surgery,
　WE 705 T183f 1993]
　RD119.5.F33T365　1993
　617.5′20592—dc20
　DNLM/DLC　　　　　　　　　　　　　　　　　　　　　　　　　　　　　　　　93-30438
　for Library of Congress　　　　　　　　　　　　　　　　　　　　　　　　　　　　CIP

1　2　3　4　5　6　7　8　9　0　99　98　97　96　95

To teachers and mentors past and present, who planted the seeds of knowledge in facial aesthetic surgery; and to our students and fellows, who challenge our concepts and energize our efforts to teach and learn.

Foreword

Two decades ago few texts existed in the specialty of facial aesthetic surgery; today a large number of publications elaborate the principles and evolving techniques useful in the surgery of appearance.

We endeavor in this book to present a visual text-atlas format of procedures currently favored in our approach to patients requesting facial aesthetic surgery. Strong emphasis and importance is placed on *proper analysis and selection* coupled with the *avoidance of significant risk*. Since patients seeking an improvement in appearance are generally well and healthy, surgery to alter and improve appearance should not render them unwell. We find the procedures described herein to possess outcome effectiveness and minimal risk, producing high patient and surgeon satisfaction. As in all forms of surgery, our surgical approaches continue to evolve and improve with continued learning, experience and careful long-term evaluation of results.

M. Eugene Tardy, Jr., M.D., F.A.C.S.
J. Regan Thomas, M.D., F.A.C.S.

Preface

Patients seeking improvement in appearance constitute a special group of individuals, distinct in many ways from those who suffer illness and seek relief or cure from the physician. Aesthetic surgery patients are generally well and healthy, wishing simply to correct an inherited facial characteristic, improve upon existing facial features or to restore and rejuvenate facial deficiencies relentlessly ravaged by the ageing process. To these essentially well patients the facial aesthetic surgeon owes a very special duty—a distinct and reliable improvement in appearance generated by procedures possessing the least possible risk of injury or untoward outcome.

A calculated balance must be struck between the most aggressive operations advocated by some and less risky procedures designed to result in a safe, clearly definable and lasting improvement. Thus a vital "risk-benefit ratio" exists in any form of aesthetic surgery, from which the experienced surgeon plans, on an individualized basis, the type and extent of procedure(s) best suited to the individual patient. The pithy question remains unanswered: do more aggressive rejuvenation procedures, clearly placing the patient at more risk for complication, produce an obvious immediate as well as long-term improvement, or do less extensive operations, undeniably occasioning less risk, impart a similar or nearly identical favorable outcome? Each position has its advocates—our philosophy lies somewhere in between these two disparate viewpoints. While most texts on aesthetic surgery exist as an advocacy for the author's preferred techniques, we intend in this description to present procedures based upon the individual anatomy encountered in each individual. Emphasis herein is placed on principles and approaches about which the authors share similar philosophies. The type, nature and extent of each procedure will necessarily vary as a consequence of the unique facial features presenting in each patient. We wish to describe our approaches and procedures which, over the years, result in favorable lasting outcomes which satisfy patient's needs and create surgical satisfaction. By no means do we suggest that herein lie the only surgical answers, or even always the best surgical approaches, but we can testify to their success, reliability and significant freedom from serious complication. The latter phrase looms all-important as a cardinal principle in all forms of aesthetic surgery: *avoid making the well patient ill in the attempt to make him look better.* The commonly repeated nostrum—"if you perform enough surgery you will inevitably encounter a wide variety of complications"—is simply not true.

In fact, facial aesthtic surgery, properly planned and executed, carries an amazingly low risk of significant complication and a high rate of patient satisfaction. To be sure the risks and potential complications encountered in all surgery must never be minimized, but happily significant surgical complications continue to be rare. To a large extent, a major premise and intent of this book is emphasize methods of avoiding complications while creating significant appearance improvement.

Unlike other surgical specialties, the visible facial signature of the aesthetic facial surgeon is on constant display for all to appreciate or criticize. Therefore the judicious siting of incisions and preservation of normal facial proportions and balance is an absolute prerequisite to success. It is an accepted truism that pure surgical technical capability will not assure favorable outcomes. A constellation of attributes must be possessed or developed for success in the practice of aesthetic surgery. The following capabilities and compulsive practices should be routine for facial aesthetic surgeons:

1. **Absolute Fastidiousness and Compulsive Attention to Detail**

2. **Sharply-Honed Analysis Skills**
   Exact diagnosis and assessment of normal and abnormal facial features is essential. The ability to develop a mental concept of the "ideal normal" and to envision the final outcome, factoring in the unpredictables of healing, must be refined.

3. **Finely-Tuned Communication and "People" Skills**
   Without question these abilities rank on an equal level with surgical skills. The successful outcome—a satisfied patient—depends as much on the surgeon's willingness to spend time talking with the patient before surgery, as it does the effort expended during surgery.

4. **Thorough Knowledge of the Principles of Aesthetic Facial Surgery and Where They Do and Do Not Apply**
   The exceptions to the rule are often as important as the rule itself.

5. **Compulsion and Resolve to Prepare, Plan and Rehearse**
   The surgical procedure must simply be the final technical reflection of the mental planning process.

6. **Discipline to Individualize Each Procedure Based Upon Precise Anatomy Encountered**

7. **Appreciation of Realistic Risk/Benefit Ratios in Planning Surgical Extent**

8. **Honesty to Recognize Surgical and Anatomic Tissue Limitations**
   The knowledgeable surgeon recognizes the limitations of procedures and does not allow personal ego to overshadow realistic expectations.

9. **Assiduous Long-Term Follow-Up of Patient Outcomes**
   No better form of continuing medical self-education exists.

10. **Willingness to Constantly Teach and Therefore Learn**

    The wise surgeon surrounds himself with younger, eager surgeons, unjaded by tradition and often brighter than the teacher. Continual re-energizing results from this valuable stimulus.

Throughout this text each subject will be considered in the following manner: diagnosis and candidate selection, surgical goals and planned outcomes, surgical techniques, results and outcomes, and sequelae and complications. Through this scheme we hope to provide a more organized disposition to catalyze the learning process for surgeons just beginning their careers as well as for those with long experience. Emphasis will be placed on the total management of the aesthetic surgery patient, including nonsurgical as well as surgical aspects. The ultimate goal of all aesthetic surgery remains clear: a happy patient and a proud surgeon.

M.E. Tardy, Jr., M.D.
J. Regan Thomas, M.D.

Acknowledgments

No volume of this magnitude is possible without the inspiration and superb assistance of many dedicated professionals. Our gratitude for their support and friendship is acknowledged herewith, highly inadequate repayment for their indispensable contributions.

Robert J. Brown, B.A., a master illustrator with few peers.

John Conley, Richard Farrior, Trent Smith, Morrison Beers, Carl Patterson, Bill Wright; inspirational teachers and mentors all.

Frank Kamer, Charles Krause, Tony Bull, Richard Goode, Roger Crumley, George Brennan, Gary Burget, Fred Stucker, Dean Toriumi, Alan Putterman, Bill Nunnery and **Normal Pastorek,** colleagues whose guidance and devotion to excellence is invaluable.

Edward Applebaum and medical photographers **Chet Childs** and **Eric Johnson** for their support and assistance in the Department of Otolaryngology-Head and Neck Surgery, University of Illinois School of Medicine.

Mary Ellen Fitzpatrick, R.N., a devoted, dedicated, uncompromising surgical nurse and medical practice associate, for her keen insight into the human condition and patient motivations, superb ability to generate patient understanding, and for a dedication to excellence.

Patricia L'Odense, who labored daily and diligently to transform our dictated and scribbled thoughts into a polished computer-generated manuscript, tolerating without complaint our many revisions and changes required.

Irene Arima, who provided invaluable contributions through constant storage and retrieval of patient photographs, charts and consent forms, cheerfully engaging with precision in the drudgery of this necessary effort.

Karen Brown, who deserves special thanks for assistance in organization and detail efforts as an invaluable "right-hand man", and gratitude for lending us her husband—the artist—during endless hours of creative illustration development.

James Heinrich and **Eric Lindbeck,** for their willingness as Fellows to review the final manuscript with a fresh and critical eye.

Karen Fell Taeyaerts, who demonstrated that no book is born without the enthusiasm and professional dedication of a talented editor, who through-

ACKNOWLEDGEMENTS

out the creative process provided encouragement and support for a finished product of excellence.

Nancy C. Baker, who with a wonderfully developed aesthetic sense provided judgement and guidance in format, composition and aesthetic development.

Eugenia Klein, who early on generated enthusiasm and encouragement from Mosby for this book, and continues to provide advice, guidance and consultation.

– and finally to our families, for their forbearance and support, and for their continuing forgiveness for the transgression of slides and manuscript drafts creating clutter in otherwise orderly homes.

M.E.T.
J.R.T.

Color Plates

Cover Art Workshop of Antonio Canova, Italian, 1757-1822, *Venus Italica*, c. 1815-22, detail, North Carolina Museum of Art, Raleigh, Purchased with funds from the North Carolina Art Society (Robert F. Phifer Bequest).

Chapter 1 Leonardo da Vinci, *Facing Profiles: A Man and a Youth*, c. 1500, Uffizi Gallery, Florence.

Chapter 2 Auguste Rodin, *La Danaïde*, S.1155 Musée Rodin, Paris, © 1995 Artists Rights Society (ARS), New York/ADAGP, Paris, Photo credit: Bruno Jarret.

Chapter 3 Gustave Courbet, *Jo, the Beautiful Irish Girl*, Photo: National Museum, Stockholm.

Chapter 4 Maxfield Parrish (1870-1966), *Sleeping Beauty*, 1912, Photo courtesy: American Illustrators Gallery, New York.

Chapter 6 Maxfield Parrish (1870-1966), *Egypt*, 1903, Photo courtesy: American Illustrators Gallery, New York.

Chapter 7 Leonardo da Vinci, *Ginevra de' Benci (obverse)*, Ailsa Mellon Bruce Fund, © 1994 Board of Trustees, National Gallery of Art, Washington.

Chapter 8 Peter Paul Rubens, *Portrait of Susanna Lunden (née Fourment)*, detail, Reproduced by courtesy of the Trustees, The National Gallery, London.

Chapter 9 SAG6261 *The Misses Vickers* by John Singer Sargent (1856-1925), Sheffield City Art Galleries/Bridgeman Art Library, London.

Chapter 10 René Magritte, *The False Mirror* (1928), oil on canvas, 21¼ × 31⅞ in. (54 × 80.9 cm.), The Museum of Modern Art, New York, Purchase, © 1994 The Museum of Modern Art, New York.

COLOR PLATES

Chapter 11 Ivan Le Lorraine Albright, American, 1897-1983, *Into The World There Came a Soul Called Ida*, oil on canvas, 1929/30, 142.9 × 119.2 cm., Gift of Ivan Albright, 1977.34, Photograph courtesy of the Art Institute of Chicago.

Chapter 12 Bartolomé Bermejo, *Santo Domingo de Silos entronizado como abad*, N° cat. 1323, ©Museo Del Prado, Madrid. All Rights Reserved.

Chapter 13 Pierre-Auguste Renoir, French, 1941-1991, *Portrait of the Artist's Father, Leonard Renoir, 1869*, oil on canvas, 24 × 18 in., The Saint Louis Art Museum, Purchase.

Chapter 14 Sir Thomas Lawrence, British, 1769-1830, *Mrs. Jens Wolff*, oil on canvas, 1803-15, 128.2 × 102.4 cm., Mr. and Mrs. W.W. Kimball Collection, 1922.4461, Photograph ©1994, The Art Institute of Chicago, All Rights Reserved.

Chapter 15 Auguste Rodin, *La Pensée (Thought)*, S. 1003 Musée dOrsay, Paris, © 1995 Artists Rights Society (ARS), New York/ADAGP, Paris, Photo credit: Bruno Jarret.

Chapter 16 Auguste Rodin, *L'Homme Au Nez Cassé*, S.755 Musée Rodin, Paris, © 1995 Artists Rights Society (ARS), New York/ADAGP, Paris, Photo credit: Bruno Jarret.

Chapter 17 Gerrit van Honthorst, Dutch (1590-1656), *Pastorale*, c. 1627, Gift of the Samuel H. Kress Foundation, The Seattle Art Museum 61.156, Photo credit: Paul Macapia.

Chapter 18 Emile Jean Horace Vernet, French, 1789-1863, *Portrait of the Marchesa Cunegonda Misciatelli With Her Infant and Its Nurse*, 1830, oil on canvas 52 × 41 in., Collection of The University of Arizona Museum of Art, Tucson, Gift of Samuel H. Kress Foundation.

Chapter 19 Diego Velasquez, *The Toilet of Venus (The Rokeby Venus)*, Reproduced by courtesy of the Trustees, The National Gallery, London.

Contents

Foreword vii

Preface ix

Color Plates xv

PART I BASIC PRINCIPLES 1

1 / Nature and Principles of Aesthetic Facial Surgery 2
  Special Characteristics of Aesthetic Surgery 8
  Patient Population 12
  Ambivalence and Uncertainty 14
  The Education Process 17
  Outcome Prediction and Success 20
  Setting 23
  Extended Follow-up 25
  Sequelae and Complications 26
  Reasoned Disengagement 30
  Suggested Reading 32

Appendix A: Plastic Surgery of the Face 33

Appendix B: Authorization and Informed Consent 48

Appendix C: Patient Instructions Following Nasal Plastic Surgery 49

Appendix D: Patient Instructions Following Facelift Surgery 50

Appendix E: Patient Instructions following Blepharoplasty 51

2 / Operating Environment for Facial Aesthetic Surgery 52
  Office-based Operating Facility vs. Hospital-based Operating Room 54
  Physical Surroundings 56
  Conclusion 63

3 / Psychological Assessment of Surgical Candidates 64
  Initial Encounter: A Personal Approach 66
  Candidate Rejection 74
  Suggested Reading 83

4 / Anesthetic Methods: Patient Comfort and Safety 84
  Premedication 87
  Intravenous Anesthesia and Analgesia 87
  Side Effects and Complications 91
  Suggested Reading 93

5 / Uniform Photography in Aesthetic Facial Surgery 94
  Office Photography 100
  Patient Positioning 100
  Frankfort Horizontal Plane 101
  Photographic Background 105

Camera Body 108
Lenses 109
Motor Drive 110
Data-back 112
Film 112
Electronic Lighting 116
Office Photography Suite 122
Summary 123
Suggested Reading 123

6 / **Aesthetics, Analysis, and Judgement** 124
Concepts of Beauty 126
Proportions of the Aesthetic Face 129
Preoperative Facial Evaluation 148
Suggested Reading 153

PART II FACIAL AESTHETIC AND LIFTING PROCEDURES 155

7 / **Forehead-lift** 156
Diagnosis and Candidate Selection 158
Surgical Goals 164
Surgical Techniques 165
Results and Outcomes 186
Sequelae and Complications 190
Suggested Reading 193

8 / **Temporal Lift** 194
Surgical Technique 198
Results and Outcomes 202

9 / **Brow-lift** 208
Surgical Technique 212
Results and Outcomes 219
Summary and Conclusions 221

10 / **Aesthetic Blepharoplasty** 222
Diagnosis and Preoperative Evaluation 227
Surgical Goals and Planned Outcome 233
Surgical Techniques 237
Results and Outcomes 284
Sequelae and Complications 291
Suggested Reading 293

11 / **The Facelift Operation: Principles and Techniques** 294
Diagnosis and Candidate Selection 296
Goals of the Operation 303
Surgical Techniques 304
Results and Outcome 347
Sequelae and Complications 355
Suggested Reading 362

12 / Secondary and Revisional Facelift *364*
   Diagnosis and Candidate Selection   *366*
   Surgical Goals   *367*
   Surgical Techniques   *367*
   Results and Outcome   *374*
   Complications and Sequelae   *378*
   Suggested Reading   *379*

13 / Aesthetic Surgery of the Ageing Neck   *380*
   Neck Rejuvenation   *383*
   Combined Submental Fat and Skin Resection   *400*
   Suggested Reading   *409*

PART III   AESTHETIC AUGMENTATION PROCEDURES   *411*

14 / Chin Augmentation   *412*
   Diagnosis and Candidate Selection   *414*
   Surgical Goals and Planned Outcomes   *418*
   Surgical Technique   *419*
   Results and Outcomes   *427*
   Complications and Sequelae   *430*
   Suggested Reading   *433*

15 / Injectable Fillers   *434*
   Diagnosis and Candidate Selection   *437*
   Goals and Planned Outcomes   *437*
   Technique   *438*
   Results and Outcomes   *440*
   Complications and Sequelae   *437*
   Suggested Reading   *450*

PART IV   RHINOPLASTY IN MIDLIFE AND AGING PATIENTS   *451*

16 / Rhinoplasty in Midlife and Aging Patients   *452*
   Diagnosis and Candidate Selection   *454*
   Surgical Goals and Planned Outcomes   *469*
   Surgical Techniques   *476*
   Evaluation of Results and Outcomes   *509*
   Complications and Sequelae   *525*
   Summary   *526*
   Suggested Reading   *527*

PART V   LIPECTOMY OF THE FACE AND NECK   *529*

18 / Lipectomy of the Face and Neck   *530*
   Diagnosis and Candidate Selection   *532*
   Surgical Goals and Planned Outcome   *534*
   Surgical Technique   *538*

CONTENTS

Results and Outcomes   555
Complications and Sequelae   562
Suggested Reading   564

PART VI ADJUNCTIVE REJUVENATION PROCEDURES   565

19 / Dermabrasion   566
Diagnosis and Candidate Selection   568
Surgical Techniques   569
Results and Outcomes   575
Complications   576

20 / Chemical Peel   578
Diagnosis and Candidate Selection   580
Surgical Goals and Planned Outcome   581
Surgical Technique   583
Results and Outcomes   589
Complications and Sequelae   594
Suggested Reading   597

Afterword   598

Index   599

PART I BASIC PRINCIPLES

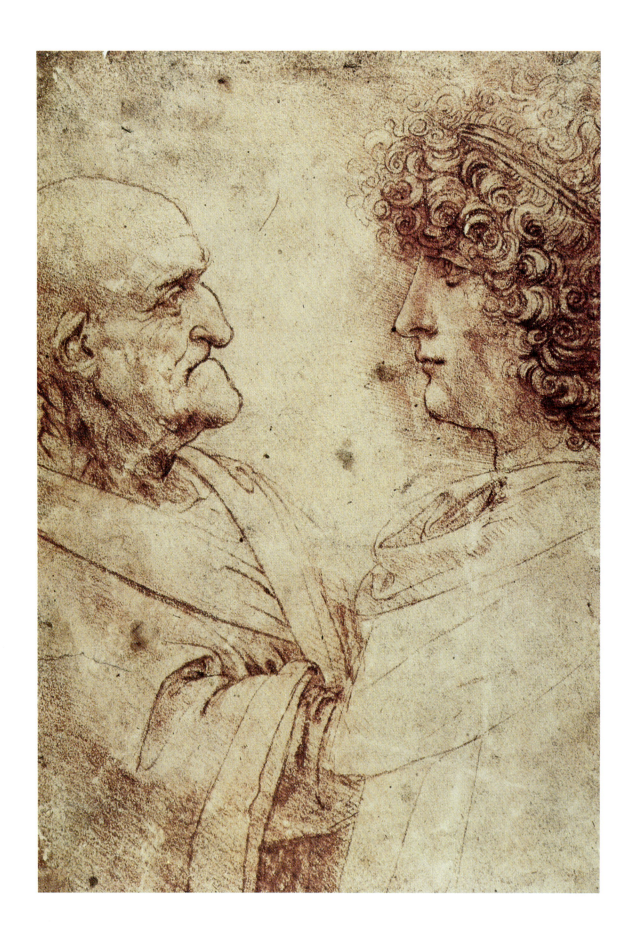

CHAPTER

1

 Nature and Principles of Aesthetic Facial Surgery

PART I   BASIC PRINCIPLES

No spring, nor summer beauty
hath such grace,
As I have seen
in one autumnal face.

John Donne

Aesthetic facial surgery—the science and techniques of improving facial appearance—occupies a unique position among related surgical disciplines: "well" patients request "unnecessary" surgery to make themselves *weller* and *happier*. The surgeon accepting this unique responsibility risks creating an "unwell" patient if a near-perfect surgical procedure and outcome do not materialize. Furthermore, unlike other forms of surgery, aesthetic procedures about the face and neck remain open for immediate and continued critical scrutiny; the surgeon's "tracks" exist as evidence of his skill at incision and scar camouflage, artistic capabilities, and attention to symmetry and proportion. Facial surgery necessarily involves a sometimes ill-defined "risk-benefit ratio" in which the patient accepts a short period of inconvenience and possible slight discomfort to gain the desirable reward of an improvement in appearance and self-image. A similar risk-reward ratio factors into the surgeon's technical plan and execution: how much risk of complication occasioned by more extensive or aggressive surgery is justifiable to obtain a potentially slightly better outcome when a similar result may be achievable by more conservative—and possibly safer—surgery?

The ideal outcome of any aesthetic facial surgery may clearly be defined as a *happy patient* and a *proud surgeon*. Technical excellence alone, however, does not ensure an ideal result. A host of nonsurgical factors as well as the unpredictables of healing factor into the final outcome equation (Fig 1–1). To be able to satisfy the patient requires experience and understanding beyond simple technical expertise. Not infrequently the judgment about when to *refuse* to operate may lead to the happiest outcome. Thus many nonsurgical factors must be considered in the overall care and management of patients seeking appearance improvement; the most successful surgeons must possess both surgical and nonsurgical judgment required for comprehensive care. The best surgeons, in our opinion, are good physicians first and skilled surgical craftsmen second.

Unique to facial aesthetic surgery is the requirement to play close attention to *bilateral symmetry* before and during corrective procedures. With few exceptions, facial plastic surgery procedures require a similar—but not always the same—technical procedure in each half of the face. This holds true even for rhinoplasty, an operation on a midline facial structure. Thus

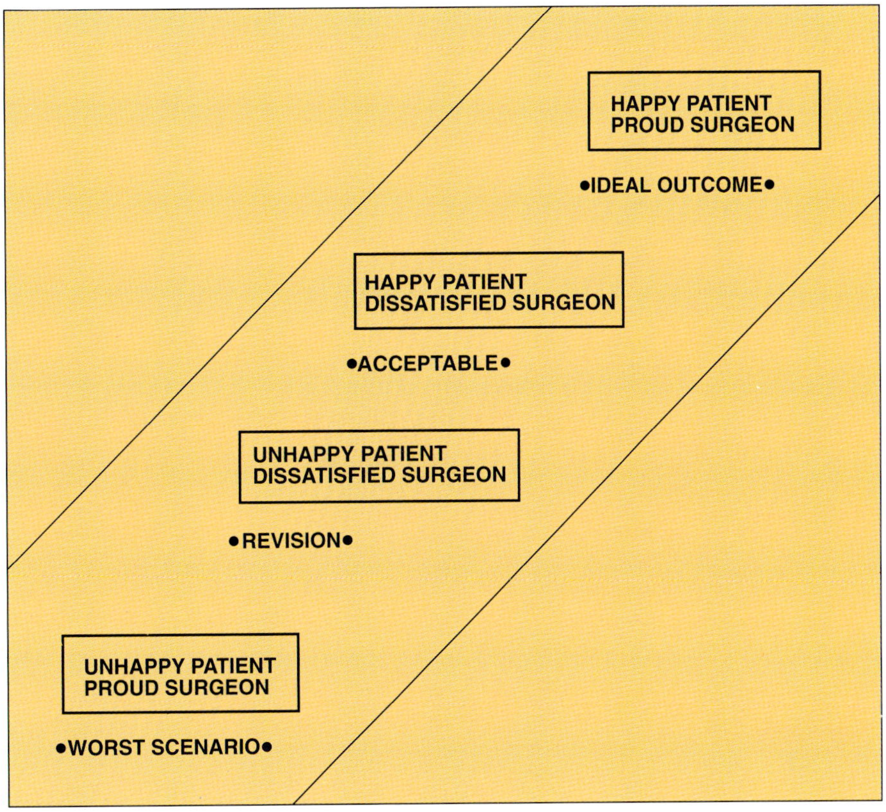

CHAPTER 1   Nature and Principles of Aesthetic Facial Surgery

Figure 1-1
Spectrum of outcomes in aesthetic facial surgery. Fortunately and appropriately, the vast majority of patients indicate extreme pleasure and satisfaction from appearance-changing surgery.

the surgeon must orchestrate a *bilateral operation,* modified as necessary to achieve postoperative *symmetry,* even when imperfect symmetry existed before surgery, a commonplace finding (Fig 1-2). It is astonishing how carefully patients assess symmetry, both in the healing process and after final healing, after being blissfully unaware of facial irregularities before surgery.

Because of its nature, aesthetic surgery is often referred to as "minor surgery," and is not considered serious by patients. This misconception is supported vigorously by lay press hyperbole, which routinely maximizes the glamour of appearance surgery and ignores its serious risks and complexities. This spurious perception, enhanced by little or no postoperative pain, all too often spawns an attitude of inattention to the details of postoperative care instructions, *a vital part of the overall treatment plan.* Patients undergoing surgery to relieve an illness or disorder tend to feel obligated to follow instructions carefully to hasten healing and relieve discomfort.

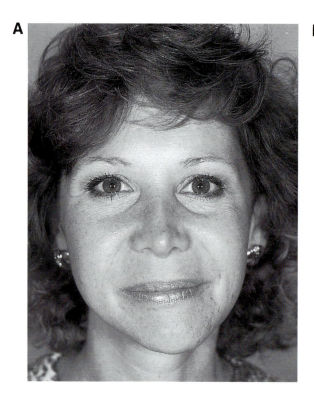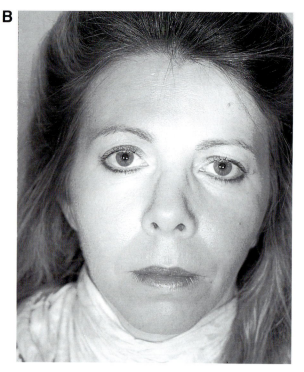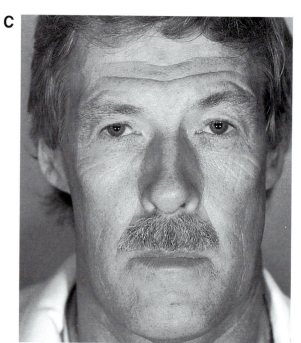

Figure 1–2

A, marked facial asymmetry in a candidate for aesthetic surgery. Mandibular asymmetries are commonplace and must be accurately pointed out and documented for patients before facial appearance surgery is undertaken. **B,** preoperative asymmetries of the jaw, mouth, midface, and nose. Note particularly the different levels of insertion of the alar lobules into the face. **C,** brow and eyelid asymmetries of the upper facial areas in a candidate for rejuvenation surgery. Eyelid asymmetries are the rule rather than the exception in the majority of patients.

CHAPTER 1 Nature and Principles of Aesthetic Facial Surgery

A significant percentage of patients undergoing facial surgery disregard or "stretch" the vital rules relating to postsurgical care and behavior. Strong emphasis must therefore be placed on shared responsibility between the patient and the surgeon for achieving the earliest and best possible outcome. We routinely engage reliable, concerned family members to assist in monitoring the vital discipline of postsurgical care.

The converse of this situation is reflected when a patient is overly concerned and plagued with untoward fear of surgery. This patient's unreasonable anxiety is triggered by isolated anecdotal reports of life-threatening and crippling effects of aesthetic surgery. Although such examples exist, they are indeed rare and are invariably traceable to poor surgical judgment by unqualified or adventuresome surgeons. The simple truth is that millions of patients undergo plastic surgical procedures yearly, with little discomfort, a predictable surgical and postsurgical course, and personally rewarding results.

In the final analysis, facial aesthetic surgery is unrivaled in the surgical disciplines for achieving so much personal satisfaction and pleasure for both the surgeon and the patient. With accurate analysis, precise surgery, and *carefully selected surgical candidates*, both short- and long-term outcomes produce profound gratification.

In his biography of Jacques Josef, the father of modern rhinoplasty, Dr. Paul Natvig reported that "On June 20, 1916 a section for Facial Plastic Surgery opened at the Royal Ear and Nose Clinic of the Charité Hospital in Berlin—the first of its kind."

As quoted in Natvig, Jacques Josef in 1917 wrote the following:

On 20 June 1916, special rooms of the Royal Ear and Nose Clinic (Geheimrat Passav), a Section for Facial-plasty—to my knowledge, the first of its kind—was opened. It was a wartime creation which owes its establishment to the vision and energetic efforts of the Surgeon-General Prof. Dr. Passow. . . .

The following brief report covers the time from 20 June 1916 and 30 June 1917. During this time I have performed 120 plastic facial operations.

As for the nature of the deformities which were treated in the Section, they were for the most part severe disfigurements of the face and, generally, cases which had previously undergone plastic surgery without any success, or with mediocre result. . . .

. . . The discharged patients have all been cured of their psychic depression which the consciousness of bodily deformity always involves. Those still under treatment are making good progress. To my satisfaction I may add that we did not have a single case of death throughout the entire year, which tallies with my experience in private practice.

From this humble beginning, facial plastic surgery has matured and developed, in several related surgical disciplines, to the point where the majority of large universities and urban communities possess aesthetic facial surgeons of high skill and integrity who employ their highly developed specialized talents to provide satisfying fulfillment to patients seeking realistic appearance improvements. Teaching and training in facial plastic surgery are currently formalized and highly structured and produce talented young surgeons of increasing maturity and judgment.

PART I   BASIC PRINCIPLES

Special Characteristics of Aesthetic Surgery

Planned Elective Surgery

The luxury of carefully and methodically preplanning the operative event sets aesthetic surgery apart, to some degree, from exploratory surgical procedures where decisions are made only after analyzing the intraoperative findings. Planning is predicated on detailed and intricate analysis of great accuracy; the inability to perceive the nuances of facial analysis precludes proper correction (Fig 1–3). Examination of the individual patient anatomy, coupled with analysis and reanalysis of standard and uniform photographs, allows repeated mental rehearsal and thoughtful evaluation of planned technical steps. Photographic review with the patient catalyzes the mutual understanding process, informs the surgeon of specific patient

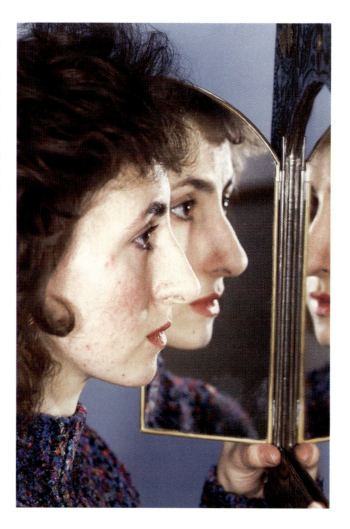

Figure 1–3
Evaluation of the face by using a three-way mirror provides patients views of the face seldom appreciated. Facial asymmetries are pointed out, differences in the two profiles are noted, and approximate degrees of improvement generated by the planned surgery can be explained and demonstrated.

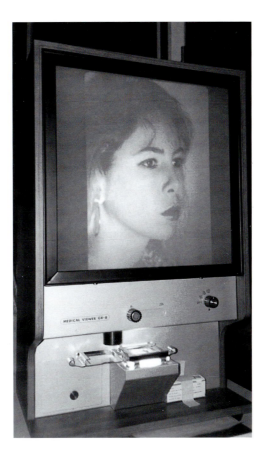

Figure 1–4
Preoperative analysis of patient photographs on a brightly illuminated view screen allows magnification of facial features to greater-than-life-size proportions. Glass screens allow instructive drawings to be made and easily erased after demonstrations to the patient.

wishes and dislikes, and allows a demonstration by the surgeon of the possibilities and limitations imposed by the individual anatomy (Figs 1–4 and 1–5). An artistic approach culminates from the process of surgeon-patient discussions as patients are made aware of previously unrealized facial deficiencies or strengths.

Few surgeons—in fact, probably none—possess the requisite skills to attend to all the skeletal, soft-tissue, dental, functional, and aesthetic changes that are necessary in certain patients. The preplanning process thus allows the luxury and unquestioned benefits of consultation and an interdisciplinary approach to comprehensive overall repair and rejuvenation. In addition to the facial plastic surgeon, the plastic surgeon, ophthalmologist, dermatologist, oral surgeon, dentist, and aesthetician can be enlisted to render valuable capabilities for comprehensive patient care.

Cultural, ethnic, and geographic considerations play a role in the surgery of appearance, an area not dominated by the healthy and wealthy alone. Increasingly, patients of more modest means seek (and certainly deserve) the opportunity to improve their appearance. Many possess a definite preconceived opinion about preserving specific cultural or ethnic features. Planning must factor in these justifiable requests.

Figure 1–5
The common cotton-tipped application serves as a convenient and safe pointer for both the surgeon and patient to identify *specific* wants and needs prior to surgical procedures.

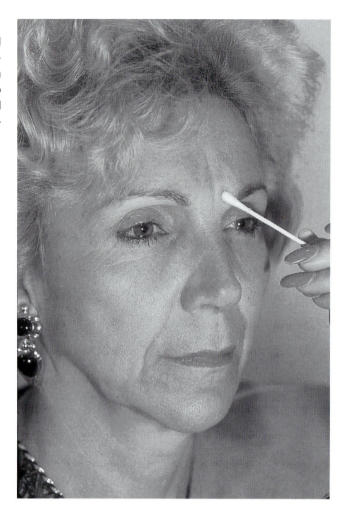

Unlike other forms of surgery, patients and surgeons commonly engage in a graduated programmed "guardian maintenance" protocol in which selective procedures are carried out at appropriate times and in appropriate sequence to best forestall the ravages of aging (Fig 1–6). Unquestionably, the majority of facial rejuvenative and lifting procedures produce the finest and most natural results when planned and carried out before skin elasticity and texture have significantly deteriorated. Generally the surgeon must take the lead in timing the maintenance procedures to reflect the patient's best interest. Chronologic age is a less important factor in determining readiness for rejuvenation surgery than the genetically programmed appearance changes occurring at various periods throughout the patient's life.

CHAPTER 1   Nature and Principles of Aesthetic Facial Surgery

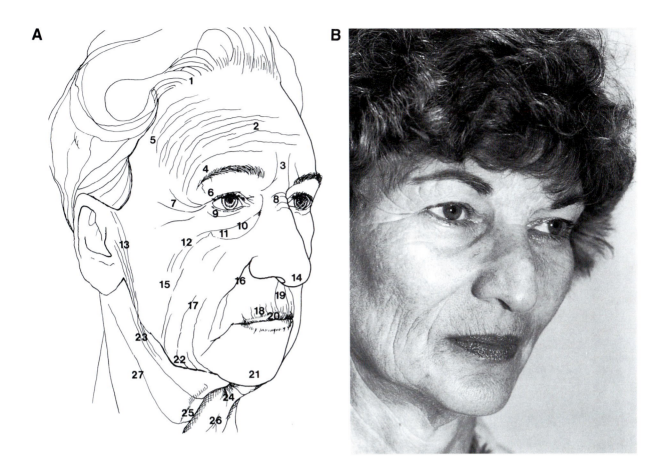

Figure 1-6
A, typical aging changes occurring progressively in facial regions, beginning initially in the orbital eyelid and brow areas and progressing to the remainder of the face and neck: *1,* thinning hair and receding hairline; *2,* forehead rhytids and ptosis; *3,* glabellar rhytidosis; *4,* brow ptosis; *5,* temple rhytidosis and ptosis; *6,* upper lid redundancy and ptosis; *7,* lateral canthal rhytidosis; *8,* nasal root rhytidosis; *9,* lower lid redundancy and rhytidosis; *10,* lower lid fat pseudoherniation; *11,* malar bag formation; *12,* cheek rhytidosis; *13,* preauricular rhytidosis; *14,* nasal tip ptosis and dependency; *15,* cheek sagging and fat atrophy changes; *16,* deepening nasolabial crease; *17,* facial rhytidosis and sagging; *18,* perioral rhytidosis; *19,* upper lip flattening and lengthening; *20,* thinning and atrophy of vermillion (red lip); *21,* chin pad ptosis and retraction; *22,* jowl formation; *23,* cervical rhytidosis; *24,* submental fat accumulation; *25,* platysmal banding; *26,* rhytidosis and midneck hollowing; *27,* submaxillary gland ptosis. **B,** aging patient revealing a constellation of facial features influenced by the aging process.

Patient Population

Surgery to improve appearance suffers from the misperception that predominantly affluent, middle-aged women seek surgery to restore youthfulness and forestall aging. In reality, persons of both sexes and all age groups share the need for improved appearance (Fig 1–7). Men constitute a significant portion of the patient population (Fig 1–8). As the population ages and patients maintain good health longer, much older patients seek to look as good as they feel. Very young patients disturbed by significant congenital problems (e.g., retrognathia, herniated orbital fat, nasal deviation) deserve restorative and corrective appearance surgery (Figs 1–9 and 1–10). Particularly in the young, procedures should be planned and designed with an eye toward the future in the realization that enhanced life expectancy may afford the young patient 60 to 70 years of healthy existence. The choice of safe and appropriate facial implants in the young is therefore vital, and rejuvenation procedures should be planned and executed to achieve a *long-term* favorable outcome (Fig 1–11).

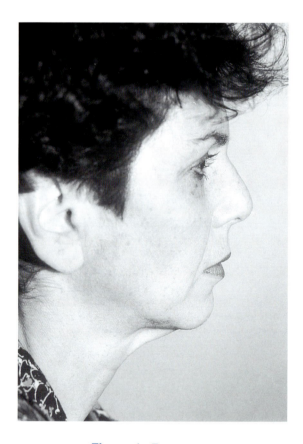
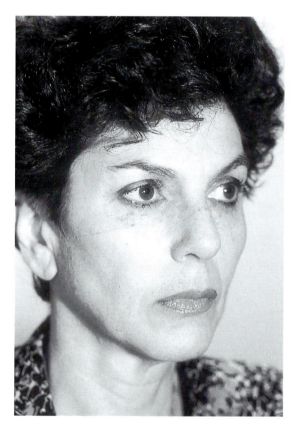

Figure 1–7
A and **B**, early aging change in an ideal female candidate for rejuvenation surgery.

CHAPTER 1 Nature and Principles of Aesthetic Facial Surgery

Figure 1–8
Typical aging characteristics in a male.

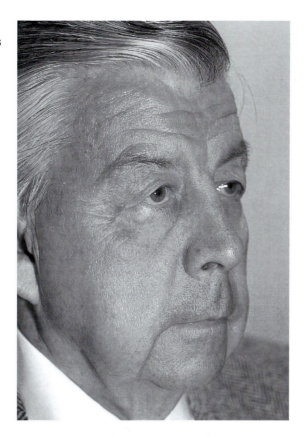

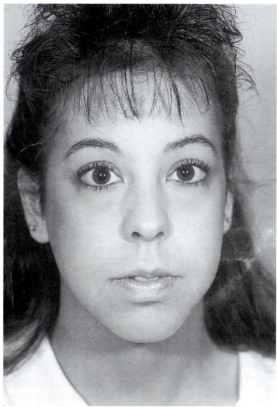

Figure 1–9
Severe familial lower lid fat herniation in a 10-year-old patient. The rejuvenation surgery indicated here is thus not always confined to older patients.

PART I   BASIC PRINCIPLES

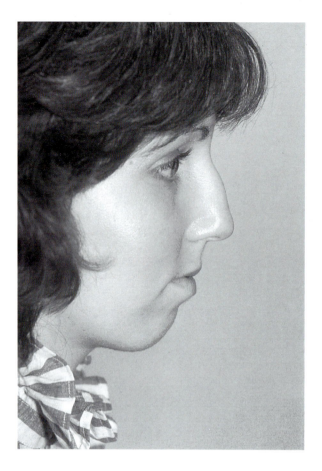
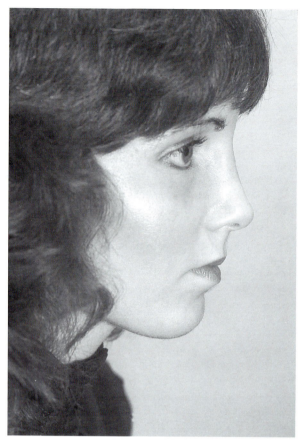

Figure 1–10
The postoperative appearance at 5 years shows significant improvement in the nose and chin of a young patient.

Prospective patients enjoying healthy "golden years" commonly take prescribed (and nonprescribed) medications that may have an unfavorable impact on anesthesia and clotting capabilities. In particular, as a significant percentage of the population consumes daily aspirin (Table 1–1), a careful, specific history and forewarning about the consequences of untoward surgical bleeding are strongly indicated.

Ambivalence and Uncertainty

Patients troubled by appearance, whether a profound abnormality or a minimal subtle deformity, are commonly bombarded by factors that create ambivalence and uncertainty about undertaking to change their appearance. An ill-informed press, family, and friends may combine to cloud the patient's judgment and justification. Spouses ("I love you the way you are

CHAPTER 1 Nature and Principles of Aesthetic Facial Surgery

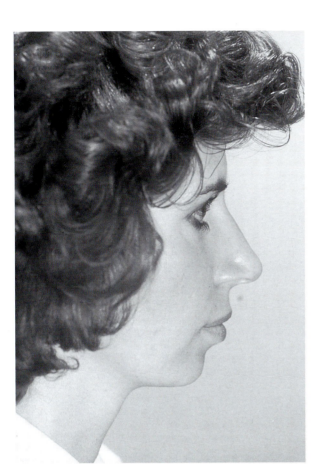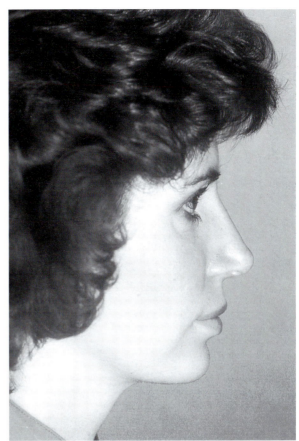

Figure 1–11
Long-term outcome of a chin implant placed in a young patient.

now") often become less than supportive of a genuine need for appearance change. Happily an open and frank preoperative discussion with recalcitrant spouses regularly dispels their concerns and often converts them into a supportive and loyal caregiver. We encourage each patient to allow us to meet and engage in solid informed consent discussions with family and friends before surgery. Significant peace of mind usually prevails after such chats for all concerned (in addition, probably no better form of ethical "marketing" exists).

All surgeons encounter patients who harbor deep-seated guilt about having "luxury" surgery when a close friend or relative is battling cancer or another serious life-threatening illness. Surgical appointment cancellations, at the last moment, may occur as an outgrowth of such forebodings. The surgeon must listen to and be sympathetic to these realistic but occasionally misplaced doubts; if quiet, reasonable reassurance fails to allay such concerns, surgery is always best postponed.

Table 1-1

Aspirin Preparations

Aspirin: oral
Aspergum
Empirin
Norwich
Norwich Extra-Strength Aspirin
Aspirin Children's
Bayer Children's Chewable Aspirin
St. Joseph Adult Chewable Aspirin Caplets
Ecotrin Caplets
Ecotrin Duentric
Genacote
Therapy Bayer Aspirin Caplets
Ecotrin Maximum Strength Caplets
Ecotrin Maximum Strength Duentric
Genacote Maximum Strength
Aspirin Delayed Release Tablets
Easprin
Maxiprin
Megaprin
8-Hour Bayer Timed-Release Aspirin
Measurin
Aspirin SR Tablets
Sloprin
ZORprin
Bayer Aspirin Caplets
Bayer Aspirin Tablets
Genprin
Bayer Aspirin Maximum Strength Caplets
Bayer Aspirin Maximum Strength Tablets

Aspirin: rectal
Aspirin Uniserts

Aspirin with buffers: oral
Buffex
Magnaprin
Arthritis Pain Formula Caplets
Magnaprin Arthritis Strength
Salagen
Ascriptin
Aspirin Tri-Buffered
Bufferin Tri-Buffered Caplets
Bufferin Tri-Buffered Tablets
Ascriptin Extra-Strength Caplets
Bufferin Extra Strength Tri-Buffered
Cama Arthritis Pain Reliever
Inlay-Tab
Alka-Seltzer Effervescent Pain Reliever and Antacid
Alka-Seltzer Flavored Effervescent Pain Reliever and Antacid
Alka-Seltzer Extra Strength Effervescent Pain Reliever and Antacid

Acetaminophen and aspirin: oral
Gemnisyn
Goody's Headache Powders
Gelprin
Goody's Extra Strength Tablets
Supac
Duradyne
Vanquish Caplets
Excedrin Extra-Strength
Excedrin Extra-Strength Caplets

Oxycodone and aspirin—oral
Percodan–Demi
Codoxy
Percodan

Propoxyphene hydrochloride, aspirin, and caffeine
Darvon Compound, 65 Pulvules
Propoxyphene Compound 65

Other aspirin combinations—oral
Fiorinal
Isollyl Improved
Lanorinal
Fiorinal with Codeine No. 3
Dihydrocodeine Bitartrate, Aspirin, and Caffeine Tablets
Synalgos
BC Powder
Stanback Powder
BC Cold Powder Non-Drowsy Formula
BC Cold Powder Arthritis Strength
Butalbital Compound
Fiorgen PF
Fiorinal
Fortabs
Idenal
Isollyl Improved
Lanorinal
Empirin with Codeine 15 mg No 2
Empirin with Codeine 30 mg No 3
Empirin with Codeine 60 mg No 4
Equagesic
Equazine-M
Mepro-Analgesic #2
Meprobamate and Aspirin Tablets
Meprobamate Compound
Micrainin
Talwin Compound Caplets
Ursinus Inlay-Tabs
Gensan
P-A-C Revised Formula
Azdone
Damason-P
Lortab ASA
Momentum Caplets
Axotal
Anacin Caplets
Anacin Tablets
Cope
Anacin Maximum Strength

CHAPTER 1   Nature and Principles of Aesthetic Facial Surgery

There still exists a negative opinion of aesthetic surgery by a small segment of family physicians and internists who fail to understand the demonstrated value of appearance surgery and strongly disapprove or counsel the patient against "tampering with what isn't sick." As Sir William Osler wrote: "It is equally important to make the patient happy as it is to make him well."

The Education Process

Patients seeking aesthetic surgery require a significantly greater investment of consultative time, both before and after surgery, than the usual medical patient. The physician unwilling to devote this added aliquot of direct physician-patient time or who relinquishes or delegates it to others undoubtedly should best seek another line of work. The patient should be made to feel that no question is frivolous or unimportant and that the surgeon is always available for answers.

The educational process in facial plastic surgery may assume much more importance than the surgery itself by alerting patients to reasonable expectations and limitations imposed by individual anatomy. (Remarkably, some of the happiest, most fulfilled and loyal patients are those who did not achieve perfect surgical outcomes but who have been educated to recognize the overall value of the improvement gained; such patients commonly become the most potent referral source.)

We find clear written information provided to patients helpful in three distinct ways:

1. It clarifies and illuminates their often sketchy personal information regarding plastic surgery as a whole and individual procedures in particular.
2. It assists the patient in formulating meaningful questions about a unique situation.
3. It reinforces, in a strongly worded way, the critical importance of paying attention to postoperative care instructions in order to prevent or limit complications of healing.

Accordingly, both before, immediately prior to and after surgery, patients are provided with clear, direct, and logical instructions (see the appendixes to Chapter 1). In reality, the patient and surgeon approach the resolution of a surgical problem as a team, each sharing responsibility for an eventual pleasing outcome.

Much has been written about the philosophy and technique of "informed consent." Clearly, providing patients with a comprehensive "laundry list" of potential complications, including death, accomplishes little. Conversely, failing to provide each individual with sufficient information to arrive at an informed personal decision is equally faulty. The proper approach, in our opinion, lies somewhere between these two extremes and necessarily differs for each patient. Such information, provided accurately and clearly to the patient's contentment, may be considered before surgery as enlightened informed consent; after surgery, it is at best an excuse. We choose to discuss with every patient, in a comfortable, unhurried, relaxed setting, the most common and frequent sequelae and complications and emphasize those that might be more common to the particular case. All questions are encouraged and painstakingly answered. Complications we have never encountered (e.g., death, blindness, paralysis) seem unnecessary to relate, and in fact inappropriate to discuss with the majority of typical patients. In short, no completely correct approach to informed consent can be formulated, because here again the *art* of medicine should prevail and individual judgment be exercised.

At the end of the initial consultation the patient is encouraged to return for further discussions if in fact more personal comfort can be afforded by so doing. Questions posed by phone are welcome and encouraged, and are answered personally by the surgeon, not an assistant. Finally, we encourage all patients, if it adds to their comfort, to seek consultations from other surgeons, provided they select surgeons of integrity and high reputation. If requested, names of highly qualified surgeons are provided. Patients appreciate this forthright courtesy.

Patients are encouraged to return for additional consultation before surgery to review in detail enlarged views of their photographs on a slide-viewing screen. Asymmetries or irregularities often never before appreciated are exposed and discussed in detail. Anatomic limitations are documented and discussed. It remains our policy not to parade a syllabus of the preoperative and postoperative photographs of other patients before an individual contemplating surgery, in the belief that, like the medical record, the photograph is confidential and remains so (specific permission is granted for publishing and teaching purposes). Patients are similarly reassured that their own picture will not be available to others. However, patients whose surgery is complex or involves multiple stages (e.g., forehead flap, scar revision procedures) may be better informed and prepared by seeing what to expect during the course of serial operative and healing events. Such patients are thus shown our published examples of the proposed procedure to prepare them for the events about to occur.

Without question, computer imaging will occupy a position of great importance in the near future. We continue to evaluate available systems, but do not presently use imaging routinely. Whereas certain patients are better informed and reassured by witnessing a computer facsimile of an intended result, others may misinterpret and, despite all admonitions, fail to understand that what appears simple to change with imaging will not always be possible with flesh and bone (Fig 1–12). As the available imaging software becomes more sophisticated and less cumbersome, computer imaging will play a useful role in surgical planning.

CHAPTER 1   Nature and Principles of Aesthetic Facial Surgery

AGREEMENT CONCERNING ELECTRONIC IMAGING

In the course of my consultation, I may have been shown or may be shown pictures on an electronic imaging device (computer). I understand that those pictures and alterations of those pictures are solely for the purposes of education, illustration and discussion in order to more completely inform me about the nature of surgical changes which may or may not be possible. I understand that the outcome of the surgical procedure is directly related to my individual characteristics, as well as personal variabilities in swelling and healing. I understand that because of the significant differences in how living tissue reacts to surgery my final surgical result may not be an exact replication of the video image results shown.

_____   _____
Patient   Date

_____
Witness

Figure 1–12
Disclaimer form recommended by some surgeons who use computer imaging in patient education techniques.

Occasionally an anxious patient can be reassured by speaking directly to a patient who has recently undergone a similar procedure. This request is judged to be reasonable and is honored by arranging a reassuring phone conversation, usually without disclosing patient names. We maintain an office list of previous patients who are willing to fulfill this kindness.

Finally, a significant portion of the preoperative educational process must be expended to respond to questions vital to the patient about nonsurgical topics. Universally patients need clear guidance about the extent and limitations of postoperative physical activities, when exercise and sports may be resumed, how long swelling and bruising may be present, when exposure to the sun is permitted, and when return to work and normal social activities is appropriate. Out-of-town patients need reassurance about travel and flying activities. Strong emphasis is placed on the need for regular and frequent follow-up to monitor postoperative progress and occasionally to make suggestions for proper and appropriate personal care. Almost all patients seeking aesthetic facial surgery request and need sound advice about skin care. We highly value the collaborative efforts of dermatologic colleagues and skin care specialists in this vital aspect of patient treatment.

Outcome Prediction and Success

Although the unpredictables of healing will always plague compulsive surgeons, the surgical outcome of aesthetic facial procedures, carried out in well-selected surgical candidates, remains highly quantifiable and predictable. Complications and untoward sequelae should be rare if careful selection and planning, compulsive surgical technique, and attentive aftercare prevail.

Less predictable is the patient's level of contentment and satisfaction with the surgical outcome. The ultimate goal, as previously indicated, is to achieve a result characterized by a happy patient and proud surgeon (see Fig 1–1). Patient contentment, however, assumes that the individual expectation level, often difficult to completely comprehend, has been achieved without compromise. Success is perceived by some as an improved appearance without significant discomfort or surgical sequelae. The majority of patients desire the development of a natural postoperative appearance without visual evidence that restorative surgery has been carried out (Fig 1–13). Others, however, tend to find success and contentment only when favorable comment occurs from friends or family; without such comments, disappointment may ensue. *Without question, the most difficult aspect of rejuvenative surgery exists in the preoperative quest to clearly define the expectation level and appropriate motivational factors prompting patients to seek appearance enhancement.* Although an operation may be a technical success, it may not always achieve the elusive, often ill-defined goal of "happiness."

CHAPTER 1   Nature and Principles of Aesthetic Facial Surgery

> *Dear Dr. Tardy,*
>
> *Here is the article I mentioned to you. You can see that I would not dare let you read it before my surgery. You may have tried to retaliate!*
>
> *It is written in the "voice" of some of my northshore clients. Surely they must come to you too!*
>
> *My face looks great...and my friends say I look better than Marilyn Monroe at 20!*

EYELIFT DIARY

Wednesday afternoon

Sure you feel a little nervous. I mean it's like going to a new beauty shop, it's the same thing. You know how you feel. You don't know if this guy is scissors happy or will get your color wrong or what.

They are so deadly serious in this hospital. I mean they take blood, do x-rays, heart stuff, like you were having an operation or something. And, they want payment in advance. Just like that doctor. What do they think you're going to die and not pay the bill or something? Well, it will be all over tomorrow and that will be a relief. My eyeshadow has been clumping on my lids forever, and let's face it, Erase is just not doing it for my bags anymore. Like I was telling my sister the other day, after 30 it's patch, patch, patch. And, I mean, as you get older, you have to take some time for yourself. I go to the health club every morning, and once in a while you have to take a whole day off to have your eyes done.

Good, I have a private room and a view. And the phone is on. Have to call the office for my messages.

Wednesday night

My girlfriend Ruthie finally arrived with the martinis and some snacks and we were sitting around laughing when this resident doctor walked in. He spoke very poor English, and he wanted to know when I first noticed my condition. I told him my eyes started falling about 40 years ago, right after I was born. These foreigners have no sense of humor. Well, I hope I can sleep. This bed is terrible.

Thursday morning

Some of these nurses really throw their weight around. One came in this morning and had a fit because I was smoking a cigarette. I mean what do they expect you to do when they wake you up banging around in the hall at 6 A.M.? This same one wouldn't even give me a cup of coffee, let alone a bit of breakfast, and at these prices. It's a disgrace.

Anyway, the anesthesiologist came in just about this time, another foreigner, but at least this one was a woman. You'd think she'd be a little more understanding. I told her, look, I am not into pain. I don't want to feel a thing, I mean, out is where I want to be for the whole thing. She said I was not having a general, which I do not remember being informed about, and if she gave me too much I could stop breathing. So, I said, just keep me breathing a little. Wow, you have to tell these people their own business. It's really something.
The guy who came with the stretcher was very rude. I tried to explain to him that I was talking to a very important client on the telephone about his third honeymoon. His new bride has asthma and it was urgent that I get them seats as far forward as possible in the nonsmoking section, but he wouldn't listen. First things first. Actually, it was just as well he interrupted me, because around this time I started to feel a little funny, maybe from the shot they gave me. I hope I didn't give him the wrong seat numbers. I'll have to recheck it later today.

On the way down to the operating room, I noticed how those walls could really use a good coat of paint and I made a mental note to mention it to the doctor when I saw him. I mean, he's on the board and I'm sure he'd appreciate my input.

> Oh, here he is. Boy, green is definitely not his color. He ought to have his colors done like I did. It really makes a difference. Hey don't push, I can move over myself.
>
> **Thursday afternoon**
>
> ...crying, can't stop crying...what time is it? Take these off...can't see, better no. I can walk myself to the bathroom, leave me alone. Mirror, who is that? What have they done? Bloody stitches...swollen ...hurts. Help me...weak.
> WHY DIDN'T SOMEBODY TELL ME THIS WAS AN OPERATION?
>
> **Thursday**
>
> I know I said I'd be in today, but I wouldn't even put my hand outside the door to reach for the mail. Let me tell you, I am a mess. I hope they got the license of that truck.
>
> Anyway, when I got home, I had my lawyer on the phone right away. He had the nerve to tell me to read what I signed. Give me a break. I have enough to read for my business as it is. I now know I made a colossal mistake. I mean, I sent this client to the Cayman Islands and she had the entire face done and she said it was a nothing. And, cheap as dirt. It was like a regular vacation. Something about the salt water healing everything up in one day.
>
> **Two weeks later**
>
> Yeah, I told you, I had my eyes done. Believe me, it is just a small procedure. A piece of cake. You really ought to think about doing it. But, call my doctor. He charges half a fortune, but I'm telling you, he's terrific. I mean you go to Loehmanns for your clothes, but not your face. Ruthie and I will come over and we'll have a party the night before, but I mean, do it. It's a NOTHING!

Figure 1–13
Amusing but amazingly insightful letter received from a wonderfully observant patient. In a short diary this individual has clearly illuminated the fears, concerns, misinformation, misunderstandings, and preconceived notions rather common to many patients undergoing aesthetic surgery. Despite herculean efforts at total informed consent, patients often fail to list or avoid contemplating the serious nature of all surgical procedures.

Again, sufficient time must be expended to reassure a patient whose expectations may have been elevated above what was surgically possible. Uniform and standardized photographs are invaluable in this situation, because comparisons of before and after photographic documents display irrefutable improvement.

Temporary disenchantment may develop in patients who undergo similar procedures on the same day and request to room together. Invariably, even though similar operations may vary considerably from patient to patient, early concern and disappointment may surface as one patient notes more or less swelling or bruising, more or less discomfort, a slightly different bandage, or even different postoperative orders. We seek to avoid setting the stage for this vexing problem by providing different rooms and individualized attention for each patient. A substantial degree of happiness and satisfaction prevails in at least 95% of carefully selected patients for aesthetic surgery, which marks this field as one of the most satisfying and rewarding in all of medicine.

CHAPTER 1　　Nature and Principles of Aesthetic Facial Surgery

Setting

Most patients profess an aversion for the traditional medical setting, often characterized by aromas of alcohol and disinfectants, polite but abbreviated interviews, spartan and primarily functional furnishings, and year-old magazines. While an opulent office setting seems as likely to "turn off" the typical patient as to inspire him or her, a degree of tastefulness and relaxed comfort must be achieved without overwhelming expense (Fig 1–14).

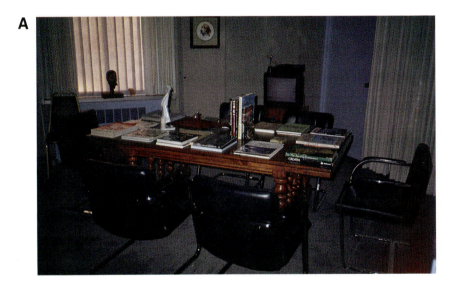

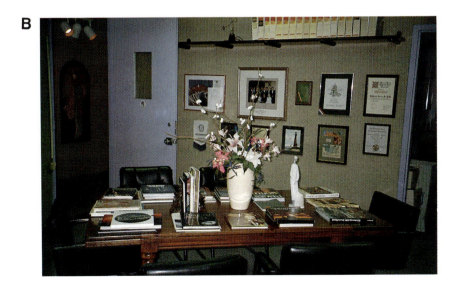

Figure 1–14
A, a comfortable, attractive, and functional but nonopulent waiting room area stocked with interesting books rather than magazines establishes a pleasant setting for patients. **B,** conference room ideal for discussions with patients and families. Facilities are provided here for projection and analysis of patient photographs during preoperative discussions in a relatively nonclinical setting.

Perhaps the most critical and vital element of the office setting remains the nonphysician employees, whose attitude, cheerfulness, sincerity, and intelligence pay high dividends in patient satisfaction and loyalty (Fig 1–15). A wise surgeon seeks the best staff available, compensates them generously, and ensures that they feel a vital part of the health care team and are devoted to achieving patient improvement and contentment.

A primary complaint of patients—and rightfully so—results from inordinate waiting periods in a busy office. Because candidates for aesthetic surgery always require an investment of time beyond that of the patient with a minor illness, great care should be taken to schedule sufficient appointment periods to accommodate this need. The patient's time is equally as important as the surgeon's. Under no circumstances should the surgeon not keep to time in a compulsive manner. In those rare instances where emergencies or unexpected delays occur, a personal apology is proper and appreciated.

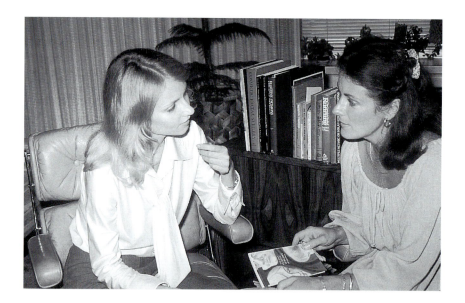

Figure 1–15
Patients benefit from and greatly appreciate discussions with well-informed and concerned office personnel. Questions and issues never discussed with the surgeon often emerge in this setting and lead to a greater degree of truly informed consent.

CHAPTER 1   Nature and Principles of Aesthetic Facial Surgery

Extended Follow-up

The tendency exists among certain surgeons engaged in aesthetic plastic surgery to regard the operative event as the end of the doctor-patient relationship, often relegating postoperative care (e.g., suture removal, photography) to office personnel. Those who engage in this questionable practice lose a valuable opportunity to personally learn from self-confrontation of the dynamics of the healing process, *a vital feedback mechanism allowing necessary modifications of surgical techniques for optimum outcome.* Attending to the "little things" concerning patients in the early and later postoperative period breeds a high level of patient contentment; relegating this responsibility to someone else is poor judgment. We encourage patients to return frequently in the first year following surgery, and for some procedures, notably rhinoplasty, where the evolution of healing continues to change for many years, a much longer follow-up at yearly intervals is encouraged. Unique and infrequently performed procedures should also require more frequent and prolonged follow-up. One of the most critical attributes to be developed by the facial surgeon is the ability to successfully and satisfactorily reassure and mollify a patient concerned about the healing process until sufficient time has ensued to allow healing to be complete. Failure to do so sets the stage for early abandonment of the surgeon; an unrealistic, anxious, and disenchanted patient, who may in fact be experiencing a superb outcome, may seek the services and counsel of another surgeon.

Frequent phone calls to patients in the early postoperative period are reassuring to patient and surgeon alike. The surgeon finds value in the reassurance that instructions are being followed to the letter, and the patient enjoys the attentive concern. With particularly anxious or difficult patients, daily phone calls combined with frequent office follow-up pay significant positive dividends. We routinely provide our home phone number for patients as an additional gesture of availability; this privilege is rarely abused.

Sequelae and Complications

Despite every best effort, unexpected complications and sequelae of surgery will develop in a small percentage of patients (the principles and techniques documented in the following chapters are principally aimed at the avoidance of complications, a vital concern in surgery performed upon healthy, well patients who seek to be better, not worse). A clear differentiation must be drawn between sequelae, which are normal after every operation (Fig 1–16), and complications, which are unanticipated detrimental occurrences (Fig 1–17). Examples of normal sequelae include temporary hypoesthesia or dysesthesia after flap undermining (facelift, foreheadlift), redness and itching of scars, swelling and ecchymosis, and in the case of rhinoplasty, temporary stuffiness. True complications of surgery are uncommon and represent an unplanned event that may disturb or delay healing, compromise the ultimate result, and even make the patient worse than before the procedure.

No matter how well informed, the patient experiencing a postoperative complication experiences to varying degrees the twin emotions of anxiety and anger. It now becomes vital that the surgeon acknowledge and explain the ramifications of the complication and develop a means of treatment to correct or minimize the complication's impact. *Ignoring or cavalierly minimizing the patient's anxiety provides a sure pathway to patient alienation.* Communication now looms even more important, with the time expended in patient conversation before surgery to cement the doctor-patient relationship becoming ever more valuable. Patients experiencing a complication should be seen and talked to by phone frequently, with even more attention to the problem than might be given to a similar problem developing after nonaesthetic surgery. The art of medicine assumes the greatest importance in this situation to minimize the impact of the complication on the patient's procedure as well as psyche.

It is always helpful, as an adjunct to appropriate postoperative care, to involve the patient in some manner, no matter how small, in his own care. Such involvement may include seemingly mundane acts: frequent gentle massage, application of ointment, specific exercises. Consultation with knowledgeable sympathetic colleagues is highly useful and demonstrates to the patient that every effort is being sought to achieve the desired improvement. High interpersonal communications skills may be necessary to convince the patient of the futility, and possible significant untoward effects, of too early interventional surgery. (Witness the common problem of the disenchanted postrhinoplasty patient who arm-twists the surgeon into repeated revisions within short periods. Invariably the ultimate outcome is compromised beyond satisfactory repair.) It is always reassuring

CHAPTER 1 Nature and Principles of Aesthetic Facial Surgery

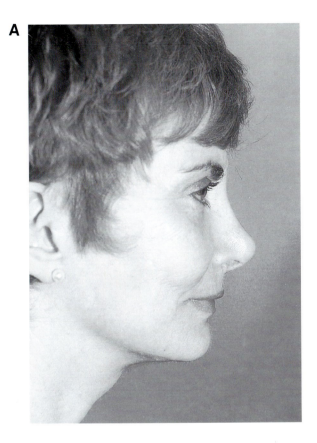

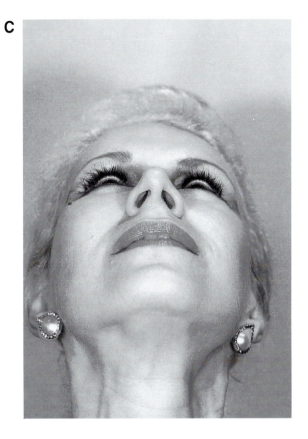

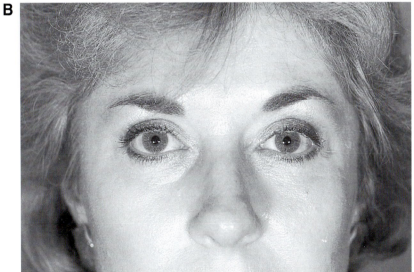

Figure 1-16
Scars represent the necessary sequelae of rejuvenation surgery and, as long as they are carefully camouflaged, are acceptable trade-offs for improved appearance. **A,** typical preauricular scars 1 year following a facelift. **B,** typical upper and lower lid blepharoplasty scars 10 months following surgery. **C,** inconspicuous submental scar 4 months after submental lipectomy.

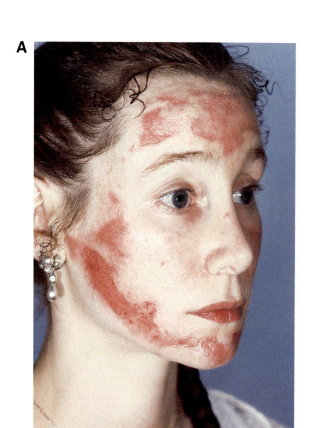
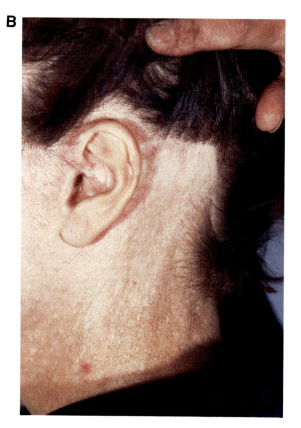
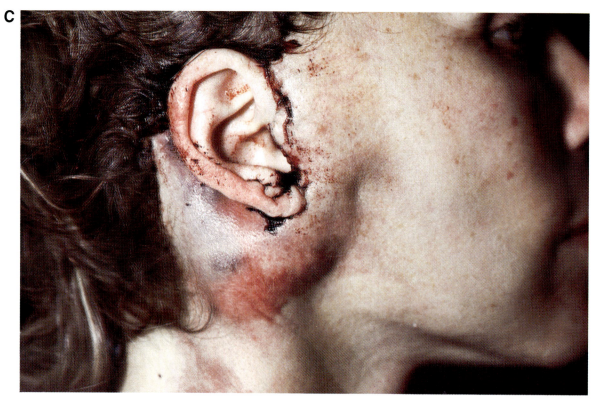

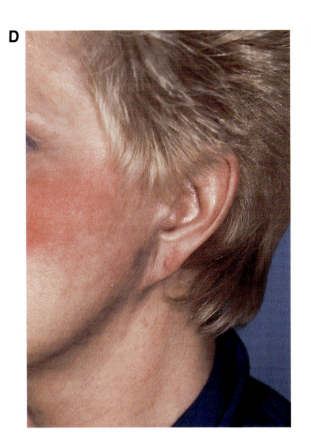
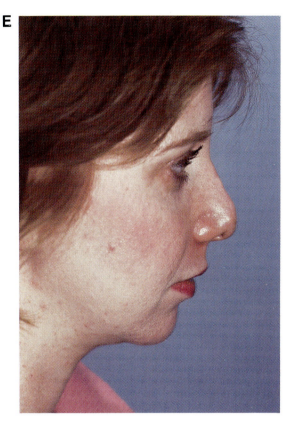

Figure 1–17

A, a patient treated elsewhere demonstrates the significant and severe complication of chemical peeling several months after the procedure. **B,** preventable complication of facelift surgery in which the treating surgeon has lifted the posterior hairline to an unacceptably high level and left unsightly and widened scars. **C,** early postoperative nonexpanding hematoma in a facelift patient. **D,** satyr ear deformity, a preventable complication having occurred here as a consequence of the treating surgeon placing too much pull on the facial skin closure with inadequate support of the underlying layer of the superficial musculoaponeurotic system (SMAS). **E,** severe nasal tip ptosis and associated nasal deformities in a patient operated on elsewhere.

to note that patients managed through a complication with sensitivity and careful attentiveness regularly become the surgeon's greatest advocate despite an unexpected and less-than-perfect course.

The significant and real dilemma of financial consequences arises when revision surgery becomes necessary. Opinions vary among surgeons as to the propriety of charging for procedures designed to correct or revise the flawed result. Some advise that not charging may give the appearance of an admission of a personal surgical shortcoming. Others make a case for reducing the fee and charging for "my time" only. We do not presume to possess the final answer to this dilemma but do feel strongly that operations performed to revise our own surgical procedures should be provided for the patient at no cost as a gesture of good will and concern. A satisfied patient is much more vital to the stature, reputation, and peace of mind of the aesthetic surgeon than the collection of a small fee.

Reasoned Disengagement

The surgeon with a busy practice will regularly encounter patients who harbor unrealistic expectations, unreasonable requests, or inappropriate anatomy for the procedure requested or, more commonly, simply are "unlikable" and even argumentative. Gentle disengagement without totally alienating such patients represents an art in itself. As the aphorism states: You make your living from patients you operate on, and your reputation from those on whom you refuse to operate. All surgeons can recall patients whose motivations were borderline or suspect, who after surgery were clearly unveiled as poor emotional candidates, demanded unreasonable results, or become increasingly unpleasant without justification. Such patients commonly provide clues to misbehavior by demeaning or degrading comments to the office staff; we rely heavily on the sensitivity of experienced staff to forewarn us about such recalcitrant individuals. Not all individuals, after all, make suitable candidates for appearance-changing surgery. To detect such individuals and to decline to operate without totally alienating them remain an art form.

Honesty is always the best policy. The person eager for surgery that is clearly not indicated should be gently informed of that fact and made to understand why. (It is not uncommon to spend more time explaining to the patient why surgery should *not* be done than in explaining what *should* be done). Insistent patients may be advised—very reasonably so—that you do not possess the skills necessary to achieve the result demanded. No surgeon should feel reluctant to admit that another surgeon may be better qualified. It is totally within reason to provide the patient with names of colleagues of high reputation whose opinion you value and suggest consultation. Although such patients may eventually ferret out a surgeon willing and eager to perform surgery, they seldom find satisfaction.

If, as occasionally occurs, we are uncertain about developing a strong and healthy relationship with a prospective patient, photographs are taken and the patient urged to return after the surgeon has had time to carefully study and contemplate the surgical possibilities. If the patient fails to return, the problem is solved. If a second visit does occur, demonstrating photographically the limitations of surgery may convince the patient of the futility of proceeding. A firm sincere discussion of the increased risk of complications and the risk-reward ratio concept may dissuade an overly eager candidate. Although this process may be time-consuming, in a sense it simply represents good judgment. It remains surprising how often patients who are politely refused surgery become prime referral sources of patients who are ideal candidates for surgery. A surgeon unwilling to expend adequate time with such patients undoubtedly will find greater fulfillment in a different specialty.

Finally, the patient whom you truly find "unlikable" (inevitable in any large practice setting) should be gently but firmly disengaged from without compromise. No surgeon, after all, has a duty to perform aesthetic surgery on every patient requesting it. It is always better to avoid surgery in this circumstance than pay the agonizing penalty sure to surface later. We simply advise such patients that the physician-patient relationship in aesthetic surgery is a bond that becomes vital in the overall management of the problem. We point out that a certain comfort level must be developed and nurtured throughout and that, for perhaps unexplainable reasons, we do not feel comfortable in proceeding with procedures either unnecessary or nonindicated. The patient is thanked for the confidence shown in consulting us and apologized to for the fact that we do not feel qualified or well suited to act as the patient's surgeon.

In the final analysis, managing patients seeking appearance improvement involves **qualifications**—the judgment and skills required to achieve a mutually satisfactory outcome, and **integrity**—the rigid adherence to a code of behavior and honesty.

Anything else remains less than ideal.

Suggested Reading

- Goin JM, Goin MK: *Changing the Body: Psychological Effects of Plastic Surgery.* Baltimore, Williams & Wilkins, 1981.
- Goldwyn RM: Aesthetic surgery: Basic principles, in Regnault P, Daniels R (eds): *Aesthetic Plastic Surgery.* Boston, Little, Brown, 1993, pp 31–44.
- Goldwyn RM: *The Patient and the Plastic Surgeon.* Boston, Little, Brown, 1981.
- Lederer W: *The Fear of Women.* New York, Grune & Stratton, 1968.
- McKinney P, Cunningham BL: *Aesthetic Facial Surgery.* New York, Churchill Livingston, 1992.
- Natvig P: *Jacques Joseph—Surgical Sculptor.* Philadelphia, WB Saunders, 1982.
- Osler W: *Aequanimatas.* New York, McGraw-Hill, 1906.
- Potts WJ: *The Surgeon and the Child.* Philadelphia, WB Saunders, 1959.
- Rees TD: *Aesthetic Facial Surgery.* Philadelphia, WB Saunders, 1980.
- Tardy ME, Klingensmith M: Refinements in facelift surgery, in Roenigk RK, Roenigk HH (eds): *Dermatologic Surgery.* New York, Marcel Decker, 1989.
- Tardy ME, Brown R: *Surgical Anatomy of the Nose.* New York, Raven Press, 1991.
- Tardy ME: *Principles of Photography in Facial Plastic Surgery.* New York, Thieme-Stratton, 1992.
- Wright MR: The male aesthetic patient. *Arch Otolaryngol Head Neck Surg* 1987; 113:724.

CHAPTER 1 Nature and Principles of Aesthetic Facial Surgery

APPENDIX

A

PLASTIC SURGERY
of the
FACE

CONTENTS

FOREWORD

FACIAL PLASTIC SURGERY—FACT AND FICTION

THE CONSULTATION FOR PLASTIC SURGERY

OUTPATIENT PLASTIC SURGERY

POSTOPERATIVE CARE

FEES

A REALISTIC ATTITUDE

RHINOPLASTY: PLASTIC SURGERY OF THE NOSE

MENTOPLASTY—CORRECTION OF OVERDEVELOPED OR
UNDERDEVELOPED CHINS

OTOPLASTY: CORRECTION OF PROTRUDING EARS

SCAR CAMOUFLAGE—IMPROVING FACIAL SCARS AND BLEMISHES

DERMABRASION—SURGICAL "SANDING"

SURGERY OF THE AGING FACE—IMPROVING APPEARANCE

BLEPHAROPLASTY—EYELID PLASTIC SURGERY

BROWLIFT—CORRECTION OF SAGGING EYEBROWS

SUBMENTOPLASTY—CORRECTION OF A "DOUBLE CHIN"

RHYTIDOPLASTY—FACELIFT

COLLAGEN (ZYDERM) AUGMENTATION

THE RISKS OF PLASTIC SURGERY

PART I   BASIC PRINCIPLES

FOREWORD

The decision to undergo aesthetic (cosmetic) facial surgery is a most personal and important one that requires the utmost in mutual understanding and rapport between the patient and surgeon. Fortunately, this form of plastic surgery is largely *elective,* thereby allowing the patient adequate time to thoroughly understand the details and ramifications of any desired procedure.

To this end I and my office staff devote a considerable amount of time and effort to each patient to ensure that all questions are answered in detail and that each patient approaches surgery with a degree of confidence and expectation born of a realistic understanding of the goals and limitations of surgery.

To prepare you for our discussions and objective evaluation of your own *individual* problems and wishes, **this monograph should be reviewed carefully in advance of your surgical consultation.** Although not all portions will apply to your particular problem or desired operation, certain *general principles apply to all facial aesthetic procedures.* A greater understanding of these principles will assist you in defining more specific and meaningful questions during our consultation and examination. As you read, jot down any questions you may have—they will always be explained and clarified to the best of our ability. Undoubtedly, there will exist individual variations between the general details discussed in this monograph and the specific recommendations to be made for your own *personal* benefit.

Finally, you should remember that the facial plastic surgeon is a highly trained, skilled, and artistic physician, not a miracle worker. *The degree of success depends not entirely on his technical skills and analysis, but often upon the limitations inherent in each patient's type of skin, bone structure, and healing capacities.* If any limitations exist in your case, they will be pointed out and explained—factually and honestly. Certain patients are simply not good candidates for surgery and may be understandably disappointed when plastic surgery is not recommended (or is delayed until a more appropriate time when results will be better).

The objective of cosmetic surgery is to make you look as good as it is possible for you to look. Surgery cannot do more than that. If you are expecting a transforming miracle from surgery, you more than likely will be disappointed. Plastic surgery is a combination of art and science and as such can be subject to unpredictables—usually minor in nature. Fortunately, the overwhelming majority of plastic surgery results are highly satisfactory and pleasing when accompanied by careful presurgical planning, meticulous surgery, and full patient cooperation. **The goal of the surgeon is to produce "natural" facial features,** thereby improving appearance and minimizing any facial abnormality. Cosmetic surgical procedures have been repeated successfully many thousands of times and are overwhelmingly dependable when carried out by experienced surgeons.

Please understand that the purpose of this informational booklet is exclusively to provide you with information and knowledge upon which intelligent decisions may be made. *No portion should be construed as implying a warranty or guarantee of any specific surgical result—a practice that no ethical or responsible surgeon would follow.*

I urge you to read this booklet carefully because it will provide you with an understanding of many of our office policies and procedures.

M. EUGENE TARDY, JR., M.D., F.A.C.S.

FACIAL PLASTIC SURGERY—FACTS AND FICTION

What Is It?

Plastic surgery is a surgical method of reconstructing and repairing deformities that are present at birth or caused by burns, injuries, wounds, disease, or aging. It is a means of restoring both function and appearance. While there is great popular appreciation for the cosmetic benefits of plastic surgery, there is much less understanding of the value of plastic surgical procedures in shortening periods of disability and improving the quality of life.

The word "plastic" is defined as "giving form or shape to matter." Medical-grade plastic materials may

CHAPTER 1   Nature and Principles of Aesthetic Facial Surgery

be required in some areas of reconstructive and aesthetic surgery. However, neither the word nor the specialty bears any relationship to commercially prepared synthetic plastic materials and products.

Papyrus inscriptions dating back to the Egyptians in 2550 B.C. suggest that plastic surgery is the oldest form of surgery known to mankind. The history of plastic surgery is intimately associated through the ages with man's wars, religious ceremonials, punishment, primitive healing, and need for recognition.

In modern times, plastic surgery has received great impetus from the demands of World Wars I and II. The practice has been stimulated further by the hazards of our fast-moving motor age and the growing desire to conform physically with the standards of appearance established by our news and entertainment media.

In our youth-oriented business world, many men and women seek cosmetic surgery to compete with a younger generation. While styles and fashions change continually, the norms of the beautiful face have changed little over the past 200 years. It is easy to understand why more people desire the relatively lasting benefits of cosmetic plastic surgery when one considers the lifetime we devote to clothes that complement us, cosmetics that allure, and hairstyles that temporarily improve our appearance.

Who Does It?

Plastic surgery is not confined to the face and neck but is performed on all parts of the body by regional and general plastic surgeons with successful results. The general plastic surgeon practices his art on virtually any area of the body, whereas the facial plastic surgeon specializes in operations about the face, nose, and neck area.

A large number of *regional surgeon specialists*, intimately familiar with their particular areas of the body, perform plastic surgery; they bring the patient the benefits of a dual insight.

Otolaryngologists (head and neck specialists), for example, perform a wide range of head and neck plastic surgery, including work on the nose and ears, cosmetic surgery of the aging face and eyelids, and facial reconstruction.

Ophthalmologists perform plastic surgery on the eye when they transplant corneas from one individual to another, reconstruct the orbit (eye socket), eradicate tumors, and repair eyelids. Ophthalmologists also perform aesthetic surgery on the eyelids.

Neurosurgeons practice plastic surgery in treating tumors and injuries of the brain, reconstructing skull defects, and closing scalp wounds.

Thoracic surgeons do a considerable amount of reconstructive surgery of the chest. A large number of *general surgeons* apply plastic surgical techniques in repairing hernias, operating on the stomach, strengthening the abdominal wall, removing tumors and ulcers, and repairing defects with skin grafts.

Orthopedic surgeons apply plastic surgery quite successfully in correcting deformities of the finger and toes and in the process of transposing and repairing tissues such as tendons, arteries, and nerves.

Urologists use plastic surgical techniques in performing kidney transplants and in the repair of various abnormalities present at birth. Vaginal plastic repair is a reconstructive procedure performed by *gynecologists*. *Obstetricians* commonly accomplish plastic repair of the birth canal. Many *dermatologists* practice plastic surgery by means of skin planing, chemical removal of the outer layer of skin, and removal of skin lesions by surgery and cautery. They, as well as other specialists, perform hair transplantation.

As a rule a competent surgeon performing plastic surgery will be certified by his respective surgical examining board and will have considerable experience in this field of medicine and surgery. Most will be a Fellow of either the American Academy of Facial Plastic and Reconstructive Surgery or the American Society of Plastic and Reconstructive Surgeons. Never hesitate to inquire of any surgeon his credentials and qualifications—any ethical surgeon will be quite willing to make you aware of his credentials and experience.

Guiding Principles

Every physician skilled in plastic surgical procedures must have a thorough knowledge of the anatomy, pathology, and physiology of the area involved. He, furthermore, must understand the reaction of tissues to surgery and how to handle them during an operation. Utmost consideration is given to the preservation of important structures, maintenance of good blood supply, prevention of hemorrhage and infection, suturing of wounds without tension, and protection of tissues with appropriate dressings. Many of these factors are under the surgeon's control, either by his skills in the operating room, medications that he may prescribe, or techniques that he may employ following the surgery. Equally important is the patient's ability to heal properly and respond to treatment.

Plastic surgery is often not the superficial "minor" operation held in popular esteem. Rather, most procedures should be regarded as major undertakings that when carefully planned result in substantial benefits to the patient.

Surgery intended to improve sagging skin or wrinkles necessarily leaves scars. Despite what you may have heard, *all surgical scars are permanent and cannot be totally erased.* They can, however, be rendered inconspicuous. The goal of the plastic surgeon is to place scars in natural lines of the face and eyelids where they are least noticeable or are more easily camouflaged by makeup or hairstyles. While such scars are permanent, they rarely are noticeable or cause any trouble.

The facial plastic surgeon is particularly skilled in the meticulous hiding of incisions in natural skin folds, existing wrinkles, and the hairline. Complete elimination of scars is impossible since they represent the natural method by which nature heals the human body.

Just as the chest surgeon cannot operate in an intelligent way without x-ray films of the chest, the plastic surgeon cannot operate on the face or eyelids without medical photographs. These photographs are not meant to flatter you, and they will show your face in every detail. Photographs aid greatly in planning in advance the meticulous details of each operation. We will photograph you in the office and in selected cases request that you obtain special photographs taken by a professional photographer. Your consent to take and use photographs for educational purposes will be requested and is a vital part of our commitment to teaching younger surgeons and colleagues.

Anesthesia

It is our policy to utilize "twilight" intravenous anesthesia for most procedures, with a physician-anesthesiologist providing an additional element of patient safety. Patients may receive preoperative medications before arriving in the operating room to relax them; intravenous medications are then given to help the patient enter a "twilight" anesthesia state found by most patients to be pleasant and comfortable. A local anesthetic is then used to numb the area of surgery. Most people have amnesia for the entire operation but are usually alert upon returning to their room. Our experience with this approach ensures that patients are up and around sooner with less likelihood of anesthetic complications.

With these modern methods of anesthesia, there will usually be no significant pain during the operation and only minor or no discomfort for a short period after surgery. It should also be understood that all of your surgical procedures will be performed by your doctor—at times assisted by a competent team of associates. During all but the most minor procedures, a skilled physician-anesthesiologist plays an active role in the comfort and medical safety of your operation and will bill you separately for the appropriate medical changes.

Finances

Since the majority of facial plastic surgery operations are elective (nonemergencies) in nature, this provides the patient with the opportunity before surgery to arrange his finances accordingly and without undue hardship.

It is therefore customary that surgical fees for elective cosmetic surgery be paid in advance. Should surgery be canceled or postponed for any reason, the fee will be refunded. My office staff will be pleased to provide any details regarding payment. In special cases other arrangements, agreeable to the doctor and patient, may be appropriate.

As a general rule, insurance companies will not entertain claims for surgery performed solely for cosmetic purposes. Sometimes they do when cosmetic improvement is the by-product of a procedure performed to improve function, relieve symptoms, or repair the effects of injury. Our office will be happy to assist you in completing your insurance claim forms after surgery and provide copies of the operative record if your company requests them. However, we would like to emphasize two things. First, we are not a party to the contract that exists between you and your insurance company. Consequently, the company is responsible to you, not to us. Likewise, patients, not their carriers, are responsible for any charges incurred. *Second, it is not possible to fill out insurance forms so that it appears the work done was not for cosmetic purposes if, indeed, it was.* This represents both an unethical and illegal practice.

Finally, it should be remembered that the foregoing discussions are general in nature only—the specific details relating to your own individual needs and desires will be thoroughly discussed with you. It may be necessary to see you on two or more office periods in order to accurately plan your operation to suit your needs. Feel free to ask any questions you may have since they may help me to better understand and analyze your needs and wishes.

Always keep in mind that following plastic surgery it frequently takes time for the intended final result to become apparent. Be patient while your body goes through the process of healing. To this end, I will ask you to return to the office at various intervals over several months to monitor your healing. Not infrequently I will be able to make suggestions for a more rapid improvement.

THE CONSULTATION FOR PLASTIC SURGERY

At your initial visit to our offices we will discuss your wishes, examine the condition you wish to have corrected or improved, and give you an idea of what can be accomplished to provide you with the desired result. Your general health will be carefully evaluated. I will need to know specifically about any drug or other allergies you may have, specific medicines you are taking (it is best to bring them), and any medical condition that may have a bearing on your potential surgery. It is helpful to make a list of all this information as well as any questions you may have—it is important to be accurate with these details. (Space is provided at the end of this brochure for your lists and questions.)

Medical photographs will be taken to assist in the analysis of your conditions and in the precise planning of surgery. These photographs show your face in every detail and are not meant to flatter you. They are invaluable in preparing for the technical details of your surgery and remain as a permanent medical record in my office.

In some cases, additional studies (x-rays, laboratory tests, etc.) may be required prior to surgery in order to ensure the safety of your operation. A preoperative checkup by your family doctor is recommended.

Patients who have a specific time schedule to meet or wish to schedule surgery at a specific time should so inform my staff at this time in order that reservations may be made in our surgical schedule and, if appropriate, at the hospital.

In some cases it may be necessary to see you in consultation more than once to more thoroughly prepare for your surgery. An additional visit(s) allows an opportunity to personally review your questions and, if necessary, to evaluate your photographs with you. (If surgery is decided upon, there is usually no charge made for this additional visit.)

OUTPATIENT PLASTIC SURGERY

If your surgery is of the type that may be performed as outpatient surgery (either at the hospital's outpatient surgical suite or at the office), my staff will provide you with detailed printed instructions that should be followed very carefully. All patients undergoing outpatient surgery should arrange for a friend or relative to accompany them to the hospital and home again after the surgery. Patients should never plan to drive themselves to or from the hospital.

A one-night hospital stay is necessary for selected procedures to ensure complete safety. For our patients' benefit the hospital has established a very favorable inexpensive charge for an overnight stay. The *safety* inherent in this overnight policy is vital to our overall patient care program.

POSTOPERATIVE CARE

Depending upon the nature and scope of your operation(s), we will ask you to return to the office at various intervals over several months to carefully monitor your healing. *Please keep these appointments.* These visits are important since I may be able to suggest methods to enhance your healing along the way. *Remember that it often takes several months to over a year for final healing to develop*—patience born of emotional maturity is a necessary prerequisite for all patients undergoing plastic surgery.

Patients living outside the Chicago suburban area should plan to remain in Chicago with friends or family for several days after surgery—we will instruct you for what period this seems necessary. My staff can provide recommendations for appropriate comfortable nearby Chicago hotels.

FEES

Consultation Fee

The fee for your consultation and preoperative analysis is based upon the amount of time required to completely evaluate your problem as well as any required photographs necessary. It is payable at the time of your consultation.

Surgical Fee

Your surgical fee will be quoted following your consultation.

Advance payment of fees is a universal policy when the patient is undergoing cosmetic or appearance surgery. Other arrangements might be agreeable to the surgeon and patient in special cases. The patient who wishes surgery in order to look better should plan well in advance to manage his finances since such surgery is not considered an emergency need.

Prepayment indicates tangibly that the patient is able and prepared to pay for surgery that is elective but not mandatory from a medical standpoint. By the same token, the patient is assured that he has paid his bill in full and will receive no unexpected further charges for the surgery just performed.

Health insurance does not ordinarily cover the doctor's fees for cosmetic surgery, nor does it generally cover hospitalization. If the operation is performed in an attempt to improve or restore function, surgical and hospitalization insurance may cover a portion of the costs. Always check with your insurance representative for your exact personal coverage.

Our fees for plastic surgery procedures are generally regarded as quite reasonable; my staff and I will be glad to discuss them with you at any time.

Finally, please remember that our best efforts will always be put forth to achieve for you a pleasing and satisfactory operative result. Feel free to ask any questions of me or my staff. With a proper understanding of your surgery, you should approach your procedure with confidence and enthusiasm.

A REALISTIC ATTITUDE

Those who expect miracles or magic from plastic surgery risk disappointment. From the standpoint of aesthetic results, improvement is a more realistic goal than is perfection. No matter how skillful the surgeon, he cannot create a silk purse out of the proverbial sow's ear, nor can he make a ravishing beauty out of a hopeful person who is basically not attractive.

In all plastic surgery, results will depend not only on the skill and experience of the surgeon but also on the age, health, skin texture, bone structure, healing capacity, and specific problem of the patient. Many patients, because of these variables and psychological considerations, do not make appropriate candidates for plastic surgery.

Any plastic surgical repair should be regarded realistically as a means of rendering the patient's deformity inconspicuous, thus minimizing attention to the deformity. The resulting improvement in appearance often produces increased self-satisfaction and self-confidence. Corrective surgery can help greatly, for instance, in minimizing the psychological harm caused by physical deformities such as protruding ears, oversized noses, birthmarks, and a myriad of facial blemishes, sags, wrinkles, and scars.

Plastic surgery, however, will not serve as a cure-all for the individual who blames his appearance for lack of success in life. Nor is there assurance that this individual will receive universal approval from family, friends, and acquaintances after he has undergone surgery. Since the goal of the surgeon is to produce "natural" facial features, friends may not notice subtle changes in appearance. They may comment how rested you look and attribute your new appearance to a change in hairstyle or even weight loss. Creating attractive changes that complement each patient's best features is the goal of every facial surgeon.

Often, in the case of facial plastic surgery, limitations exist in satisfying the exact expectations of the patient. Sometimes the patient's goal is surgically unattainable. No surgical procedure should be taken lightly. A slight but real risk is involved in all surgery. The patient must receive medications prior to, during, and following surgery. While they are uncommon in cosmetic plastic surgery, reactions could occur. Therefore the patient should enter into such surgery with the realization that she is consulting a surgeon and not a beauty salon. You should now proceed to the following portions of this booklet that particularly interest you.

RHINOPLASTY—PLASTIC SURGERY OF THE NOSE

Plastic surgery of the nose is an exciting and challenging branch of surgery—for the patient as well as the doctor. Rhinoplasty is clearly the most elegant and sophisticated of all facial plastic surgical procedures. With modern surgical refinements, uniformly better results are obtained than were possible in past decades.

Now that you have made the decision to improve the appearance and the function of your nose, there are some facts regarding rhinoplasty surgery that I would like to share with you. Remember that although not all of the following information applies to each and every patient, nonetheless, the following thoughts should help you become more informed and therefore more confident about the details of your surgery.

Please be assured that no question that you may have is ever unimportant or irrelevant—I welcome any questions that will allow you and your family to become more informed and confident about your particular problem and its correction. Understanding and communication between you and myself are important to the successful and happy outcome of your surgical procedure.

General Information

Rhinoplasty surgery is a highly delicate and technical form of plastic surgery and enjoys a very high rate of success and patient satisfaction. Although usually performed on the younger age groups, excellent results may be obtained on patients in their fifties and sixties.

Patients who are emotionally mature and realistic can and should approach their operation with enthusiasm and excitement.

Let's begin then with several important facts regarding nasal surgery:

The goal of your surgery is an improvement in appearance, not absolute perfection. Every effort is expended to create near-perfect results, but expectations of total perfection are unrealistic and usually reflect an immature personality. The surgeon is a doctor—not a magician. The degrees of success certainly depend not only on his skill and experience but equally upon the age, health, skin texture, bone structure, and anatomy of each particular patient.

Rhinoplasty surgery is performed from inside the nose by using special delicate instruments. The bone, cartilage, and soft tissues of the nose are reduced in size, rearranged, or sculptured to obtain a desirable natural-appearing result. No external scars are left, unless excessively large nostrils require reduction in size. If any external incisions are necessary, we will discuss them with you and camouflage them through tiny incisions in natural skin creases.

The resulting improvement in appearance may be psychologically beneficial, almost always bringing increased self-satisfaction and self-confidence. Patients, however, should not always expect universal approval from all of their family members, friends, and acquaintances following surgery since they may not be aware of your reason and motivation for a change in your appearance. It is more important that you and I be pleased with the eventual surgical outcome.

Ethically no surgeon can guarantee the results of *any* cosmetic surgery—he can only promise to do everything possible to do his best to correct the patient's problem.

Plastic surgical correction of the nasal deformities should never be performed without contemplating and analyzing the surrounding facial features. In our discussions I will explain to you how we can best accomplish the changes you desire, always keeping in mind the need to keep the nose in harmony with your particular individual facial features. At times, as your surgical advisor, I may recommend other subtle changes in your chin contour, hairstyle, etc., to help you look your very best following surgery.

All surgical procedures carry some degree of risk. Fortunately, the risk factors in rhinoplasty surgery are quite small. The vast majority of patients undergo surgery and postoperative healing with no significant complications of any kind. Rarely and infrequently, complications such as some degree of postoperative bleeding, delayed healing, and small irregularities and slight asymmetries of the nose can occur, since not all of these factors are under the control of the surgeon.

It is reassuring, however, to understand that these complications occur very rarely. In some patients with badly deformed noses (severely twisted, badly fractured, etc.) it is not always possible to correct all nasal deformities in one single operation; occasionally a second "touch-up" minor procedure might be required several months following the initial major operation to improve the result and/or correct inappropriate healing. Generally, small "touch-up" procedures do not require hospitalization and under most circumstances will be performed as an outpatient procedure.

Finally, it is generally wise to be sure to arrange your financial affairs relating to your surgery in advance. Since rhinoplasty surgery is an *elective* type of operation, it should be planned so that it does not represent a personal financial hardship to you. My staff will provide as many details as we are able for you and advise you of the surgical fee.

My staff will likewise help you with forms and operative reports for your insurance company, but *please remember that your arrangements with your insurance company are strictly your own*, just as the doctor-patient relationship between you and me is strictly unique and personal.

Please do not ask us to submit incorrect or falsified reports to insurance companies or to employers since this unethical and illegal activity has no place in our practice.

Certainly if you have any problems relating to surgical costs or finances, my staff and I are always happy to help you resolve them. I think you'll find our fees quite reasonable.

Preliminary Steps to Surgery

After you and I have agreed on the need for your operation, I will personally take photographs of your face and nose in various positions to assist in the very careful planning of your own individual personalized operation. I will ask your signed consent to take these important photographs and must have your permission before surgery is planned. No two noses are ever quite alike, and no two operations are ever done exactly in the same manner. Your new nose should fit you as an individual and not necessarily be a carbon copy of someone else's nose.

Plans will be made for your admission to the hospital the morning of your surgery for a general physical examination by the house doctor, appropriate blood tests, and occasionally nasal and sinus x-ray films. These are certainly important and necessary preoperative studies to ensure your well-being during surgery.

Almost all patients are discharged the morning following surgery feeling quite comfortable and generally free of pain.

CHAPTER 1   Nature and Principles of Aesthetic Facial Surgery

You will find your operation essentially a comfortable experience, generally with little or no discomfort. We are fortunate to have superb physician-anesthesiologists who will administer intravenous sedatives and tranquilizers during the operation to keep you very comfortable. Chances are you will remember little or none of your surgery since a "twilight" intravenous anesthetic technique is employed.

For 1 or 2 hours following your surgery you will be attended to by highly competent recovery nurses who will attend to any need you may have to ensure your comfort.

Happily, little if any pain occurs after rhinoplasty. Pain medication, however, is always available should you find it necessary.

Upon return to the hospital room from the recovery room, most patients enjoy a light lunch or dinner and are able to have visitors in moderation.

The small bandage protecting the outside of the nose remains in place for 5 to 8 days, and all internal nasal dressings placed at surgery are ordinarily removed the morning after surgery by my staff or me. We rarely use any nasal "packing."

Postoperative Care

I will provide you with a detailed list of "do's and don'ts" to optimize your postoperative course. Please follow these instructions carefully—*don't take chances.* Never hesitate to call me immediately if anything concerns you. *Take no aspirin*—it may precipitate bleeding—and take great care to not hit your nose in any way and to keep the nasal splint bandage dry. I need your help and cooperation to give you the very best possible result. Upon your discharge from the hospital you may be given medications to help in the healing of your nose and to help diminish what little swelling you may have.

At approximately 1 week from the date of your surgery, we will ask you to return to the office where your nasal splint will be removed by my staff or myself. Photographs will be taken and further instructions given regarding the care of your nose. Generally patients are able to return to normal activities such as work or school at this time. Strenuous sports, exercises, swimming, or other physical activities should be curtailed for approximately 3 to 6 additional weeks. We will advise you individually about any question you may have.

Although the new shape of your nose is apparent rather quickly after removal of the splint, remember that it takes several weeks for the majority of the swelling to disappear and shrinkage of the new nasal configuration to occur. This is a gradual process that cannot be hurried. Small, subtle, and generally favorable changes take place over a period of several months, and we never consider a nose totally healed until at least 1 year following the date of surgery.

It is important to your proper healing that we see you from time to time during that year, during which time additional photographs will be taken to document the changes and the final postoperative result. These office visits are necessary and important to the very best possible improvement in appearance.

Finally, please read and understand all of the printed material that I will provide for you before and after your surgery. This material is valuable to your understanding of your operation because it emphasizes the *facts* surrounding nasal surgery. Very often we see patients who have had relatives or friends undergo nasal surgery in other parts of the country, and there often seems to develop a good deal of misunderstanding and sometimes nonfactual stories regarding this generally most pleasant kind of surgery. I feel that it is important that you and I spend sufficient time together to develop a clear understanding of what is possible to be done to improve the appearance of your nose and to allow you to understand exactly how your surgery and your medical surgical care is to be performed.

If you keep all of these things in mind, I think you can look forward to a very pleasant and exciting experience that will have meaning and value to you for your entire life.

MENTOPLASTY—CORRECTION OF OVERDEVELOPED OR UNDERDEVELOPED CHINS

Correction of an underdeveloped (or "weak") chin may be accomplished as an individual procedure, in conjunction with rhinoplasty, or in some instances, coincident with facelift surgery. A chin of appropriate size and configuration is necessary to achieve overall facial balance and harmony and provide a more natural and youthful appearance.

The surgery may be performed under local or twilight anesthesia from the time of adolescence onward. The augmentation of the chin may be performed in one of two fashions, either by placing the implant through an incision in the mouth or by making a tiny incision in the crease beneath the chin, which is well camouflaged in this position. When performed in conjunction with rhinoplasty or a facelift, this procedure adds only a few minutes to the surgery and does not require additional hospitalization. When performed as an isolated procedure, the patient may undergo mentoplasty as an outpatient procedure.

For minor chin deformities, a medical-grade inert implant is utilized to increase the chin projection. This same type of material is used constantly and safely in medicine to make artificial heart valves, to repair retinal tears inside the eye, and for many other purposes in surgery of every part of the body.

For major deformities of the chin, it may be necessary to modify the shape of the bone structures. For more complex operations, orthodontic or oral surgical consultation may be required.

Rarely, the body may not tolerate the presence of an implant and necessitate its removal.

OTOPLASTY—CORRECTION OF PROTRUDING EARS

Many children (and adults) with large, outstanding ears are often subjected to unkind teasing and taunts because of their deformity. Emotional distress, self-consciousness, hostility, and rejection may all be present or develop in varied degrees. These concerns may not always be overtly apparent to the parents.

Since the ear is almost fully developed by the fourth to the sixth year, surgical correction can be effectively performed at this age to avoid later emotional trauma. Adults may be operated on at any age. The patient should remember that *no two ears are ever perfectly symmetrical and therefore minor degrees of variation (that are seldom noticeable) are often present after correction.*

Incisions are hidden on the back part of each ear and thereafter not apparent. Children are usually hospitalized for 1 day and undergo surgery under general anesthesia. Many adults can enjoy the cost-saving benefits of outpatient surgery and return to work within a day or two following correction. A protective dressing is applied to protect the ear following surgery and removed in the office after 48 to 72 hours.

The psychological benefits of this highly successful operation provide a high degree of patient satisfaction.

SCAR CAMOUFLAGE—IMPROVING FACIAL SCARS AND BLEMISHES

The appearance of unsightly or disfiguring scars or blemishes may be improved by well-planned and carefully executed surgery, but there are important facts that patients contemplating such procedures should know.

Surgical treatment implies that incisions will be made to cut out the scar or blemish. Each cut made into the skin, regardless of where it is placed, who makes the cut, or whether it is deliberate or accidental, heals in the same manner. That is, it produces scar tissue, nature's method of healing itself. This simple fact is frequently forgotten or ignored by the public who have the impression that scars can be removed without leaving any evidence that they ever existed.

In reality, *the surgeon's goal is to replace an unsightly or disfiguring scar with a better scar,* one that is fine-lined, is level with the surrounding surface, is about the same color as the adjacent skin, and causes no distortion or pull on the surrounding structures—in short, one that is as inconspicuous as possible. The actual healing of the scar and its final appearance depend on many factors, one of which is the patient's own healing capability.

Maturation of scars takes anywhere from 6 to 18 months. Initially, a freshly repaired scar usually looks very good. Commonly it then becomes reddened and possibly somewhat raised above the surrounding skin and is frequently hard in consistency. Gradually the hardness and redness lessen, disappear, and leave a soft scar that is level with and somewhat paler than the adjacent skin. Patients seeking scar or blemish removal should therefore be prepared to accept two things: first, removal will result in a further, although optimally, much improved scar since there can be no complete removal of all traces of a scar. Second, the final appearance will not be evident for 6 to 18 months.

Understandably, most people with recent scarring want repair immediately, if not sooner. Ideally scar revision, except in selected cases, should not be undertaken too soon. The passage of time is the best, the kindest, and in the long run, the easiest treatment for most facial scars of recent origin since most will improve if given the time to do so. As mentioned above, it may take 6 to 18 months to reach maximum improvement. Most scars should become soft and smooth before surgical revision is undertaken. By that time less work may have to be done because of the improvement that has occurred. However, scars that cause distortion of normal structures (for example, eyebrows, lips, eyelids, nostrils, etc.), those that spread widely or produce deformity by contraction, and U- or J-shaped scars may be repaired earlier since no improvement of the basic problem can be anticipated as a result of the passage of time.

When treating a scar or blemish by excision, the surgeon makes every effort to place the line of incision as nearly as possible in or parallel to one of the normal crease lines in the face. Sometimes it may be necessary to change the direction of the scar so that it will approximate these lines. Excisions of large scars or blemishes may require multiple operations over a period of time that shift the surrounding tissue to fill the defect or skin grafting.

Finally, some areas of the body consistently heal with less noticeable scars than others. Certain scars about the nose, chin, jaw, shoulders, chest, upper part of the back, and extremities are apt to spread in spite of everything that may be done to prevent it.

To recapitulate, as in all other types of cosmetic surgery, *the expectation in the treatment of scars and blemishes should be an improvement and not perfection. Patients who are not able to accept this should not undertake treatment.*

DERMABRASION—SURGICAL "SANDING"

Irregularities of the surface of facial skin are commonly improved by a surgical procedure known as dermabrasion or skin "sanding." Acne or scar pitting, irregular scars, and selected facial blemishes can often be effectively improved with careful dermabrasion. A small surgical rotating wire brush or diamond wheel is utilized to remove the sharp edges of scars or pits in order to blend them more uniformly with surrounding skin.

Dermabrasion may be combined with facelift procedures to smooth and render inconspicuous the fine, small, shallow wrinkles that form around the mouth and temples. We find it additionally helpful as a final "touch-up" following scar camouflage operations because it blends the new camouflaged scar more uniformly into the surrounding facial skin.

Exposure to direct sunlight without the use of a total sun-blocking agent within 10 to 12 weeks following dermabrasion may result in unfavorable discoloration. We will advise you about sun exposure and effective sun-blocking agents.

SURGERY OF THE AGING FACE—IMPROVING APPEARANCE

Aging changes in the face do not occur suddenly—they evolve slowly and involve different regions of the face at different stages. Improving appearance surgically often requires a *series of planned operations* designed to forestall the inevitable signs of aging rather than one major all-encompassing operation.

For example, the earliest signs of aging generally become apparent around the eyes as the eyelids become baggy, "crow's-feet" form, and upper eyelid skin and eyebrows tend to sag. When adequate rest no longer diminishes these changes, the time has arrived for correction of baggy eyelids and drooping brows—often the initial operation necessary to improve appearance in an aging face. In some families these changes become troublesome in the mid-twenties or early thirties.

Aging changes in the face proper generally occur later as elastic tissue decreases and facial bones and skull actually thin and become smaller. The overlying skin "envelope" thereby becomes excessive and creates skin and muscle sagging and pouching along the jawline ("jowls"), under the chin, and at the corners of the mouth. Gravity exaggerates these changes and leads to a "tired" look when the patient actually feels vigorous and healthy.

Not generally appreciated are the aging changes that develop in the nose: it tends to become sharper, less well defined and actually longer in relation to other facial features. Lifting and conservatively sculpturing the drooping nose is one of the most effective of operations to improve appearance.

Currently patients no longer need to wait until hanging folds or almost irreversible changes of aging have occurred to seek improvement; improved operations have shifted preference for corrections to the early forties (or earlier in some circumstances), when planned limited corrections can often be made to maintain a youthful appearance for an extended time.

The final surgical results are almost always better when aging skin problems are corrected at an earlier age.

BLEPHAROPLASTY—EYELID PLASTIC SURGERY

Blepharoplasty is the broad medical term applied to operations designed to lift, remove, and reposition sagging and bulging tissues around the eyes. Many of the earliest signs of a fatigued, aged appearance occur in the eyelid area. Bulging fat in the lower eyelids ("bags") commonly occurs in certain families at very early ages (late teens to mid-twenties), while sagging skin and eyelid wrinkles make their appearance as early as the late twenties.

Correction of these aging eyelid problems provides one of the most dramatic improvements possible with aesthetic facial surgery. Although blepharoplasty is often performed as an individual procedure at an early age, it is frequently combined with the facelift (rhytidoplasty) operation in middle-aged patients.

During the eyelid operation the surgeon removes excess skin from the upper lid and camouflages the incision in the upper lid skin fold. (In certain patients correction of a sagging brow complements the upper eyelid blepharoplasty.) The lower eyelid incision is hidden immediately below the eyelash line; excess skin is removed, weak muscles are tightened or smoothed, and bulging fat is corrected. Although some temporary bruising may be expected for several days, little or no pain ordinarily results from blepharoplasty.

It is wise policy to undergo a current eye (ophthalmologic) examination prior to eyelid plastic surgery to ensure the absence of any current need for visual care by your ophthalmologist.

Patients with very dark or pigmented skin around the eyes find that this condition will persist after surgery; improvements are most dramatic when excess skin and bulging fat are responsible for the predominate aging and "tired" appearance.

Blepharoplasty operations do *not* totally eradicate pronounced or fine creases ("crow's-feet," "laugh lines") lateral to the eyelids since these wrinkles continue to be influenced after surgery by underlying facial muscles and animation.

Properly carried out, blepharoplasty is one of the most permanent and dramatic of the operations designed to minimize the aging process. The improved results are generally beneficial for many years.

CHAPTER 1   Nature and Principles of Aesthetic Facial Surgery

BROW-LIFT—CORRECTION OF SAGGING EYEBROWS

In both men and women a fatigued and tired appearance caused by drooping of the outer margins of the eyebrow is often one of the earliest signs of aging. The eye appears crowded and smaller than normal, with abnormal fullness of the upper lids.

This condition may be dramatically improved by the upper facelift operation or by removing a carefully planned segment of skin just above the eyebrow and repositioning the eyebrow at a more normal level. A small permanent scar results that is camouflaged within the eyebrow or in favorable lines.

The brow-lift operation may be effectively combined with the blepharoplasty (eyelid) or facelift operation or may be performed independently as an outpatient procedure.

SUBMENTOPLASTY—CORRECTION OF A "DOUBLE CHIN"

Gravity and aging adversely affect the graceful curves and firm lines of the neck and jawline during aging; the condition is commonly worsened by the deposition of excess fat beneath the chin and jaw that creates the so-called "double chin." "Wattles" and a "turkey gobbler" appearance ensue and are accentuated by drooping folds of muscle in the neck region.

A properly performed facelift and neck-lift will improve these aging phenomena, but not uncommonly a separate inconspicuous incision is required beneath the chin to adequately tighten excessive skin and remove fat deposits. Generally a more graceful and pleasing chin and neckline are immediately apparent after repair.

Liposuction (suctioning out localized fat deposits) may be extremely beneficial in selected patients to improve the neck and face appearance. Once removed, the submental fat rarely returns as before unless significant excess weight is gained.

RHYTIDOPLASTY—FACELIFT

The facelift operation is designed to improve the various areas of loose, sagging skin and muscle folds of the face and neck that are a consequence of aging. Facelift operations have several variations in design, depending upon the anatomy and degree of aging in individual patients. The skin, muscle, and fatty tissues of the face and neck are elevated and tightened to result in an improved appearance. Incisions may vary slightly from patient to patient in order to best correct the most prominent deformities.

Increasing numbers of men as well as women are experiencing the benefits of a facelift; as the general population ages, many older individuals who continue to work and enjoy good health wish to look as good as they can by diminishing the signs of aging.

Although age is not as important as the specific appearance of the patient, two groups of patients can benefit from a facelift: (1) younger individuals, usually around 35 to 45 years of age, who wish to forestall the signs of aging and maintain a youthful appearance and (2) older individuals who wish a dramatic correction in more severe facial and neck sagging. *The best results are usually obtained in those patients in the younger age group in whom tissues and muscles have not been almost irreversibly stretched and sagged.*

Commonly other surgical procedures are combined with a facelift to correct specific aging problems (eyelid surgery, double chin removal, dermabrasion, etc.). Increasingly, older patients are benefiting from correction of the aging nose (rhinoplasty) since one of the effects of aging may involve an elongation and drooping of the nose and lead to an interference with breathing.

Naturally, everyone contemplating the operation is interested in how much improvement they can expect and for what duration the improvement will be apparent. The amount of improvement depends upon the degree of wrinkling present and the patient's predetermined genetic predisposition. If it is marked, results may be dramatic. If sagging is early and the operation is being done to attempt to keep the patient looking young, the improvement may be more subtle—remarks will be made that the face looks less tired and more "alive."

The duration of improvement cannot be accurately predicted in all cases. If wrinkling is severe, it will obviously take a longer time after surgery for the condition to become as bad as it was before surgery. If the degenerative process of the skin is very rapid, the wrinkling and sagging will occur more rapidly. In a face that is simply fat, it will be improved for only a short time. In ideal cases, however, the duration of improvement is often from 5 to 10 years. No operation can permanently prevent aging, but the individual can expect to appear younger than if the operation had not been performed.

A realistic approach to understanding the results of facelift surgery may be illustrated by considering identical twins. If only one twin undergoes facial aesthetic surgery, he or she will of course continue to age but will always look better than the twin who did not choose to realize the benefits of facial rejuvenation surgery.

The following facts related to the facelift operation specifically and the aging process in general should be understood:

1. A satisfactory facelift performed by an experienced surgeon is a major operative procedure that requires 2 or 3 hours of surgery. So-called mini facelift procedures generally result in only a "mini" effect and have little or no lasting value.
2. Facial creams, cosmetics, muscle exercise, and chin supports all have little or no effect on the aging process and cannot be substitute for a needed facelift where facial sagging and poor muscle tone exist.
3. The incisions required for a facelift, meticulously camouflaged in pre-existing wrinkles and within the hairline, are generally inapparent shortly after surgery.
4. Some patients will experience a variable degree of bruising and discoloration in the face and neck following surgery that generally subsides in 1 to 3 weeks. Ordinarily there is surprisingly little discomfort associated with facelift surgery.
5. A temporary numbness in and around the facelift incisions and ears is normal; sensation returns gradually within several weeks.
6. Finally, it should be understood that the facelift operation will not eliminate the small vertical creases about the lips, bulging or excess skin about the eyelids, or horizontal creases of the forehead—these disfigurements require separate procedures that may be combined with the facelift.

Secondary Facelift Procedures

Often after a facelift a secondary procedure may be performed on individuals whose tissues are particularly prone to sag again. Usually the "tuck-up" is not necessary for 1 to several years following an adequate initial facelift, but with patients who are overweight, have heavy faces, or have waited until wrinkling or sagging are extreme prior to the lift, the "tuck-up" may be beneficial if performed earlier and give a more lasting result. This type of less extensive facelift requires much less surgery than the initial procedure and is often done as an outpatient surgical procedure. The incisions and scars are in the same general areas and are camouflaged as in the initial operation, but the recovery period is much shorter, and discoloration and swelling are minimal.

COLLAGEN (ZYDERM) AUGMENTATION

Fine wrinkles, deeper facial creases, and depressed scars are generally improved by the office injection of a purified collagen material known as Zyderm or Zyplast.

Common facial areas improved by collagen injections include the forehead "worry lines"; crease lines around the lips, mouth, and cheeks; and depressed soft facial scars.

A small skin test placed on the patient's forearm is necessary to ensure the absence of any allergy to the collagen protein, a rare finding. After a wait of 4 weeks, collagen injection may be safely employed as a rapid office procedure. An immediate improvement in wrinkles and creases is apparent.

Since the human body slowly and gradually absorbs the injected collagen, repeat "touch-up" injections are required at 6 to 18 months for optimum appearance enhancement.

THE RISKS OF PLASTIC SURGERY

Aesthetic plastic surgical procedures designed to improve appearance have been safely and effectively accomplished many thousands of times by competent surgeons. The risks of elective cosmetic surgery are therefore not great.

Surgical risks are lessened even further when a thorough understanding exists between the patient and surgeon regarding preoperative preparation, the precise details and ramifications of surgery, and compulsive postoperative care.

All anesthetics carry a slight degree of risk. We prefer carefully administered intravenous anesthetics rather than general anesthetics because of their safety and relative lack of side effects. If any drug or anesthesia you have received in the past has bothered you in any way, you must so inform your doctor(s) so that appropriate safeguards may be taken. *Any allergies of which you are aware or any drugs currently being regularly used are important to us.*

Any surgery carries a risk of bleeding in the postoperative period. *No aspirin* or drugs containing aspirin should be taken for 2 weeks before or after your surgery because it can affect your blood clotting capability. Any bleeding episode following your surgery, if it should occur, is ordinarily of minor consequence *but should be reported to my office immediately.* Only rarely does a bleeding episode require more than a change of bandage.

The risk of injury following surgery is minimized by bandages applied in the hospital. Caution is required on your part, however, to avoid heavy lifting, vigorous activities, or minor bumps from children, family, or friends. Please follow carefully the *specific* instructions my staff and I provide for you.

Plastic surgical procedures in the facial and nose areas carry very little risk of infection. If you should notice any of the cardinal signs of infection (pain, swelling, excess heat in the operated area, or unexpected drainage), they should also be reported promptly.

Whenever a person's appearance is changed, there exists a slight risk that the final result might fall short of his or her expectations. Since plastic surgery procedures affect individuals in a different way, it is vital to reach a clear understanding with your surgeon regarding *realistic expectations.* Electing to undergo formal surgery is not like going to a health club or beauty parlor. You must expect some temporary swelling, bruising, and minor discomfort, and you must realize that plastic surgery is an art, not an exact science. The overall level of success depends not only on your surgeon's skills but equally importantly on your age, health, skin quality, bone structure, and general expectations regarding appearance improvement.

NOTES

Questions I Want To Ask My Surgeon During My Consultation

_____
_____
_____
_____
_____
_____
_____
_____
_____
_____
_____
_____
_____
_____
_____
_____
_____
_____
_____

APPENDIX B

M. Eugene Tardy, Jr., M.D., F.A.C.S.
Head and Neck Plastic Surgery, LTD.
Chicago, IL 60657
St. Joseph Hospital
Chicago, IL 60657

AUTHORIZATION AND INFORMED CONSENT

_____
(Patient's Name)

1. I request and authorize M. Eugene Tardy, Jr., M.D. (the "Doctor"), to perform an operation upon me (or my _____) entitled (description of procedure):
_____
_____

2. The nature and effects of the operation, the risks, ramifications, and complications involved, as well as alternative methods of treatment have been fully explained to me by the Doctor, and I understand them.

3. I authorize the Doctor to perform any other procedure that he may deem desirable in attempting to improve the condition stated in paragraph 1 or any unhealthy or unforeseen condition that may be encountered during the operation.

4. I consent to the administration of anesthetics by the Doctor or under the direction of the physician responsible for this service. If an anesthesiologist assists in my surgery, I understand that the anesthesiologist will take full charge of the administration and maintenance of the anesthesia and that this is an independent function of the surgery.

5. I have been thoroughly and completely advised regarding the objectives of the operation. Since I understand that the practice of medicine and surgery is not an exact science and therefore that no reputable surgeon can guarantee results, I acknowledge that imperfections might ensue and that the operative result may not live up to my expectations. I certify that no guarantees have been made by anyone regarding the operation(s) I have requested and authorized.

6. I understand that the two sides of the human body are not the same and can never be made the same.

7. For the purpose of advancing medical education, I consent to the admittance of authorized observers to the operating room.

8. I give permission to M. Eugene Tardy, Jr., M.D., to take still or motion clinical photographs with the understanding that such photographs remain the property of the Doctor. If, in the judgment of the Doctor, medical research, education, or science will be benefited by their use, such photographs and related information may be published and republished in professional journals or medical books or used for such publication or use. I shall not be identified by name.

9. I understand that if Dr. Tardy judges at any time that my surgery should be postponed or canceled for any reason, he may do so.

10. I hereby affirm that the information furnished to Dr. Tardy by me during my diagnostic evaluation is correct.

11. I agree to follow the instructions given to me by Dr. Tardy to the best of my ability before, during, and after my surgical procedure.

I certify that I have read the above authorization, that the explanations referred to therein were made to my satisfaction, and that I fully understand such explanations and the above authorization.

Signed _____
(Patient or person authorized to consent for patient)

Witness _____ Date_____

APPENDIX C

M. Eugene Tardy, Jr., M.D., F.A.C.S.
Head and Neck Plastic Surgery, LTD.
St. Joseph Hospital
Chicago, IL 60657

PATIENT INSTRUCTIONS FOLLOWING NASAL PLASTIC SURGERY

A. **INTRODUCTION**

Please read and familiarize yourself with these instructions both <u>before</u> and <u>after</u> surgery. By following them carefully you will assist in obtaining the best possible result from your surgery. If questions arise, do not hesitate to communicate with me and discuss your questions at any time. Take this list to the hospital with you, and <u>begin observing these directions on the day of surgery</u>.

B. **INSTRUCTIONS**

1. Do not blow your nose until instructed. Wipe or dab your nose gently with tissue if necessary.
2. Change the dressing under your nose (if present) until the drainage stops.
3. The nasal cast will remain in place for approximately 1 week and will be removed in the office. **Do not disturb it; <u>keep it dry</u>**.
4. Avoid foods that require prolonged chewing. Otherwise, your diet has no restrictions.
5. Avoid extreme physical activity. Obtain more rest than you usually get, and avoid exertion, including athletic activities and intercourse.
6. Brush your teeth gently with a soft toothbrush only. Avoid manipulation of the upper lip to keep your nose at rest.
7. Avoid excess or prolonged telephone conversations and social activities for at least 10–14 days.
8. You may wash your face—carefully avoid the dressing. Take <u>tub baths</u> until the dressings are removed.
9. Avoid smiling, grinning, and excess facial movements for 1 week.
10. Do not wash your hair for 1 week unless you have someone do it for you. **DO NOT GET THE NASAL DRESSINGS WET.**
11. Wear clothing that fastens in the front or back for 1 week. Avoid slipover sweaters, T-shirts, and turtlenecks.
12. Absolutely avoid sun or sunlamps for 6 weeks after surgery; heat may cause your nose to swell.
13. Don't swim for 1 month since injuries are common during swimming.
14. Don't be concerned if following removal of the dressing your nose, eyes, and upper lip show some swelling and discoloration—this usually clears in 2–3 weeks. In certain patients it may require 12–18 months for all of the swelling to completely subside.
15. Take medications prescribed only by your doctor(s).
16. Do not wear regular glasses or sunglasses that rest on the bridge of the nose for at least 4 weeks. We will instruct you in the method of taping the glasses to your forehead to avoid pressure on the nose.
17. Contact lenses may be worn within 2–3 days after surgery.
18. After the doctor removes your nasal cast, the skin of the nose may be cleansed gently with a mild soap or Vaseline Intensive Care Lotion. <u>Be gentle</u>. Makeup may be used as soon as the bandages are removed. To cover discoloration, you may use "Erase" by Max Factor, "Cover Away" by Adrien Arpel, or "On Your Mark" by Kenneth.
19. <u>Don't take chances!</u> If you are concerned about anything you consider significant, call me at 312-472-7559.
20. When we remove your splint, your nose will be swollen and will remain so for several weeks. In fact, <u>it takes at least 1 year for all swelling to subside</u>.

APPENDIX D

PATIENT INSTRUCTIONS FOLLOWING FACELIFT SURGERY

The following instructions apply to patients who have undergone facelifts. Since no two patients are ever exactly alike in their surgical needs, the type of surgery performed, or the rate of healing, we may elect to individualize the following guidelines for each patient. In such instances, we will so instruct you. Otherwise, we urge you to follow the advice below very carefully in order to accelerate your healing and maximize your surgical outcome.

1. Since you have just undergone a _major_ surgical operation, use good common sense in the first 14 days after surgery in restricting your normal activities, exercise regimens, and any activity requiring heavy lifting or straining.
2. You may be up and around the day after surgery, but some natural fatigue may persist for 2–3 days because of the normal effects of the anesthesia and surgical procedure.
3. When you move, stand, or change positions, do so deliberately and carefully for the first 7 days. In turning your head, move the head and shoulders deliberately as a single unit.
4. You may eat a normal diet the day following the surgery. In moderation, talking and smiling are perfectly acceptable.
5. Your head should be elevated on at least two pillows during sleep for the first 14 days in order to keep your head higher than your heart to facilitate the resolution of swelling. Sleep on your back or side, not face down.
6. Do not take any aspirin or aspirin-containing medicines for 14 days, and then only on the advice of your personal physician. Other routinely taken medications may be taken as necessary.
7. Any unexplained development of pain, facial swelling, or fever should be reported to us immediately.
8. Some facial and neck swelling and bruising are normally present after facelifts, but the degree of each varies widely from patient to patient. Do not be concerned if you have more or less than others who have undergone the "same" operation. Generally, most patients appear quite sociably acceptable within 10–14 days after surgery.
9. You may _gently_ cleanse the incision lines twice daily with 3% hydrogen peroxide and cotton (or Q-tips). Apply the ointment provided _sparingly_ twice daily to the incision lines in order to avoid excessive crusting of the incisions and to accelerate the reduction of incision redness. Do not apply any other ointment or medications unless we prescribe it.
10. You may _gently_ shampoo your hair 72 hours after surgery but avoid any strong rubbing or combing trauma to the incisions in the hair and around the ear. Do not blow-dry for 5 days, and postpone any planned permanent waves or hair coloring for 4 weeks following surgery.
11. Your earlobes and portions of the face that have been lifted and repositioned will be slightly numb for several weeks; sensation will then return as healing progresses. Do not wear heavy or tight earrings for 6 weeks, and avoid prolonged exposure to extremely cold temperatures.
12. It is acceptable to do some light walking 72 hours after surgery. Jogging and light noncontact exercise should not be resumed until 3 weeks, and strenuous sports require 6 weeks of healing before being safely resumed.
13. Excessive exposure to sun (including sun-tanning parlors) in the first 3 weeks after surgery may result in prolonged facial swelling and injury to the skin. Thereafter, you should always protect your skin with a strong sunscreen containing PABA (para-aminobenzoic acid) in order to decrease the inevitable aging effects of the sun on your skin.
14. Finally, it is _**very important**_ to your well-being that you completely follow all instructions given you by this office and that we check your progress regularly following surgery.

We greatly appreciate the confidence you have shown in us by allowing us to assist you in improving your appearance and health, and you may be assured of our very best efforts to achieve the most satisfactory surgical result possible for your particular individual anatomy and condition.

APPENDIX E

PATIENT INSTRUCTIONS FOLLOWING BLEPHAROPLASTY (EYELID SURGERY)

1. Sleep on your back or side with your head elevated.
2. Blepharoplasty usually causes little if any postoperative pain. If you notice significant sharp or dull pain that persists, notify my office immediately.
3. Cold compresses (ice-cold wash cloths) may be used over your eyes for 20–30 minutes six times per day if you wish. Ordinarily, however, no cold compresses are necessary or of great value.
4. <u>Take no aspirin or aspirin-containing pain medications. Tylenol, Darvocet N-100</u>, or other mild pain relievers prescribed are safe if needed.
5. You may use your eyes for reading or TV viewing as frequently as you wish.
6. Apply the ointment provided to the incision twice a day. Use <u>sparingly</u>, and place only a <u>tiny amount</u> on the incision lines.
7. Do not use contact lenses for at least 2 weeks. Pulling on the eyelids while inserting or removing the lenses may interfere with precise incision healing. Glasses may be used at any time.
8. Do not use mascara, eyeliner, or eye shadow until approved by us (usually 10–14 days). Minimal makeup applied to any bruising of the lower lid is acceptable at any time, but do not pull on the lids or incisions.
9. Any apparent redness of the whites of the eyeball is only a form of bruising and will subside during the early healing process.
10. Do not engage in vigorous exercise or sports for at least 3 weeks or until approved by us.
11. Stitches are removed at different times after surgery depending upon the extent of surgery carried out, the type of stitches, and the type and quality of your skin. We will advise you accordingly.
12. It is not abnormal to feel slight itching and tightness of the eyelids during the early healing period.

We greatly appreciate the confidence you have shown in us by allowing us to assist you in improving your appearance and health, and you may be assured of our best efforts to achieve the most satisfactory surgical result possible for your particular individual anatomy and condition.

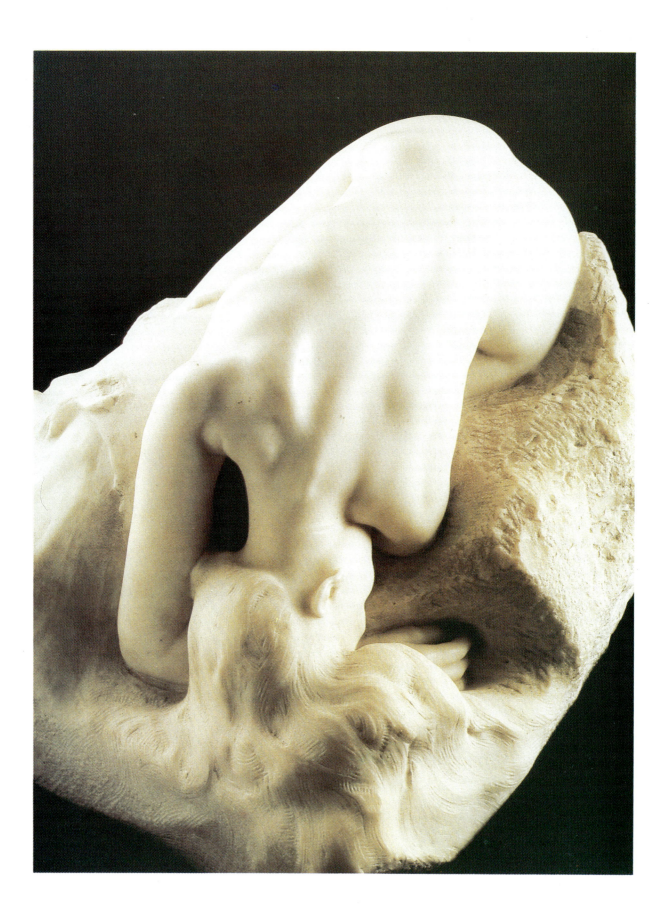

CHAPTER 2

Operating Environment for Facial Aesthetic Surgery

*Nothing but stillness can remain
when hearts are full
of their own sweetness,
bodies of their loveliness.*

William Butler Yeats

The proper operating room for facial plastic surgery must be more than simply a room where operations are performed. Likewise, it should provide more than the required surgical and aesthetic equipment and hardware. Ideally, the entire environment confronting the patient should be attuned to providing a safe, comfortable, and precisely controlled surgical event. This should incorporate the personnel, the surroundings, the medications, as well as the requisite equipment.

Office-based Operating Facility vs. Hospital-based Operating Room

Over the past decade tremendous growth in the amount of office-based surgery has occurred. Definite advantages can accrue to the patient and surgeon alike from utilizing the office-based surgical facility. Generally costs to the patient can be reduced, while the surgeon benefits from more streamlined and convenient surgical scheduling. Significant procedures requiring other than simple local anesthesia demand an office facility equipped and staffed in a manner comparable to a hospital operating room.

Most patients agree that an office surgical experience is less intimidating, more comfortable, and generally more convenient for them and their families. Preoperative conditioning of the patient must provide firm emphasis, however, that "office surgery" must not be equated with "minor surgery." Undergoing surgery in an environment where every person and each policy and procedure have been designed strictly for the comfort and safety of the patient undergoing facial plastic surgery eliminates much of the psychic trauma often generated by the hospital. The privacy of an office facility is a beneficial advantage to the patient who may wish to keep the surgical event confidential.

The surgeon benefits by designing an environment where the operating room, office facility, and its personnel exist under his direct control (Fig 2–1,A); this results in flexibility of scheduling and elimination of time-consuming travel between the office and one or more hospital operating

CHAPTER 2 Operating Environment for Facial Aesthetic Surgery

rooms. Data suggest that the risk of postoperative nosocomial infection is less than that reported in hospital facilities.

A hospital-based operating room possesses the significant advantage of overwhelming backup and life support systems, if ever required. Instant access to additional anesthesia and nursing expertise, state-of-the-art life support systems, and immediate knowledgeable medical consultation represent significant advantages of surgery performed in hospitals. If, as is the ideal, the hospital has designed and devoted a dedicated operating and ambulatory surgery facility with specialty nursing staff for the care of patients undergoing facial plastic surgery, the very best operating environment can be realized (Fig 2–1,B). As more hospitals compete for the

Figure 2-1
A, hospital operating suite specifically designed to care for the surgical needs of ambulatory surgical patients. The suite is ideally spacious, attractive, and functional and possesses the whole spectrum of safety equipment and operating essentials for anesthesia. **B,** office operating suite emulating the environment and safety features found in a traditional hospital operating room.

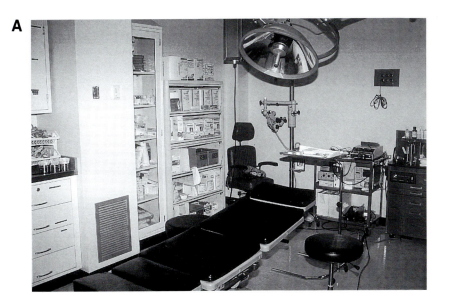

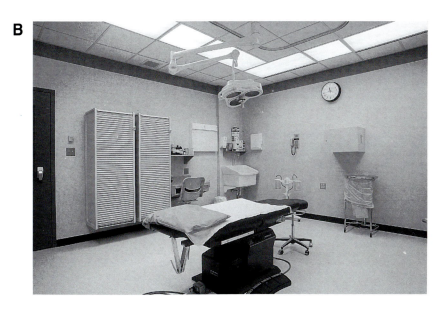

loyalty of patients, realizing that it makes good business sense to provide optimum care and facilities for patients undergoing planned, elective, and largely risk-free procedures, facial plastic surgery will occupy an even greater role in hospital-based patient surgical care.

Many patients enjoy the security of knowing that their surgery is planned under the protective setting of a reputable hospital, and even request this privilege. The surgeon practicing his art in a hospital setting enjoys the camaraderie and related expertise of his medical colleagues, is available to them for consultation and plastic surgical advice, and remains free of the potential pressures exerted by the financial and administrative responsibilities of a personal office surgical facility.

Various regulatory bodies have established guidelines and mechanisms of accreditation to ensure high standards for hospital operating rooms. Bodies such as the Joint Commission for Health Organization (JCHO) make additional demands for hospital accreditation. Regulations for office surgical facilities vary by state. Several groups exist that can provide support, guidance, and accreditation to office facilities, such as the Accreditation Association for Ambulatory Health Care, Inc. (AAAHC), and the American Association for Accreditation of Ambulatory Plastic Surgery Facilities (AAAAPSF).

Physical Surroundings

The best operating room environment, whether established in the hospital setting or office facility, is designed to provide support for the psychological concerns of the patient by instilling confidence and allaying untoward anxiety. Pastorek has described the loss of respect and dignity experienced by a patient with facial trauma in the emergency room as a situation where "the wound becomes the patient." In spite of the seemingly routine nature of the patient's planned procedure, it represents a unique, significant, and potentially traumatic event for that patient. Attention to the needs and fears of the patient throughout the perioperative experience avoids the diminished persona of a "rhinoplasty attached to a body."

Operating Room

The operating room for facial plastic surgery should be well organized, without the all-too-common cluttered and stacked environment that exists in most hospital operating rooms. The patient, already in an insecure state, does not see a cluttered and disorganized room; he sees (and is concerned by) cluttered disorganized medicine.

Surgical instruments and other "frightening" equipment should not be in the direct view of the patient. The patient should be kept warm and comfortable at all times. Quiet, soothing background music is helpful in calming the patient and sets a pleasant environment for medical personnel (Fig 2–2). Bright lights should be diverted from the patient's eyes, and frequent gentle touching or hand-holding by appropriate staff is reassur-

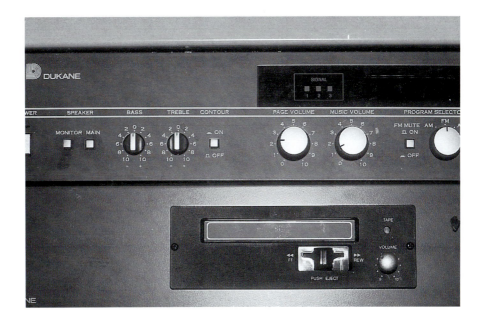

Figure 2–2
A built-in music console provides a soothing background environment for patients undergoing appearance surgery.

ing (Fig 2–3). The usual noise of the operating room must be eliminated to maintain an aura of calm and quiet reassurance. Conversation, particularly frivolous or potentially disturbing comments, must be avoided lest it be misunderstood or misinterpreted. In this regard communicative hand signals between the scrub nurse, surgical assistants, and surgeon streamline the operative process.

Proper colors in the operating room have always been an area of debate. Strong feelings have been expressed on the side of "functional" color schemes that allow complementary colors requiring visual accommodation of the surgeon's eyes in comparison to the operative field. Other concerns have been raised about the "emotional" impact of vivid colors upon patients (warm vs. cold colors, etc.). Office-based surgical facilities may provide more latitude in designing a pleasant suite for surgery by incorporating decorative features such as art work and soothing wall coverings.

The operating room represents a special environment that should reinforce to the patient the feeling that serious, dedicated activities are performed there in a professional, "no-nonsense" manner. Patients tend to harbor a preconceived concept and level of expectation of professional medical attitudes: the operating room and its staff should reflect this professionalism.

Finally, equal attention must be devoted to the preoperative and postoperative care provided the patient.

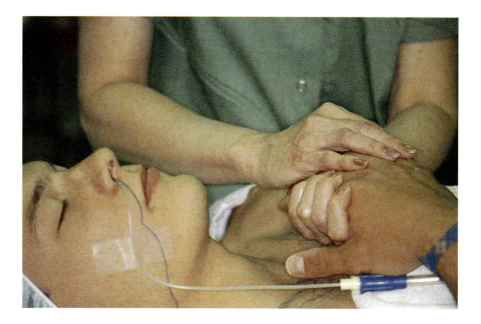

Figure 2-3
For the duration of all procedures the patient's hand is held by a dedicated anesthesiologist or a designated assistant. Patients regularly and gratefully comment about the overwhelming sense of security this seemingly small gesture provides as local anesthesia and/or intravenous sedation ensues.

Although the attentive concern of ancillary medical staff is vital, nothing is as reassuring and comforting to an anxious patient than personal attention by the surgeon, who should maintain a highly visible profile in the care of the patient immediately before as well as immediately after the procedure. Patients deserve and appreciate the courtesy of continuous nontruncated care and attention by the surgeon to whom they have entrusted their face.

Equipment

Mentioned here are only a few items of the vast array of equipment requirements for a properly prepared operating room. These represent a few areas of special concern to reflect the state of the art and technical requirements for surgical procedures in the head and neck region.

Along with other mandatory and traditional vital sign monitoring equipment, the *pulse oximeter* plays a vital role, particularly in a patient receiving intravenous analgesia. By providing continuous oxygen via a nasal silicone catheter, oxygen saturation levels may be maintained at 98% to 100%, even in deeply sedated patients (Fig 2–4).

CHAPTER 2 Operating Environment for Facial Aesthetic Surgery

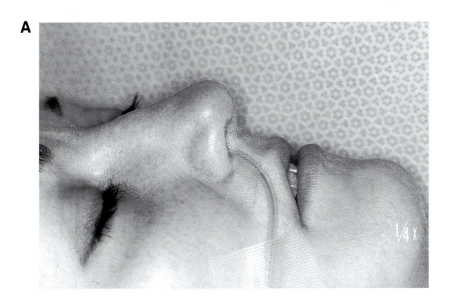

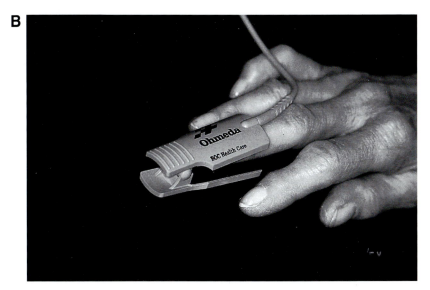
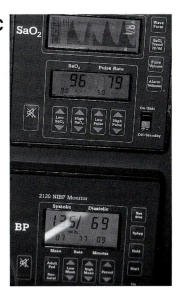

Figure 2-4
A, a small 8 F silicone catheter delivers 1½ L of oxygen to nasopharynx during all intravenous sedation procedures. Arterial oxygen saturation is thus maintained at high levels in even deeply sedated individuals. **B,** pulse oximetry plays an important role in monitoring arterial oxygen saturation, both during and after the surgical procedure. **C,** oxygen saturation percentages, constantly monitored, should be in full view of all members of the operating team during surgery.

Proper light sources for facial surgery may be different from sources adequate for abdominal or other surgery. Fiber-optic illumination with minimal heat production and high intensity should be available (Fig 2–5). The fiber-optic headlight supplements the facility's overhead light, significantly increasing the illumination of small cavities and hard-to-reach areas.

Continuous display of preoperative photographs plays a vital role in comparing erect patient anatomy with that visualized in a recumbent patient. We maintain a slide projector in the operating room and project the images on an appropriate wall surface for continuous comparisons and teaching activities during the course of the operation. The greater-than-life-size image thus displayed adds significant refinement to the surgeon's judgment skills (Fig 2–6).

Medical Personnel

The individuals with whom the patient comes into contact significantly impact on the patient's response to the surgical event. Appropriate appearance, grooming, and demeanor is important, especially for patients in the elective outpatient environment.

Operating room personnel should be schooled in proper demeanor and behavior around the patient. Conversation about other patients, operative procedures, call schedules, etc., are to be avoided when around the patient. Even during anesthesia, inappropriate comments may be misinter-

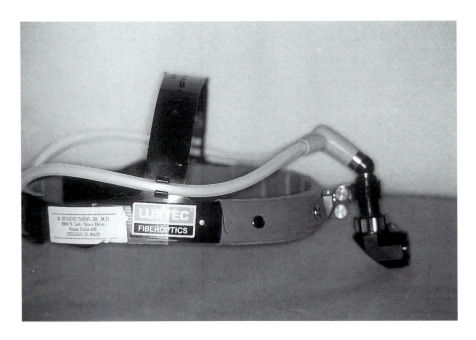

Figure 2–5
For all rejuvenation procedures requiring surgical dissection in cavities or under flaps, fiber-optic headlighting provides an extra measure of security through improved visualization.

CHAPTER 2 Operating Environment for Facial Aesthetic Surgery

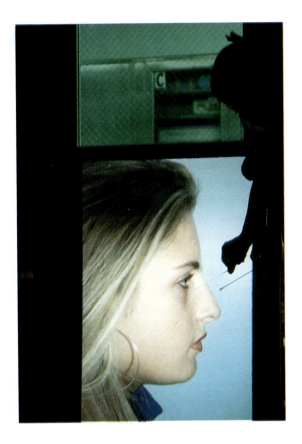

Figure 2–6
We prefer the considerable advantage of having the greater-than-life-size patient image(s) projected on the operating room wall during all surgical procedures. Refinements in analysis, judgment, and teaching techniques all benefit from this policy.

preted. To an anxious, frightened patient inappropriate joking, laughter, or boisterous behavior is often misinterpreted as relating unfavorably upon their surgery. The patient should be given the courtesy of knowing that all activities in the operating room are centered on the surgery at hand and that all involved share a personal concern for the patient's well-being. There should exist a feeling that all is under control, but no sense that it is simply an "assembly line" routine.

Instrumentation, particularly needles and syringes, should be kept out of view of the patient. All monitoring equipment utilized for patient safety should be explained, along with explanations of what to expect (tightening of automated blood pressure cuffs, the burning sensation of certain intravenous medicines, the beeping noises of the monitor).

Anxiety-producing conversation must be avoided. For example, requesting a no. 15 or 11 instead of using the word "knife" or "blade" and asking for more "local" instead of more "injection" have less chance of increasing anxiety.

Finally all involved should emphasize *gentleness with the patient*. Any touching or movement of the patient must be accomplished with a light touch. Too often the operative table or headrest is moved with forceful, jarring inattentiveness. The sterile drapes and equipment are often firmly affixed to the patient without enough concern for the comfort (and even claustrophobia) of the person underneath. Ask frequently whether the patient is comfortable, and warn them before they are abruptly moved. Always remember that there is a sensitive, often frightened person in an unfamiliar, sometimes dignity-diminishing situation. A sensitive staff treats the patient in the manner suggested not only because it is a necessary appropriate courtesy but also because it is good medical care.

Any patient who has an operation requiring more than a minor local anesthetic, including intravenous anesthesia, requires the same attentive nursing surveillance employed in any professional recovery room. Vital signs, levels of consciousness, alertness, absence of confusion, and general recovery from intravenous medications must be monitored and recorded. Within relatively short periods (45 to 90 minutes), patients are assisted to a special comfortable "step-down" recovery area where they sit or recline in semirecumbency in large lounge chairs (Fig 2–7).

When recovery is essentially complete and the patients fully alert, those for whom an overnight stay is planned (a preference of the senior author) are transported to their hospital room for "minimal overnight observation" until discharge by the surgeon early the following morning.

Those patients returning home or to nearby hotels after recovery is complete must do so in the company and care of a responsible family member or friend who has also been briefed on the essentials of postoperative care.

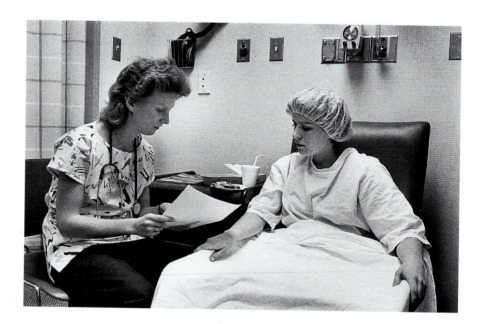

Figure 2–7
For both hospitalized and ambulatory patients, a "step-down" recovery area supplied with recliner chairs provides an ideal environment for monitoring patient recovery following surgery.

Patients are required to provide us with a location and phone number(s) where they plan to be in the early postoperative days in order that frequent phone checks may be made on a routine basis to monitor progress and reinforce the discipline of following postoperative instructions fully. Written postoperative instructions must be provided and thoroughly explained since aesthetic facial surgery patients, especially when their postoperative course remains pain free, too often tend to "stretch the rules."

Involving an operating room–patient care coordinator or similar person can be a major help with the family as well as ensure a comfortable and safe "flow" of the preoperative and postoperative activities.

Conclusion

Surgery is an activity that is never experienced without trepidation by the patient. Even if the procedure is elective and the patient looks forward to the eventual result, the event itself is inevitably anxiety producing.

Minimizing the anxieties and risks surrounding surgery remains the responsibility of the entire surgical team.

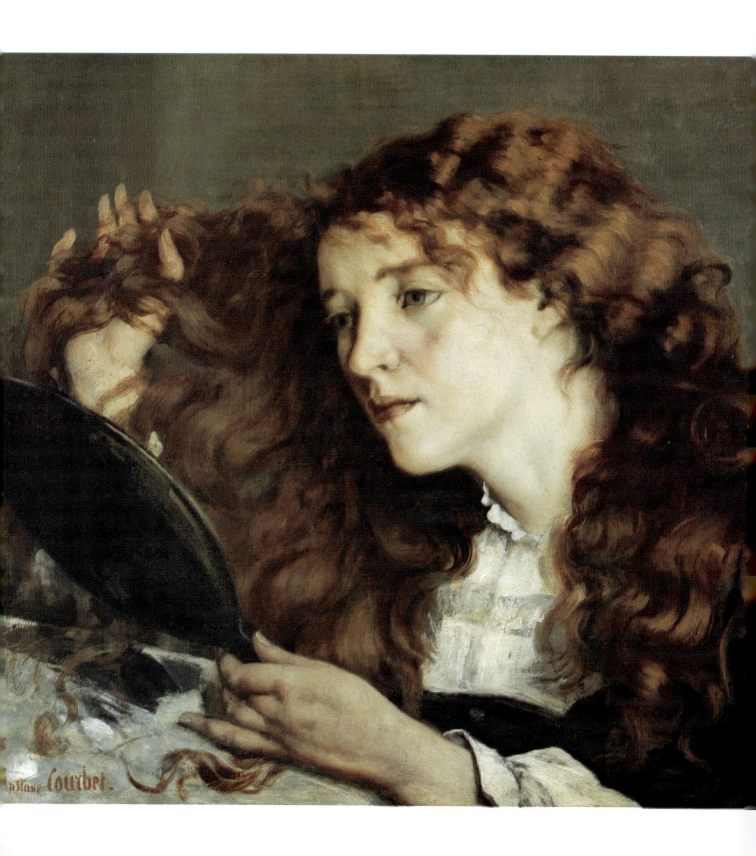

CHAPTER 3

 Psychological Assessment of Surgical Candidates

PART I   BASIC PRINCIPLES

Every man contemplates an angel in his future self.

Ralph Waldo Emerson

Initial Encounter: A Personal Approach

Patients arrive as potential candidates for facial plastic surgery for a wide variety of reasons; motivational factors must be ascertained and thoroughly evaluated by the surgeon. Unlike an organic illness where a suggestive list of symptoms and findings portends a specific diagnosis, patients seek aesthetic surgery to change their personal image for a wide variety of reasons. No checklist exists (or probably ever will exist) to compute the psychological makeup of individuals. Helpful guidelines certainly are available, but in the final analysis the surgeon must integrate all of the facts and psychological indicators available by sorting and sifting through impressions gained via the communication process to arrive at a single vital decision: *Does this patient have sufficient motivational and psychological stability (ego strength) to predict with a reasonable degree of certainty that a satisfactory surgical outcome will result in a patient who is happy?* Nothing else assumes quite the importance of this latter observation, because even an anatomically and technically excellent result is a failure if the patient is not pleased and content. Realistic motivations and expectations are mandatory prerequisites for patients seeking appearance surgery.

It is therefore essential to gently guide the patient to a form of self-analysis and awareness of the interdependent structures of the face and to assist the patient in defining true motivations. This exercise will assist in understanding the scope of the deformity and operation as well as the *limitations* imposed on the procedure by the existing imperfect anatomy, while clarifying the less well defined issue of inner wishes and feelings.

The overwhelming majority of individuals seeking facial plastic surgery possess satisfactory motivation and ego strength to withstand the temporary physical and emotional trauma of surgery. Most find significant fulfillment in the eventual surgical outcome and become strong supporters of others contemplating a similar appearance change. A small percentage of individuals request surgery either for totally unrealistic reasons or for more subtly inappropriate justifications. The former generally are not difficult to sort out, but the latter group may conceal their true motivation from the surgeon with great skill and cunning. Therefore the facial plastic surgeon must develop communication and diagnostic skills beyond the requisite technical skills of surgery in order to assiduously avoid operat-

CHAPTER 3   Psychologic Assessment of Surgical Candidates

ing on patients who may be made psychologically worse as a consequence of inappropriate surgery.

Although each initial patient encounter is different, it is helpful to establish an examination routine to ensure thoroughness. Each patient is personally escorted to the examination room by the receptionist after having signed the comprehensive photographic consent form. Our preference is to always inquire of the patient, with nonspecific open-ended questions, why he or she has sought consultation, never assuming that an obvious large nose, baggy eyelids, or sagging face is the source of concern. Before focusing on the facial examination, a review of the medical and social history, taken in preconsultation discussion with the office staff, occurs. Specific attention is centered on significant allergies to medicines or inhalants, daily medication used (particularly aspirin), previous facial surgery or trauma, chronic or recurrent illnesses, and previous plastic or reconstructive surgery. If other plastic surgery procedures have been performed, it is always instructive to learn why the patient is seeking another surgeon.

During this initial dialogue the surgeon continuously observes the general appearance of the patient, in particular assessing overall facial balance, symmetry and proportion, hairstyle, quality of skin and general facial animation, and habits of dress and personal confidence revealed by speech and "body language."

This early phase of the initial encounter thus forms the basis for "impression management," a process by which the patient and physician get to know each other in a professional but friendly setting. The patient is always thinking "can I trust my face to the doctor," while the surgeon is constantly assessing the feasibility of the patient's expectations and the potential for a positive happy ultimate outcome. A two-way verbal and mental assessment augmented by facial expression, verbal intonation, and body language thus occurs between two strangers. Within a matter of minutes, a mutual appraisal of vital significance has occurred in which each individual's impression of the other is cemented, confirmed, or doubted. For our part, the elements of interaction must, when summated, result in a simplistic judgment about whether we "like the patient." If any doubt at all exists regarding this fundamental principle, further probing assessment is indicated, or gentle disengagement is necessary. One must always hold the principle paramount that the majority of patients seeking facial surgery are "well" patients who seek to be "weller" (happy); the surgeon has the opportunity to make them sick (unhappy). Initial open-ended questions, such as, "How can I help you?" "What changes would you like to see made?" "What changes will make you happy?" or "Tell me a little bit about why you've come here today," will often put a nervous patient at ease and allow substantive dialogue to occur. What the candidate for aesthetic surgery says is important; what he or she is really thinking is critical. These two sometimes disparate concepts must be appreciated and occasionally separated in patient evaluation.

Open-ended questions should lead inevitably to a discussion of specific desires and needs. These are best described with the patient viewing himself in a three-way mirror. Exact concerns and desired changes should be elicited by the surgeon with the aid of a Q-tip as a convenient pointer (see Fig 1–3). The patient is urged to demonstrate in the reflected image precisely what is displeasing. The surgeon in turn should continue the education process by pointing out positive and negative anatomic features, limitations as well as possibilities, anatomic asymmetries, and liabilities as well as advantages and should attempt, insofar as is possible, to educate the patient about what possibly can and cannot be safely accomplished. Surgical confidence on the part of the surgeon is clearly important, but an unrealistic air of omnipotence or arrogance is clearly a reflection of poor judgment.

An aura of concerned cautious optimism is perhaps ideal, never "overselling" the operation or promising an extraordinary result.

This education process is facilitated by assessing the patient's appearance in the three-way mirror, supplemented by a detailed review of accurate photographs to provide a more thorough understanding of facial aesthetics. This is often done at a second preoperative visit. The aim is not to totally convert the patient's aesthetic values to those of the surgeon, but rather to expose him to the accumulated experience and developed artistic sense of the responsible surgeon. Reviewing stylized line art illustrations and even "ideal" photographs may be helpful in clarification; however, each patient's anatomic limitations must be constantly reemphasized and recorded as such. Fashioning an "ideal" result by drawing on a lateral-view photograph may carry the risk of "implied guarantee," a significant hazard in today's litigious climate. In the final analysis, however, any graphic process that will cement the patient and surgeon's understanding of the desired outcome, limited by the realistic *range* of possible results, is useful.

Assuming to this point that the initial encounter has been a mutually positive experience, a systematic facial examination is begun. The transition between a verbal discussion and the actual physical examination must be one that flows almost imperceptibly, never abruptly touching the face or exploring the nasal interior with a cold speculum.

We always explain to the patient what we are about to do and that it will not hurt or be uncomfortable and reinforce that notion by ensuring that the first touch of the patient's face by the examining physician's fingers is the gentlest possible. Inconsiderate or less than gentle manipulation of the face and nose invariably casts doubt in the patient's mind about the artistic surgical capabilities of their potential surgeon.

After gaining a general idea of the patient's concerns and level of understanding, we prefer to examine the patient's facial and nasal features first, followed by a repeat review of his specific concerns in a three-way mirror. Some degree of mental organization assists in the discipline of examination, although variations might be necessary because of individual anatomy, surgical requests, and patient reactions. Visual examination and finger palpation are equally important in the nasal evaluation. Throughout the evaluation a mental image of the potential outcome and surgical limitations inherent in every individual is being visualized.

During the comprehensive facial and nasal examination, we prefer to

CHAPTER 3 Psychologic Assessment of Surgical Candidates

make few specific comments regarding the face, instead electing to await discovery of the patient's specific voiced concerns.

The hand-held three-way mirror is now positioned before the patient, and specific questioning is carried out. At this juncture it is vital to ferret out exactly what features are disliked or in need of change or preservation and what expectations are harbored. A surprisingly large number of individuals are initially unable to define *exactly* which anatomic aspects of the nose troubles them and which modifications are preferred. Many are predictably unsophisticated regarding subtle (and even overt) variations and asymmetries in facial anatomy and require reassuring self-education during this phase of the interview. Again, what the patient says is one thing, whereas what he or she is actually thinking is quite another.

Not uncommonly patients will arrive with photographs of desired facial features from fashion magazines. This sometimes unrealistic quest can be turned to the surgeon's advantage in several ways: it provides an evaluation of the patient's aesthetic sense and values, thus improving patient-doctor communication, and it provides the opportunity to point out the limitations of surgery because of the raw materials with which the surgeon must work, that is, the patient's own personal anatomy.

Once the patient has completed the mirrored demonstration of desires and expectations (during which the surgeon listens and occasionally prompts), the surgeon may now take charge of the discussion and painstakingly point out, while the patient holds the mirror, the positive and not-so-positive aspects of the individual nasal and facial anatomy. Concentration is initially brought to bear on the major deformities and patient's primary concerns, then focused on subtle deformities, asymmetries, and disharmonies that often have eluded the patient. Sites of external scars and areas requiring reduction, augmentation, or reorientation are shown precisely. The benefits of improving previously unrecognized facial deficiencies such as chin augmentation, if indicated, are detailed, recommended, but not made mandatory. These decisions are best left to the *informed* patient and family.

Throughout the initial evaluation the anatomic limitations encountered are emphasized and reemphasized to lay the foundation for the development of reasonable outcome expectations. Aesthetic surgery is always best "undersold" because even though significant appearance improvement is routine, a truly spectacular transformation is less common.

Revealing a photographic series of outstanding operative results of facial surgery to a prospective patient is probably unwise and even somehow unfair unless a general *range of results* is reviewed. We decline to show patients operative results obtained on others and point out that no two faces are ever alike, that our patients' records are confidential—as theirs will likewise be—and that one cannot "choose" a face or nose as one would select a new car. The overwhelming majority of patients appreciate this ethical approach. Situations do arise, however, in which the patient education process can be enhanced by pointing out photographically the effect of correcting an unusual problem foreign to the patient's understanding (augmenting a recessed midfacial deformity, correcting a significant retrognathia, balancing pre-existing asymmetries, etc.). Caution should immediately be exercised if agreement between the patient and surgeon seems at all difficult to reach. A second and even third interview may be advantageous to thoroughly cement the surgeon-patient relationship; at that point, if any major doubts persist, the operation is probably best not performed.

As the next step in the interview process, we personally record a full series of uniform preoperative facial photographs. This requires less than 90 seconds of valuable consultation time, ensures that the proper standardized views are obtained, and allows a further opportunity to evaluate the patient's personality and level of maturity. The individual incapable of striking and holding a required pose, who is frivolous or uncooperative during photography, or who questions the need for a full series of photographs may in fact be an individual unlikely to carefully follow important preoperative and postoperative instructions. The psychological evaluation process thus goes forward even during the short period required for photodocumentation.

Computer imaging for effective patient evaluation and education holds great promise for the future but does not yet fulfill its potential. The systems personally evaluated still fall short of the clarity and fine detail of color transparencies, which are preferred for demonstrating major and more subtle anatomic details to patients. Currently, computer imaging systems are expensive to acquire and involve a substantial expenditure of time and "busy work" to record, modify, and evaluate the patient's appearance, time that we prefer to spend in more vital discussion with aesthetic surgery candidates. Despite disclaimers to the contrary, computer image modification may raise the expectation of certain individuals beyond what may be reasonably accomplished, because the computer is incapable of divining the vital aspects of the limitations imposed by thick skin–subcutaneous tissue elements and possesses no capacity for predicting appearance changes wrought by the dynamics of healing over time. Regrettably, this promising imaging tool lends itself currently to unscrupulous marketing techniques by less-than-ethical surgeons who play on the public's penchant for computer techniques to attract the gullible patient.

A valuable approach in patient education regarding rhinoplasty combines the effort of the surgeon and capable office staff. After agreement about the indications and reasonable expectations for surgery has been reached with the surgeon, a further detailed, sympathetic discussion of the operation and the circumstances surrounding its performance is carried out by the surgical nurse, the patient's counselor and companion throughout the process (see Fig 3–1). In essence, the surgical nurse becomes the patient's "best friend" and ombudsman before, during, and after the operative event. Commonly a strong bonding occurs between the nurse and patient. This approach amplifies the understanding and education process and allows the patient ample opportunity to have every question, however seemingly mundane, answered clearly. Areas of concern left unresolved by the surgeon and patient will often surface and be recon-

CHAPTER 3 Psychologic Assessment of Surgical Candidates

ciled with a sensitive and sympathetic nurse. In the patient education process no question is ever considered too unimportant or redundant. Since it has been well documented that patients remember only a variable fraction of what has been discussed, this dual approach has value in its reemphasis of important details.

At this juncture the patient is encouraged to view a short slide/tape presentation that underscores and amplifies the fundamentals of the operation and the events surrounding it and highlights the responsibilities that must be shared by the patient and surgeon to maximize the possibilities of an intended excellent result. This short audiovisual presentation is not a highly technical one, but rather an information-giving device to visually augment the discussions with the surgeon and nurse.

Patients uniformly appreciate this educational approach to the understanding and planning of facial aesthetic surgery, and as important, misunderstandings are clearly minimized. Involving the immediate family or close friends in these processes is advantageous. It is truly astonishing how many misconceptions and myths have grown up around the operation of rhinoplasty over the decades.

If in the surgeon's judgment realistic motivation and understanding are present, plans are made to schedule the desired operation. If any doubt exists, it is propitious to schedule a second interview and consultation prior

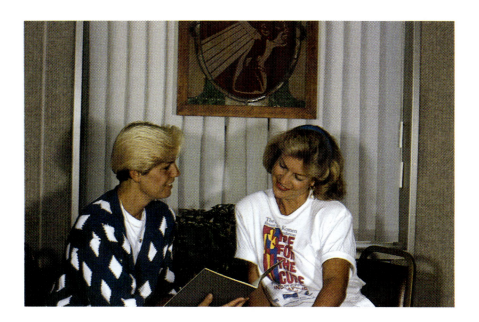

Figure 3-1
The vital communication process between the surgeon and patient is vastly improved by the close relationship developed between the involved surgical nurse and the patient. Patients often feel more comfortable asking "less important" questions from someone other than the surgeon, a factor helping to solidify the informed consent.

to any firm decision for surgery. This allows a period of reflection and contemplation on the part of the patient. We routinely suggest that a second opinion may be helpful and comforting to them, provided that they seek surgeons of high reputation and honesty. The majority of patients requesting facial surgery in our offices are highly motivated, are reasonably knowledgeable about the operation, and can be judged so during the first encounter. Thus, it is unnecessary to routinely require a second interview. Further discussions are of value, however, if any doubt exists (in the mind of the patient or the surgeon) and if a complete mutual understanding regarding what the patient really wants and what the surgeon can realistically provide has not been reached. Second interviews are particularly valuable to review photographs of the patient and outline facial relationships and limitations from various photographic views not commonly seen by the patient. Disproportionate features, inadequate or excessive tip projection, a cervicomandibular angle in need of definition, and subtle facial asymmetries are more thoroughly understood and accepted if these abnormalities can be viewed on uniform standardized photographs of high quality.

Once the decision for surgery is established, the consent forms for the precise surgical procedure as well as for photography are signed and witnessed (Fig 3–2). These consent forms are personal ones retained in the office file. Similar forms are signed by the patient on admission to the hospital so that a duplicate set of consent records are always available. Patient information booklets (see Appendix A in Chapter 1), if not already possessed, are personally provided to the patient to augment his understanding of the procedure and its appropriate aftercare. These are fairly detailed in nature and designed to further catalyze the education process and clearly outline the patient's responsibilities in the quest for the most favorable result. Again, patients appreciate these small courtesies and uniformly fare better when verbal instructions are supplemented by written guidelines.

As the final event in the initial consultation, we sit down with the patient and family in a comfortable, nonclinical setting and listen while the patient is encouraged to ask any further questions and voice any fears. We try to again dispel any myths and reiterate exact expectations and limitations. Our method of anesthesia is reviewed thoroughly. This final step in the initial consultation allows the patient the third of three opportunities (two with the surgeon, one with the nurse) to become realistically educated about facial surgery and to develop an informed eagerness about the changes in facial appearance about to be enacted.

At this point we emphasize the patient's responsibilities in the mutual quest for an ideal procedure and outcome. A section of the informed consent form in which the patient agrees to accurately follow all vital postoperative instructions is completed. Phone numbers where the patient may be reached after surgery are recorded. Patients commonly "hide out" with friends or family after surgery and frustrate physician attempts to check with them regularly by phone.

The common and reasonable complications that might be expected

CHAPTER 3 Psychologic Assessment of Surgical Candidates

M. EUGENE TARDY, JR., M.D.
HEAD AND NECK PLASTIC SURGERY, LTD.
Chicago, Illinois 60657
St. Joseph Hospital
Chicago, Illinois 60657

–AUTHORIZATION AND INFORMED CONSENT–

_____
(Patient's Name)

1. I request and authorize M. Eugene Tardy, Jr., M.D. (the Doctor) to perform an operation upon me (or my _____) entitled (description of procedure):
_____
_____
_____

2. The nature and effects of the operation, the risks, ramifications, complications involved, as well as alternative methods of treatment, have been fully explained to me by the Doctor and I understand them.

3. I authorize the Doctor to perform any other procedure he may deem desirable in attempting to improve the condition stated in paragraph 1 or any unhealthy or unforeseen condition that may be encountered during the operation.

4. I consent to the administration of anesthetics by the Doctor or under the direction of the physician responsible for this service. If an anesthesiologist assists in my surgery, I understand that the anesthesiologist will take full charge of the administration and maintenance of the anesthesia, and that this is an independent function of the surgery.

5. I have been thoroughly and completely advised regarding the objectives of the operation. Since I understand that the practice of medicine and surgery is not an exact science and therefore that no reputable surgeon can guarantee results, I acknowledge that imperfections might ensue and that the operative result may not live up to my expectations. I certify that no guarantees have been made by anyone regarding the operations(s) I have requested and authorized.

6. I understand that the two sides of the human body are not the same and can never be made the same.

7. For the purpose of advancing medical education, I consent to the admittance of authorized observers to the operating room.

8. I give permission to M. Eugene Tardy, Jr., M.D., to take still or motion clinical photographs with the understanding that such photographs remain the property of the Doctor. If, in the judgment of the Doctor, medical research, education, or science will be benefitted by their use, such photographs and related information may be published and republished in professional journals or medical books or used for such publication or use. I shall not be identified by name.

9. I understand that if Dr. Tardy judges at any time that my surgery should be postponed or cancelled for any reason, he may do so.

10. I hereby authorize that the information furnished Dr. Tardy by me during my diagnostic evaluation is correct.

11. I agree to follow the instructions given to me by Dr. Tardy to the best of my ability before, during and after my surgical procedure.

I certify that I have read the above authorization, that the explanations referred to therein were made to my satisfaction, and that I fully understand such explanations and the above authorization.

Signed _____
(Patient or person authorized to consent for patient)

Witness _____ Date _____

Figure 3–2
Current patient surgical consent form completed by each patient at the time surgery is scheduled.

from facial surgery are reviewed; no attempt is made to supply a long "laundry list" of every possible complication, a valueless process. Fortunately, contemporary aesthetic surgery carries with it a paucity of complications.

The overall intent of the initial consultation is relatively simplistic: regardless of whether an operation is scheduled for any particular patient, we wish him or her to leave the office setting with the feeling that a concerned, thorough effort has been made to understand and analyze the problem, honestly discuss individual possibilities and limitations, and educate the patient insofar as is possible about the precise details of the operation itself. If nothing else, the public relations fallout from this approach benefits not only the patient and public but the profession as a whole.

No guarantees of surgical outcomes are possible or ever given; rather a sincere promise that every effort will be made to provide the finest result possible within the limitations of patient anatomy is offered. The second interview is commonly sought by a relatively small percentage of patients seeking facial aesthetic surgery, but is offered to all.

Candidate Rejection

All experienced facial surgeons appreciate the critical importance and the extreme difficulty of selecting patients with appropriate motivation and expectations. The anatomic indications for aesthetic surgery are easier to judge than the psychological considerations. Surgical residents in training quickly and accurately learn the physical characteristics favorable for aesthetic surgical correction, but the experience and judgment to assess emotional motivations are less readily acquired. An experienced surgeon can predict the reasonable anatomic and aesthetic outcome of a surgical procedure; forecasting the patient's reaction to that outcome is an altogether different matter. A good surgical outcome does not always satisfy every patient. Since the functional end point of aesthetic surgery is a happy patient, every effort must be made to develop a sixth sense about patient expectations and motivation.

Being a good listener helps to provide valuable insight into the many reasons why patients seek aesthetic surgery. Patients with particular personality disorders may not realize a favorable psychological outcome despite a near-perfect surgical result. Some patients, described in the following section, have been encountered frequently enough over the past 25 years that the aesthetic surgeon should more closely evaluate them prior to surgery:

- The patient with unrealistic expectations
- The obsessive-compulsive, perfectionistic patient
- The "sudden whim" patient
- The indecisive patient
- The rude patient
- The overflattering patient
- The overly familiar patient
- The unkempt patient
- The patient with minimal or imagined deformity
- The careless or poor historian

CHAPTER 3 Psychologic Assessment of Surgical Candidates

- The "VIP" patient
- The uncooperative patient
- The overly talkative patient
- The surgeon shopper
- The depressed patient
- The "plastic surgiholic"
- The price haggler
- The patient involved in litigation
- The patient whom you or your staff dislikes

Although patients who fit into one or more of these groups may, on further evaluation, be good surgical candidates with suitable motivations, many make entirely unsuitable patients. It is the surgeon's responsibility to exercise forbearance in the latter instance, either postponing or tactfully refusing a surgical procedure.

Patient With Unrealistic Expectations

Often patients do not understand or, many times, may not wish to understand the limitations of aesthetic surgery. High expectations honed by mass media and current medical marketing hype imply that the surgeon can "remove" a scar or sculpt a "perfect face." On occasion patients produce magazine photographs of the highly angular, "chiseled" faces of photogenic models and expect the surgeon to replicate that facial type. Such individuals fail to understand the limitations of their thick skin or coarse facial features.

In the same category are patients requesting a radical change that would appear disproportionate when balanced with other facial features. These patients may have their minds made up and do not wish to compromise their flawed expectations with gentle reason and surgical judgment. Common among these are surgeon shoppers who seek out a surgeon willing to accept their unrealistic goals.

Obsessive-Compulsive, Perfectionist Patient

These patients possess unrealistic expectations but exhibit several typical personality characteristics that differentiate them. Perfectionists are often immaculately dressed and groomed. Facial makeup and other cosmetic enhancements are liberally applied and typically overdone.

The perfectionist is often overly compulsive when arranging the initial consultation; he may send detailed letters regarding his wishes and the timing of office appointments and surgery and even stipulate ground rules for the surgeon and staff to follow. Complaints about other surgeons who have treated the patient (usually "unsuccessfully") are often detailed or at least implied.

Overly perfectionistic patients frequently arrive with long, detailed (and at times unrealistic and inappropriate) questions and insist upon precise responses in advance of the natural interchange between the physician and patient, which is the hallmark of the plastic surgery consultation. It is precisely because of their self-proclaimed need for a "perfect" surgical outcome that satisfaction with any surgical result is unlikely. Any slight imperfection or asymmetry will be magnified out of proportion with its importance postoperatively, followed by demands for immediate and even repeated revision surgery.

"Sudden Whim" Patient

Some individuals who insist that surgery be performed immediately feel no need for routine systematic evaluation and surgical preparation. They place an unrealistic time frame on the surgeon. These patients may be improperly motivated by a sudden whim. Reasons for the expressed urgency for aesthetic surgery are often unclear and, if stated, are usually unrealistic and triggered by a friend's adverse comment or an abrupt life-style change. These patients can be identified through routine screening by the surgeon's office staff because they demand appointments immediately and try to circumvent the orderly sequence of preoperative evaluation. Characteristically these patients have little patience with the surgeon's efforts to completely evaluate, discuss, and inform; instead they wish to schedule surgery immediately and show little concern for surgical hazards, complications, or even outcome. A search for some significant psychological event in such patients may often reveal a causal relationship.

Indecisive Patient

This patient characteristically requests a plastic surgical procedure but cannot clearly explain why. Typically the patient may seek several consecutive consultations and yet may remain uncertain whether a procedure should be done. Unsure of specific anatomic problems and the desired surgical outcome, the patient often prefers to allow the surgeon to make all of the decisions and implores him to "just do whatever you think best" or states "I'll just leave it up to you."

This category includes patients who may be seeking surgery at the behest of a relative, close friend, or in the case of actors, performers, and models, overzealous photographers and career advisors. Vagueness about what would make this patient happy is a characteristic hallmark, and surgery is sought precisely for the wrong reasons. Disenchantment and even depression may ensue when the requested surgery fails to bring happiness, favorable comment, and professional advancement. These patients typically schedule surgery, cancel, and reschedule, only to cancel again for obscure and indefinite reasons.

Rude Patient

Although initially pleasant and deferential toward the surgeon as an authority figure, a rude and disrespectful patient is usually exposed when he or she exhibits an unpleasant "pushy" and even demeaning behavior toward the office and hospital staff. Unrealistic requests for preferential treatment may be made, with little regard for the rights and privileges of other patients. Playing by the rules is usually outside the understanding of such patients, and impatience with "the system" is a common characteristic. These unpleasant traits are usually easy to discover during the evaluation process because inappropriate, unpleasant behavior surfaces repeatedly.

Overflattering Patient

The patient who excessively praises the surgeon's skills, reputation, and omnipotent surgical abilities sets a tempting trap for the surgeon unable to resist this false adulation. Delicate questioning may reveal the patient's previous visits to other colleagues with unsatisfactory consultations or even surgical outcomes. Demeaning comments may be expressed about other surgeons. Such patients may often travel great distances to "be treated by only the best," but may in reality possess little first-hand knowledge of the surgeon's actual skills and surgical results. Overflattering patients may be quick to turn on the surgeon if the surgical outcome is even slightly imperfect and replace excessive praise with anger and outrage.

Overly Familiar Patient

Typically such patients show little respect for the formal confines of the physician-patient relationship. An excessively familiar attitude is taken with both the office staff and the physicians. A first-name intimacy may be assumed inappropriately, and the term "Doc" is used repeatedly. Such patients may show little regard for the office furnishings, instruments, records, and accoutrements and help themselves to whatever strikes their fancy. These inappropriate intimacies may extend to ingratiating or seductive behavior in order to gain favor or preferential treatment.

Unkempt Patient

Patients seeking an appearance and self-image change must, for ideal results, be attentive to a favorable overall facial and bodily appearance. Correcting an unattractive nose without enhancing the remainder of the factors contributing to a positive appearance will inevitably fall short of the desired improvement. Rhinoplasty candidates occasionally appear who are totally unkempt and disheveled in appearance and dress, as manifested by an unattractive hair condition, inappropriate makeup, sloppy or dirty clothing, and even an overly unclean appearance. In such individuals it is unlikely that even a perfect rhinoplasty outcome will contribute a positive self-image improvement and provide a valuable enhancement to the quality of life. A slovenly appearance may also provide the first clue to an underlying psychological disturbance.

Patient With Minimal or Imagined Deformity

Although patients with minimal deformities may constitute superb candidates for the benefits of subtle rhinoplasty, a fine distinction must be drawn between these patients and those who significantly overemphasize the importance of or imagined existence of a truly minor problem. Commonly such patients may have the perception of a "perfect" nose, which in reality would fit poorly with the surrounding facial features. It is not unusual for individuals operated on elsewhere to request revision rhinoplasty for insignificant additional changes or corrections when in fact the initial result is quite satisfactory. The surgeon performs a service for both the patient and himself by avoiding surgery on individuals in this category, who are unlikely to ever be completely satisfied.

Careless or Poor Historian

The frequency and safety with which contemporary aesthetic surgery is performed have spawned a cavalier attitude in patients regarding the risks and intricacies of these delicate operations. Individuals who express impatience with or who provide inaccuracies in the detailed medical history constitute a group unlikely to carefully follow the preoperative instructions and postoperative guidelines critical to the ideal surgical outcome. These patients may manifest evidence of immaturity and inappropriateness, often arriving late for scheduled appointments, ignoring or forgetting specific directions provided by the office staff, and generally trivializing the orderly process important in the physician-patient relationship.

"VIP" Patient

Individuals in the public eye or in positions of importance (or assumed importance) frequently seek appearance surgery, and generally represent a highly desirable group of surgical candidates. Occasionally a patient possessed of inappropriate self-importance will expect to receive special or unique treatment to the potential detriment of an ideal surgical outcome. Requests are commonly made for special nursing care, avoidance of important preoperative laboratory testing, premature splint removal, exemption from standard postoperative guidelines, and a myriad of other forms of special treatment.

Although small and appropriate courtesies are clearly justifiable, a wise surgeon remains firm in his insistence that the "routine" of the events surrounding and accompanying nasal surgery be respected. Patients (VIP or otherwise) who rebel against the gentle insistence that a certain order in the perisurigical period remains vital to an ideal outcome and is clearly in the patient's best interest are best avoided. The temptations to pacify the patient of importance are profound; the remorse associated with a less-than-ideal result as a consequence of "cutting corners" can be immense.

Uncooperative Patient

This patient type manifests many of the characteristics described in the above two categories. He simply cannot be bothered to carefully follow vital verbal or written instructions, ignores the rudiments of the proper patient-physician relationship, is late for or fails office appointments, is reticent to follow important admonitions provided by the office staff, and

CHAPTER 3 Psychologic Assessment of Surgical Candidates

ultimately cannot be trusted to adhere to postoperative guidelines. Commonly this individual is first detected by the receptionist or staff person because an uncooperative and even disdainful attitude manifests itself from the very first contact with the medical office. Almost routinely deferential and courteous to the physician, such patients tend to treat non-physician personnel shabbily and without proper respect. If any pattern of uncooperation is detected by any member of our office staff, I generally avoid operating on patients with this dangerous attribute.

Overly Talkative Patient

Loquaciousness is not uncommon in patients seeking aesthetic surgery, and by itself is not a disqualifying defect. In any busy practice, however, patients are encountered who tend to verbally dominate each and every professional encounter. They routinely interrupt inappropriately, fail to listen to and comprehend important instructions and surgical limitations, and are almost impossible to provide comprehensive informed consent for. Such individuals must be assessed for marked or latent insecurity, for the need to dominate every encounter and interactive experience, and especially for traits of manic-depressive personalities. If doubt exists, a longer preoperative evaluation process by means of serial office discussions will usually provide the surgeon with a clear comprehension of whether such patients are reliable and appropriate candidates.

Surgeon Shopper

At the conclusion of the initial consultation for aesthetic surgery, we routinely suggest to the patient that a second opinion sought from another surgeon of high reputation may be useful in making an informed decision regarding surgery. Patients seem to appreciate this courtesy, and most return to schedule a date for surgery. It is not uncommon, however, to encounter an individual seeking rhinoplasty who has visited with several or many surgeons to find assurance of a preconceived outcome, the most favorable fee, or a guarantee that "my insurance will pay for it." The surgeon should regard these individuals with caution; they are often insecure, excessively demanding, and unlikely to be satisfied with even the best outcome. Often their visits to many surgeons will be unveiled during the consultation by the wording and nature of the questions asked, obviously spawned by the analysis and comments of previous physicians. Occasionally they fall into the category of the overflattering patient by asserting that "you are the only doctor I'd let touch my nose." Regularly such individuals attempt to dictate the details of the planned operation and demand that the surgeon carry out the nasal correction in a manner other than what may be medically and aesthetically appropriate.

Depressed Patient

The overwhelming percentage of individuals seeking aesthetic surgery are well adjusted and manifest clearly appropriate justifications about their interest in changing the appearance of the face. Depression is a common finding in any large patient population and is ordinarily not difficult to sense during a careful discussion of the patient's well-being or lack thereof. The initial clue may surface from the medication history since the periodic or regular use of antidepressant medication is becoming more common. Older individuals appear more likely to have depression (or manic-depressive) symptoms, and may appear shortly after the death of a family member, a divorce, or similar disruptive events. Tearfulness, frequent sighing, and even a lack of humor and lightheartedness during the consultation may provide clear clues to an ongoing depressive state.

Surgery may, by improving a bodily part offensive to the depressed patient, accomplish a temporary raising of the spirits and improved body image; however, seldom does the underlying cause of the depression evaporate as a result of rhinoplasty. The assistance of a therapist knowledgeable about facial plastic surgery may be invaluable in the decision to undergo or to defer surgery, and in fact this is appreciated by the patient. Preoperative counseling is occasionally useful and reassuring to mildly depressed individuals; the suspicion by the therapist of a significant manic-depressive or even paranoid personality is generally a contraindication to aesthetic surgery.

"Plastic Surgiholic"

The patient who seeks repeated (usually inappropriate) plastic surgery procedures on a multiplicity of body parts is a poor candidate for aesthetic surgery. These individuals most commonly come for revision rhinoplasty and give a history of having seen many different surgeons. Seldom can they be satisfied, even though the anatomic indications for rhinoplasty may be perfectly appropriate and the surgeon confident of a satisfactory appearance outcome. This category of patient should be clearly differentiated from two vastly different groups in whom surgery is clearly helpful: (1) those who are in earnest need of revision rhinoplasty following one or more unsuccessful procedures elsewhere and (2) patients who have sought timely surgical rejuvenation procedures in the calculated and appropriate task of forestalling the ravages of the aging process. This latter group is characterized by generally complete contentment with the outcome of their various surgical procedures, while the plastic surgiholic is constantly discontent.

Price Haggler

Persons who regard aesthetic surgery as a commodity and attempt to negotiate the best possible price lack comprehension for the professional nature of the surgical undertaking. They somehow assume that a well-performed operation is a negotiable item and commonly surgeon-shop (often initially by phone) to "make the best deal." Such patients, if unable to understand that paying more or less for surgery does not translate into a better or lesser result, are best avoided.

Into this same category fit individuals who insist (or not so subtly suggest) that the surgeon "be sure to word the operation properly so that insurance will pay for it." This vexing and constant problem, occurring with even the best candidates for surgery, is handled by gently informing the patient that absolute honesty is vital in the relationship between the patient, surgeon, and insurance carrier. It is my policy to estimate, after a thorough nasal examination, what percentage of the procedure will be devoted to aesthetic changes and what percentage will be occupied by functional surgery. This estimate is provided to the patient at the very outset so that no misunderstanding exists. Most patients appreciate a frank and honest approach to financial considerations, which is not uniformly provided in every rhinoplasty surgeon's office. To underscore our policy, I point out to the recalcitrant patients that sending fraudulent information to insurance companies through the mail is a felony, and although I will exert my very best efforts in their surgical care, I do not wish to go to jail for them. Most understand and are sympathetic. Those who choose to seek another surgeon are welcome to do so.

Patient Involved in Litigation

In any surgical practice involving large numbers of revision or secondary cases, patients will be encountered who are involved in (or who are considering) litigation against their original (or successive) surgeon(s). Some have legitimate complaints; others do not. It is my policy to religiously refrain from making any judgmental comments about the previous surgery; instead I prefer to begin an evaluation at the patient's present baseline condition. No useful benefit derives from rehashing actual or perceived errors occasioned by previous surgery. If I feel that further revision surgery is likely to correct or improve the patient's appearance and/or nasal function, the exact details and *limitations* of the proposed corrections are chronicled while pointing out that no surgeon is infallible or can exert complete control over the healing process, especially when perverse scar tissue from previous surgery must be battled.

Patients who dwell persistently on the inadequacies of their previous surgeon(s) are generally best to avoid, because they come to you already angry, disillusioned, and less likely to find happiness in even the best of revision outcomes. Those who ask (and even demand) that you document the inadequacies and "mistakes" of the previous surgeon and insist that you participate in their litigation process are all firmly refused.

Patient Whom You or Your Staff Dislikes

The overwhelming majority of patients seeking appearance surgery are pleasant, happy, and well-adjusted individuals who are a joy to know and care for. Rarely, individuals are encountered who are of such a disagreeable nature that it simply is impossible to be assured that surgery will transform them into a satisfied and grateful patient. A perceptive office staff provides the most important front-line defense against such individuals and should be trained to notify you when they suspect that a problem patient may be encountered. Included in this category of patients are those who are routinely late for or fail office appointments, denigrate the office staff while flattering the surgeon, ask for inappropriate consideration or favors, use offensive language, show disrespect for other patients and staff, refuse to follow the important routine of instructions surrounding the surgical event, inappropriately question the photographic or operative consent form, write an unusually long and detailed letter prior to the initial consultation, and produce a sketch or photograph of *exactly* what they wish to look like following surgery.

Extra care must be taken to ferret out from such patients an understanding of whether they can be relied upon to be trusted partners in a surgical undertaking. Among them will be rare individuals who simply are unlikable, often for reasons that are not always overtly apparent. An alert office staff provides invaluable assistance in interpreting the first clues that manifest themselves in such patients. Disagreeableness preoperatively seems more likely to convert to hostility postoperatively if the patient perceives the result as flawed in even minor ways. Since aesthetic surgery is an elective procedure, a wise surgeon disengages from these individuals as quickly and gently as possible.

As Wright pointed out, an aesthetic surgeon need not diagnose overt psychiatric pathology in order to recognize a patient who is a psychological risk. Clearly the primary diagnostic symptom of the patient at risk stems from the surgeon's awareness of feeling intuitively uncomfortable, thereby making a conscious decision not to operate. An undisputed fact of facial plastic surgery is that all patient difficulties develop because the surgeon fails to fulfill the expectations of the patient. The truism persists: the surgeon makes a living from the patients he or she operates on, and a reputation from those he or she refuses to operate on.

Suggested Reading

- Goin JM, Goin MK: *Changing the Body: Psychological Effects of Plastic Surgery.* Baltimore, Williams & Wilkins, 1981.
- Tardy ME: Aesthetic rhinoplasty, in Cummings CC, et al (eds): *Otolaryngology—Head and Neck Surgery.* St Louis, Mosby, 1992.
- Goldwyn RM: *The Patient and the Plastic Surgeon.* Boston, Little, Brown, 1981.
- McGregor FC: *Transformation and Identity: the Face and Plastic Surgery.* New York, Quadrangle Times Books, 1974.

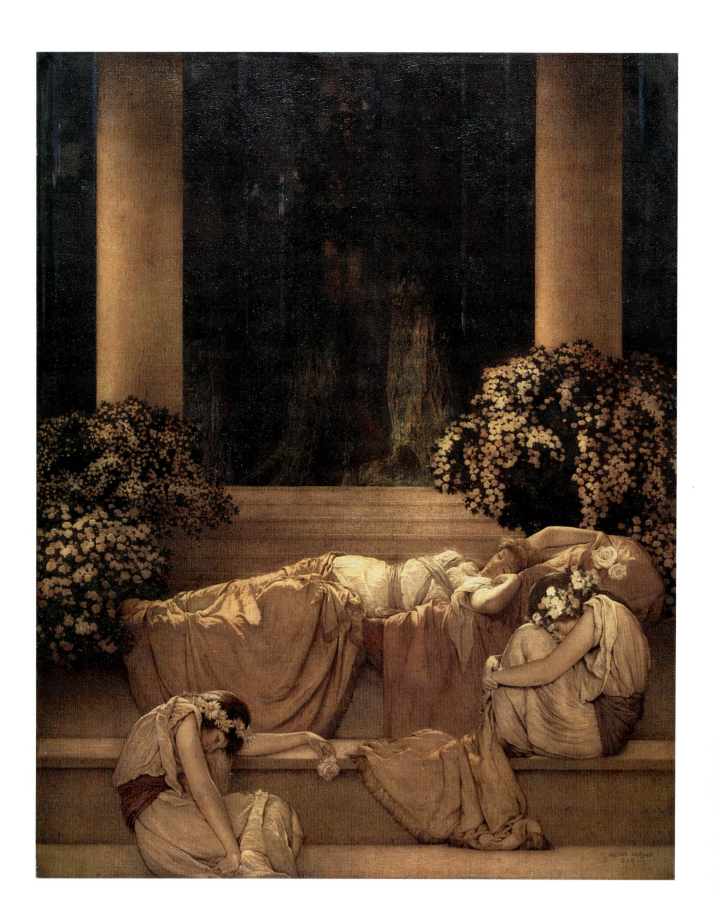

CHAPTER 4

 Anesthetic Methods: Patient Comfort and Safety

PART I BASIC PRINCIPLES

There is no joy but calm.

Alfred Lord Tennyson

An interesting facet of the concerns expressed by patients anticipating facial plastic surgery is that a greater fear exists of the anesthesia than of the surgery itself. Patients commonly pose specific and pointed questions about the risks and variabilities of operative anesthesia while minimizing or expressing far less concern regarding the planned operation and its ramifications. In patients undergoing facial plastic surgery, the provision for comfort combined with safety takes precedence over all else. These individuals, after all, are essentially well patients seeking to look better or correct a deficiency; it is vital that the anesthetic techniques used to accomplish desired surgical improvements not leave them unwell.

It is truly remarkable that among well-known, respectable, and renowned facial surgeons no single best anesthetic regimen can be agreed upon as ideal. Rather significant differences in anesthetic preferences as well as style exist. The gamut ranges from surgeons who prefer to render the patient entirely unconscious (general anesthesia) to others who prefer a semiconscious, comfortable patient who is arousable and responsive to appropriate commands and suggestions. Each surgeon must therefore find his own personal "comfort level", consistent with patient safety.

For the majority of facial plastic procedures, our decided preference is to achieve, with the use of reliable intravenous anesthesia methods carried out by experienced, skilled anesthesiologists, a comfortable but not totally unconscious patient who is arousable and able to participate in maneuvers assisting in the orchestration of the procedure. Occasional short conversations with the patient play a vital role in assessing his or her well-being and level of consciousness and are reassuring to the surgeon in reinforcement of the data provided by the monitoring devices employed. We wish to ensure freedom from pain and full or partial amnesia for the operative events. Rapid recovery from the anesthetic event, with postoperative freedom from nausea and pain, is equally important, particularly if an outpatient procedure is planned.

To accomplish these goals, we avoid the use of many different drugs, and instead prefer use largely reversible drugs given intravenously in small increments. Constant verbal reassurance feedback is given to the patient by the surgeon throughout to relieve anxiety, allay fears, and promote confidence. When deeper temporary levels of unawareness are required (anesthetic injection, rhinoplasty osteotomies, etc.), small doses of ultra-short-

CHAPTER 4 Anesthetic Methods: Patient Comfort and Safety

acting barbiturates (thiamylal [Surital] or methohexital [Brevital]) or propofol provide admirable short-term comfort.

For more than two decades, we have favored the use of intravenous anesthesia and analgesia (IAA) as a rapid, safe, predictable, and effective method of bringing a conscious, anxious patient to a state of relaxed comfort for surgery. An ideal intravenous anesthetic system should produce patient comfort and amnesia with minimal risk; involve drugs that are rapid acting, predictable, and reversible; and eventuate in rapid, comfortable recovery free of significant side effects.

Premedication

The goal of premedication, to the benefit of the patient and surgeon alike, is to achieve relief of anxiety and render the patient calm yet cooperative. Influencing the selection of drugs for premedication are the needs of the individual patient and the ultimate sedated state desired. Both factors are modified by the specific requirements of the surgical procedure (duration of the operation, need for patient cooperation and facial animation), the environment in which the operation is to be performed, and the need for rapid postoperative recovery and ambulation.

Suitable premedication is designed to attain most or all of the following objectives: sedation, diminution of secretory activity, amnesia for perioperative events, reduction in the postoperative incidence of nausea and vomiting, analgesia, suppression of cardiovascular reflexes, facilitation of the chosen anesthetic technique, and good patient acceptability. In our facility, premedication is provided intravenously by the anesthesiologist approximately 30 minutes preoperatively. Well-premedicated patients generally require less intraoperative medication to achieve satisfactory levels of anesthesia and analgesia, thus increasing the safety of the anesthetic event and promoting more rapid recovery.

Intravenous Anesthesia and Analgesia

In the early history of IAA it was anticipated that one universal drug would emerge that possessed all the favorable characteristics desired: produce sleep, provide amnesia, and effect satisfactory analgesia during and after the surgical procedure. However, it soon became clear that dangerously large doses were required to provide satisfactory and adequate anesthesia, with intolerable respiratory and cardiovascular depression the invariable result. With experience, research investigators and pioneering anesthesiologists demonstrated the efficacy and safety of *combining* various intravenous drugs to provide improved comfort with much less risk.

Intravenous drugs useful for IAA may be categorized according to their pharmacologic class and exhibit certain reliable clinical characteristics. The *barbiturates*, superb hypnotics, lack analgesic properties and provide short, unpredictable amnesia. The *opioids* are excellent analgesics but are poor hypnotics and possess unreliable amnestic properties. The *benzodiazepines* provide excellent amnesia but lack analgesic properties and are unpredictable hypnotics. Reversal of effect is possible with flumezenil, a specific benzodiazepine antagonist that can reverse all the central nervous system effects, including sedative-hypnotic, amnestic, muscle relaxant, and electroencephalographic (EEG) effects. The *butyrophenones* (specifically droperidol) possess no analgesic effects but produce a favorable neuroleptic syndrome characterized by psychomotor slowing, emotional quieting, and affective indifference. The patient appears drowsy, content, and indifferent but responds to commands and is arousable. An ideal anesthetic management plan may thus be formulated that incorporates the favorable characteristics of two or more intravenous drugs while minimizing the undesirable side effects of each. The syndrome of *neuroleptanalgesia*, characterized by apathy, immobility, and analgesia, is thus induced prior to the infiltration of local anesthetics for surgical manipulations. Various degrees of *retrograde amnesia* and *positive antiemetic effects* favorably complement the major characteristics of neuroleptanalgesia induced with a variable combination of fentanyl (opioid) and droperidol (butyrophenone). Small increments of an ultra-short-acting barbiturate (Surital or Brevital) or propofol, administered to produce transient hypnotic sleep during moments of potential discomfort or apprehension (local anesthetic injection, rhinoplasty osteotomies, etc.), add invaluable finesse to balanced neuroleptanalgesia.

Over two decades and many thousands of facial plastic surgery cases, the anesthesiologist team working with the senior author has utilized the above method of IAA without a single serious anesthetic complication. Even so, the scheme is not yet perfect. Patients, as would be expected, display individual differences in predicted pharmacologic responses and side effects. Automated monitoring devices (Fig 4–1), although vital, do not and will never replace an attentive anesthesiologist (Fig 4–2) (and surgeon as well) in recognizing, minimizing, and promptly correcting potential pharmacologic side effects or idiosyncratic reactions. Without exception risks are minimized during IAA by the *slowly titrated* administration of *small incremental doses of medications*, followed by a period of observation sufficient to accurately observe the patient's individual response to these potent drugs. Once this is confidently determined, incremental doses may be added throughout the procedure to ensure comfort, sedation, and cooperation.

CHAPTER 4 Anesthetic Methods: Patient Comfort and Safety

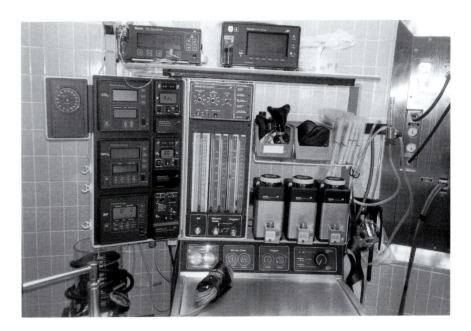

Figure 4-1
Automated monitoring of a variety of vital patient functions increases the safety of all anesthetic regimens. Although essential, such systems simply augment the fundamental monitoring carried out moment to moment by the anesthesiologist, surgeon, and operating room assistants. Each member of the operating team must assume responsibility for remaining alert to the patient's well-being.

Invaluable monitoring devices routinely involved include constant electrocardiography (ECG) and pulse rate, automated blood pressure, and pulse oximetry (see Fig 4-1). Peripheral arterial saturation levels of 97% to 100% saturation result in a sedated patient from the intranasal positioning of an 8 F soft silicone catheter delivering oxygen at 1½ L/min. The catheter effectively provides an oxygen-enriched atmosphere in sedated patients but is small enough to avoid interference with nasal and other facial plastic surgery procedures. Normal P_{O_2} levels throughout the operation are indeed reassuring and without question increase the safety of IAA.

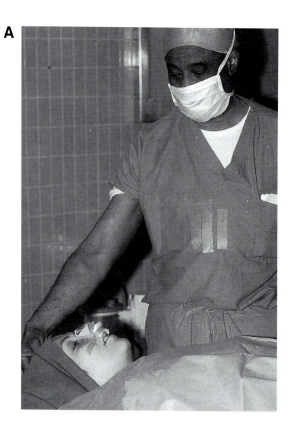

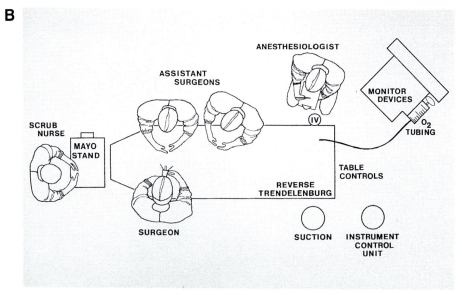

Figure 4-2
A, anesthesiologist monitoring the administration of intravenous anesthesia and analgesia. Titrating and adjusting the intravenous medications in the most effective and safe manner are truly components of an acquired art form, often more difficult than general anesthesia administration. **B,** most frequent positioning of operating team during facial plastic surgical procedures. All members of the team should be able to easily view the monitoring equipment.

CHAPTER 4 Anesthetic Methods: Patient Comfort and Safety

Side Effects and Complications

As in any form of anesthesia, the surgeon-anesthesiologist team must be constantly alert to the moment-to-moment well-being of the patient and be prepared to instantly minimize, counteract, or reverse any impending pharmacologic side effects.

Droperidol

The action of droperidol begins within 3 to 10 minutes after intravenous administration and lasts 2 to 4 hours. A neuroleptic syndrome is produced that is characterized by a placid drowsy patient displaying affective indifference, emotional quieting, and the appearance of sleep. The patient, however, remains arousable and responds to commands.

Very occasionally, droperidol produces initial restlessness, jitteriness, and visible anxiety. The patient may appear frightened and even ask to cancel the procedure. Calm reassurance allays these transient feelings of disquiet. In rare cases this subliminal free-floating anxiety condition persists for several hours after surgery.

Infrequently, extrapyramidal dyskinetic side effects may become apparent several hours following completion of the operation. These include dyskinesia of the facial, neck, and pharyngeal muscles, with speech difficulties, grimacing, trismus, oculogyric spasm, and even torticollis. Occasionally at the outset of administration of droperidol, a generalized shivering and a feeling of chilliness will occur. All of these peculiar symptoms are more frightening than serious and respond promptly to the intravenous or intramuscular administration of antiparkinsonian agents including diphenhydramine (Benadryl) and benztropine (Cogentin). All health care personnel participating in the postoperative care of patients receiving IAA must be aware of these potential side effects so that they may be promptly recognized and corrected. Some evidence exists that the concurrent administration of small amounts of diazepam or midazolam will significantly decrease the incidence of these droperidol side effects. It should be emphasized, however, that these untoward effects occur very infrequently and are readily reversible.

Fentanyl

The analgesic effects of fentanyl last 30 to 60 minutes, much shorter than the effect of droperidol. Respiratory depression occurs routinely with narcotic administration and is to be expected. Patients must be calmly and repeatedly encouraged to breathe deeply, although nasal oxygen administration effectively maintains high arterial saturations levels. Rarely, mask-assisted ventilation is necessary for an initial interval until spontaneous respiration returns. Immediate reversal with narcotic antagonists (naloxone [Narcan] or levallorphan [Lorfan]) should be employed if unexpected profound narcotic depression occurs.

Transient chest wall rigidity accompanied by a sensation of suffocation is rarely witnessed but can be controlled by reassurance and assisted ventilation if necessary. Fentanyl-induced bradycardia responds promptly to vagolytic doses of atropine.

After induction of neuroleptanalgesia, analgesia should be maintained with supplemental small increments of fentanyl to avoid overtranquilization and prolonged recovery. A significant advantage of neuroleptanalgesia derives from the favorable persistent postsurgical analgesia.

Patients undergoing facial plastic surgery rarely complain of significant pain and routinely require minimal if any postoperative pain medication.

In selected patients small intravenous doses of *midazolam (Versed)* smooths the anesthesia regimen and provides increased anxiolysis, sedation, and amnesia. The onset of action is rapid, and recovery occurs quickly in the postoperative period. These properties of midazolam make it ideal for shorter procedures, and it may be used alone very effectively in much older patients and in patients undergoing shorter outpatient procedures.

In younger and teenage patients midazolam may produce an unwanted paradoxical effect, leading to restlessness, greater anxiety, and agitation. We therefore avoid its use in the young.

The virtues of the nonopiod anesthetic propofol have been appreciated in recent years because it is an extremely effective but short-acting hypnotic. Propofol demonstrates a half-life in the body of less than 1 hour, thus aiding in rapid patient recovery. Recovery side effects are least common with propofol when compared with the other effective nonopioid intravenous anesthetics.

Thus the favorable clinical application of neuroleptanalgesia with droperidol and fentanyl, enhanced occasionally by transient increments of either Brevital or propofol and midazolam, provides for analgesia, calmness, cardiorespiratory stability, and antiemetic action (Fig 4–3). Constant intraoperative and postoperative monitoring is essential, and the judgment of an experienced, sympathetic anesthesiologist familiar with IAA is irreplaceable. Consistently remarkable is the gratitude of the patient for the simple act of having a hand held by the anesthesiologist or nurse while entering and in the state of IAA (see Fig 2–3). No little contentment derives from this seemingly minor reassuring human contact. We use it as a routine.

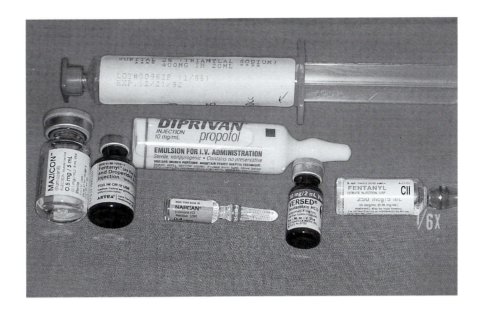

Figure 4–3
Pharmacologic agents most useful and safe in intravenous analgesia: droperidol, fentanyl, methohexital (Brevital), flumazenil (Mazicon), and midazolam (versed).

Suggested Reading

- Viljoen JF: Preoperative medications. *Otolaryngol Clin North Am* 1981; 14:579–585.
- Barash PG, Cullen BF, Stoelting RK: *Clinical Anesthesia*. Philadelphia JB Lippincott, 1989.

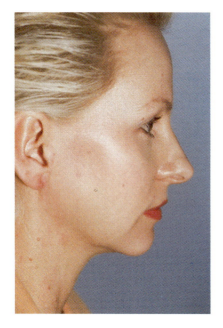
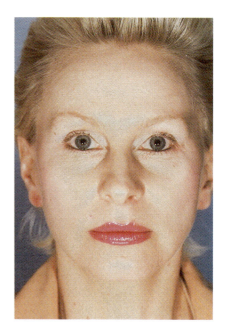
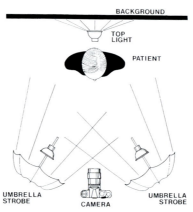
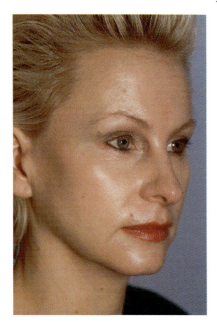
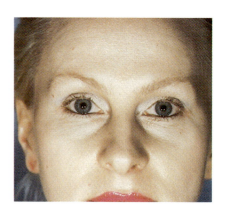

CHAPTER

5

 Uniform Photography in Aesthetic Facial Surgery

> *STANDARD. An acknowledged measure of comparison for quantitative or qualitative value; criterion; norm.*
> *UNIFORM. Consistent in appearance; having an unvaried texture, color, or design.*
>
> **American Heritage Dictionary**

Standardized, uniform patient photographs are as essential to the facial plastic surgeon as radiographs are to the orthopedist, audiograms to the otologist, and electrocardiograms to the cardiologist. Vivid, clear, and uniform preoperative and postoperative photographs allow the surgeon to plan surgery carefully and assess eventual outcomes accurately. Excellent photographs assume major importance in the head and neck region because the surgical outcome is highly visible for appreciation as well as criticism. In all fields of modern medicine, documentation for accurate record keeping, medicolegal purposes, and medical insurance coverage has been elevated to a level of importance surpassed only by uncompromising care of the patient. Standard and uniform photographs are no longer simply a pleasantly aesthetic adjunct to proper treatment; they are *mandatory*.

Of special value to the facial surgeon are the self-teaching, self-confrontational aspects of long-term standardized photographs. Sequential photographic comparison of the progressive phases of healing and postsurgical evolutionary changes provides the surgeon with an unparalleled, dispassionate assessment of his own skills and a clear record of how the dynamics of healing influence the "final outcome." No better method of continuing medical *self-education* exists. In a sense, the surgeon's attention to photographic detail provides an important clue to his surgical skills and commitment to excellence, and he is not uncommonly judged accordingly by his peers.

The purpose of this chapter is to document practical guidelines and techniques, in a simplified and straightforward manner, for creating standard and uniform photographs of consistently high quality. The approaches and recommendations contained herein are all in current use, and of equal importance, they work.

In medical photography the recorded image should reflect as precisely and faithfully as possible exactly what is seen by the observer's eye. Unlike fashion, impressionistic, and artistic photography, where intriguing and interesting illusions, shadows, and clever angles are intentionally created, medical photography for precise record keeping should reveal only the exact, unembellished image (Fig 5–1). Although some artistic license

CHAPTER 5   Uniform Photography in Aesthetic Facial Surgery

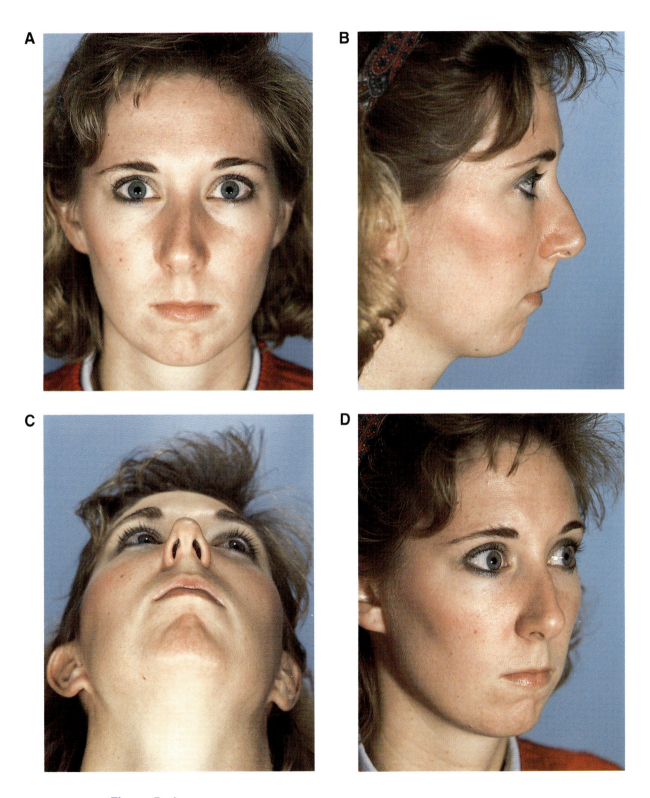

Figure 5–1
A–D, example of standard and uniform preoperative photographs taken in different head positions prior to carrying out rhinoplasty. All future photographs should incorporate similar principles of uniform positioning and lighting.

can be exercised in the development of slide presentations and medical exhibits, the photographic images most often recorded and referred to—the preoperative and postoperative photographs—should be absolutely standard and uniform in lighting, positioning, size, and color (Fig 5–2). Within the limitations of varying film emulsions and processing variations, this goal is entirely possible and should be the aim of every surgeon engaged in any form of plastic and reconstructive surgery of the face and neck. By establishing and religiously following certain standard, simple guidelines, uniformly excellent medical photographs can be achieved by anyone willing to be as compulsive about his photographic results as he surely is about his surgical results.

The question of whether or not the surgeon should become his own photographer is one for which there is no simple answer. For the most part, this chapter is presented to provide some routine guidelines for the physician who wishes to improve the quality and uniformity of the photographs he utilizes. The surgeon is encouraged to become expert in the various aspects of medical photography since special and unique additional information can be learned about the patient during photography carried out by the surgeon. For example, it is constantly a source of amazement that defects, asymmetries, and irregularities, undetected or overlooked during even the most careful physical examination, expose themselves blatantly when the patient is viewed through the camera lens. Accurate preoperative diagnosis and evaluation are thus facilitated and even enhanced. Further important psychological information is frequently revealed during the photographic sitting. A patient unable or unwilling to strike and hold an indicated pose during photography or who behaves in an uncooperative or frivolous manner may in fact be a less than ideal candidate for appearance-changing surgery. This vital information is likely to be unappreciated if the photographs are recorded by an office assistant or professional photographer.

Finally, situations arise on a regular basis in which the surgeon may require special, nonroutine views of interesting patients and problems in addition to the standardized series; unless this information is precisely conveyed to the photographer, the opportunity to record an important preoperative condition in a special, more instructive or revealing way may be lost forever.

An equally strong case may be made for assigning the responsibility for preoperative and postoperative photographs to either a professional photographer or an interested office assistant. Although personally recording a complete preoperative photographic series of the patient requires only 90 seconds, assuming the responsibility for all photography imposes an additional, albeit minimal burden on the surgeon's time. If professional assistance is available and convenient, there is much to recommend it.

CHAPTER 5 Uniform Photography in Aesthetic Facial Surgery

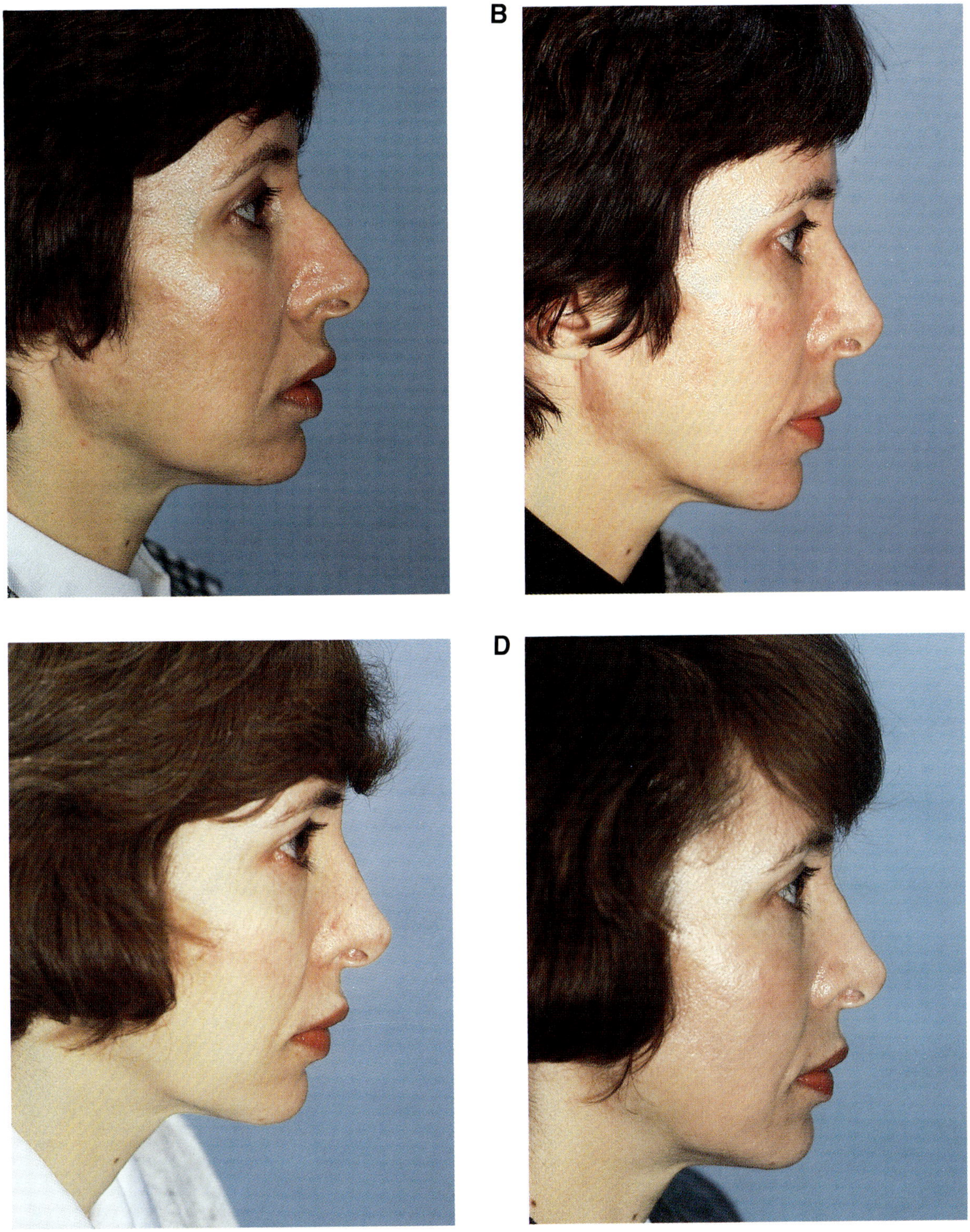

Figure 5–2
A–D, serial and consecutive views taken of a patient before and at various periods following surgery. Standardized positioning and lighting should be maintained from sitting to sitting.

Office Photography

Recording precise preoperative and postoperative facial photographs should not represent a burdensome photographic task for the surgeon, because a near-foolproof system can be developed that requires only that the same protocol be followed from sitting to sitting and most variables eliminated. Since the lighting, background, camera-to-subject distance, and lens opening remain the same, the only requirement imposed upon the photographer is to align the patient's face and head properly according to the positioning guidelines recommended.

Strict rules must be applied to composition and positioning techniques that are mandatory for uniform preoperative and postoperative photographs. For an accurate comparison of surgical results, both by an audience of learners as well as by the surgeon himself, precise reproducible positioning rules must be followed religiously. With the possible exception of aberrant lighting, erratic positioning of the patient's head is the single most common transgression in facial photography.

Patient Positioning

The patient should be seated comfortably on a small rotating stool at an elevation that will allow the feet to touch the floor, a stabilizing and security measure (Fig 5–3). A small, short back on the stool is helpful to support and maintain an erect posture, but it should not be high enough to be visible in the photograph. Although the stool may be on rollers for ease of movement, it should be capable of stabilization so that the camera-to-subject distance always remain constant, as does the distance from the patient to the light source.

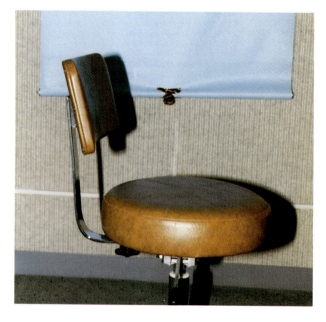

Figure 5–3
Typical swivel stool utilized for rapid and accurate positioning during facial photography.

Frankfort Horizontal Plane

The Frankfort horizontal plane is an imaginary line parallel to the horizontal. This imaginary line runs from the cephalic margin to the tragus through the infraorbital rim (Fig 5–4) and must be the constant, stable positioning factor ever present in the photographer's eye and mind. As long as the patient is positioned with the Frankfort line parallel to the horizontal floor, the major variable factor in sequential positioning is made uniform and constant. The use of a grid-type (architectural) viewing screen in the camera body is an immeasurable aid in proper patient alignment (Fig 5–5).

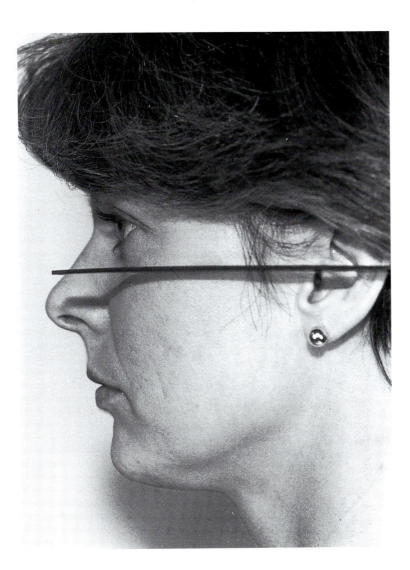

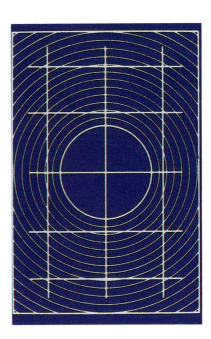

Figure 5–5
Example of the architectural grid viewing screen incorporated into a camera viewfinder to assist in establishing accurate head positioning.

Figure 5–4
The Frankfort horizontal line is an imaginary plane connecting the superior aspect of the tragus to the infraorbital margin and should be kept parallel to the horizontal in all head positions.

On frontal and base views, the midsagittal plane becomes a vital imaginary line (Fig 5–6). If in positioning, the face deviates from this important plane, which is perpendicular to the horizontal, vital information may be lost, obscured, or misrepresented. Symmetrical ears may look asymmetrical, the nose may seem deviated, and the two sides of the face may not be accurately compared.

The positioning guidelines provided by the Frankfort horizontal line and the midsaggital plane must therefore be conscientiously respected by the surgeon-photographer.

Additional positioning factors must be appreciated when obtaining *oblique* and *base* views; these involve positioning of the nasal tip. To ensure uniformity, the vertical center grid line should intersect and connect (or be aligned parallel to) the inner canthus with the oral commissure on oblique views (Fig 5–7), and for base views, the nasal tip should be positioned precisely at a horizontal line passing through the interbrow areas (Fig 5–8). Although the extent of tip projection may change slightly following rhinoplasty surgery, particularly when overprojected noses are repositioned or underprojected tips are augmented and rotated, in actual practice the difference is slight enough to create little appreciable variation in preoperative and postoperative uniformity of photograph positioning.

Figure 5–6
Example of the midsagittal plane, which is important when recording frontal and basal views.

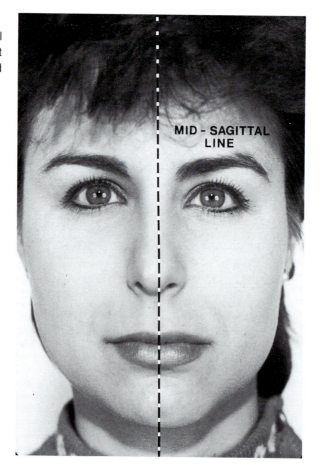

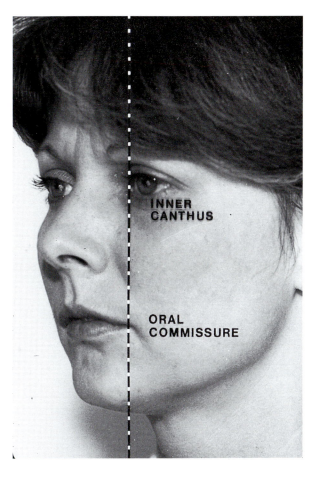

Figure 5–7
On the oblique view, a useful guide is the vertical gridline connecting the inner canthus with the oral commissure.

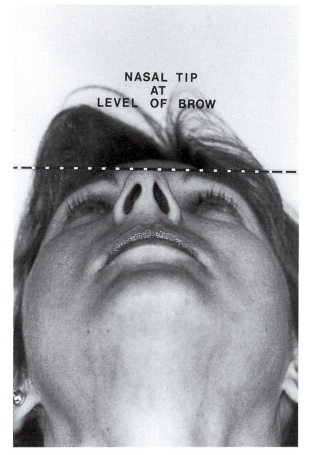

Figure 5–8
On basal views, uniformity is served if the nasal tip is positioned at a horizontal line passing through the interbrow area.

Many otherwise acceptable facial photographs are reduced in their value by a failure to control the patient's hair (Fig 5–9). Hairstyles that obscure vital portions of the patient's facial anatomy often confuse the diagnostic and record-keeping process, reduce the quality of the image by absorbing large quantities of light (or in the case of very fair individuals, reflecting too much light), obscure the desired background, and hide vital portions of the face. Simple measures may be taken to reduce these possibilities. Hair clips, combs, elastic headbands, and barrettes can be used during the photographic sitting to hold the hair away from the face temporarily (Fig 5–10). Colored elastic headbands are particularly effective in controlling the hair during photography for otoplasty (Fig 5–11). Either method will allow the ear to be visualized during rhinoplasty and facelift photography, allow all vital features to be appreciated, and allow the Frankfort horizontal line to be accurately sighted.

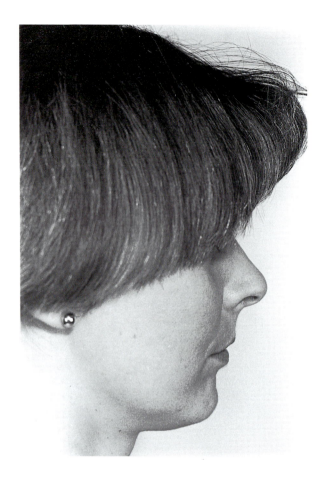

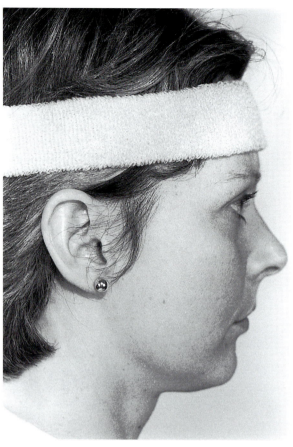

Figure 5–9
Uncontrolled hair obscuring portions of the face reduces the value of the recorded image and well as diagnostic capabilities.

Figure 5–10
Control of the hair by various implements provides an improved image for a diagnosis and comparison. Hair may be quickly and easily controlled with the use of elastic headbands of a variety of colors. This method of hair control is particularly useful in recording preoperative and postoperative photographs for otoplasty.

CHAPTER 5 Uniform Photography in Aesthetic Facial Surgery

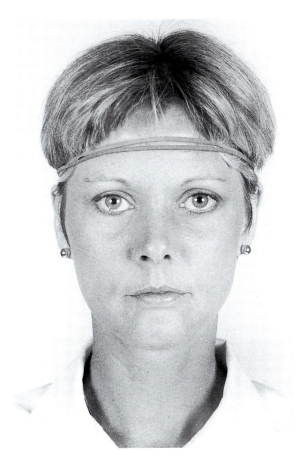

Figure 5–11
Control of hair with a common elastic headband.

Photographic Background

The appearance of a distracting, nonuniform background compromises many otherwise acceptable medical photographs. Improper backgrounds can distort the image, conceal vital information, disturb equal lighting, and distract from the main purpose of the photograph.

In practice, light shades of blue or gray complementary to skin tones serve best for the background (Fig 5–12). The finish of the background should preferably be a matte or dull appearance that partially absorbs and does not reflect light. It should be crease and seam free for perfect uniformity. No discernible pattern should be apparent to distract from the patient image.

It is ideal if the light reaching the background is augmented by a ceiling-mounted, slave-triggered electronic flash (the "key" light or "kicker") to illuminate shadows and facilitate the impression of depth in the photograph (Fig 5–13). In addition, a top-mounted flash may slightly backlight the patient and further improve the illusion of depth and three dimensions.

Figure 5–12
A light blue background free of shadows complements the recorded facial image in an ideal way.

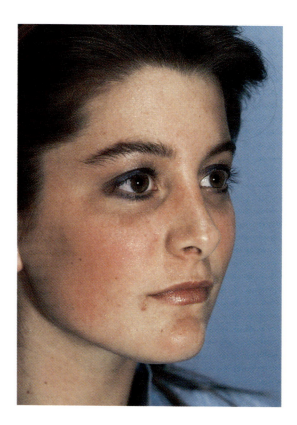

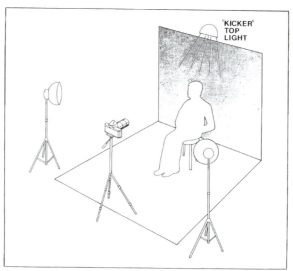

Figure 5–13
A "key" slave-triggered electronic flash positioned above the patient's head washes the background and in addition provides the illusion of increased depth perception.

CHAPTER 5 Uniform Photography in Aesthetic Facial Surgery

Black and very dark backgrounds are poor choices in medical photography of patients. Light is "swallowed up" to an unpleasant degree, the appearance of depth or three dimensions is sacrificed, and the patient image seems to be absorbed into the background. In profile views especially, the precise detail of the profile line is harder to distinguish. When converted into black-and-white prints for publication, photos taken with a black background are less distinct and contain less visual information than those with lighter backgrounds.

A pleasing light blue background can be achieved in a variety of ways. In large photo studios, seamless paper rolls of the desired color can be mounted above head height and unrolled to floor length. The paper is relatively inexpensive, and when soiled or in need of replacement, the mounted roll is simply unfurled further. In similar fashion, a suitable large section of this paper may be framed and mounted on the office wall as a stationary background. The background office wall itself may be painted the appropriate background shade, an inexpensive and practical alternative. Even simpler is the purchase of a simple plain-finish window shade of the proper size and color (Fig 5–14) to be mounted on the wall as the photographic background.

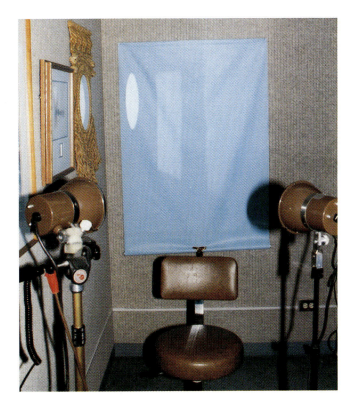

Figure 5–14
A simplistic photographic background incorporates a light blue window shade of proper size and color.

PART I   BASIC PRINCIPLES

Camera Body

Sophisticated 35-mm camera systems that possess capabilities for alternatives in photographic recording far beyond the needs for most medical photographers are available at very reasonable costs. Small, compact, lightweight, and durable camera bodies are produced by almost all major camera companies (Fig 5–15); such units have obvious advantages in terms of weight, portability, durability, and ease of operation.

The important functions of the camera body in the overall photographic system include holding and transporting the film, providing an accurate viewing image of the subject, and finally recording the appropriate image when the shutter is released. Single lens reflex (SLR) cameras offer the most extensive system of lenses and accessories and allow flexibility plus professional results. In order to establish a system of office photography in which the possible variables are reduced to a minimum, a camera body incorporating manual controls is preferable to one incorporating a large array of "automatic" features.

Our preference is for the Nikon system of cameras and lenses.

Durability and sturdiness are essential in any camera body used daily for literally thousands of exposures; in our experience Nikon products have endured well. Similar high-quality camera bodies from Canon, Olympus, Pentax, and others are available. The only defects experienced with camera bodies in the past decade have included breakage of the film advance lever mechanism (albeit after thousands of exposures; this problem can perhaps be minimized by using a motor drive accessory) and "sticking" of the mirror mechanism (this can be minimized by avoiding exposure of the camera to dust and dirt and with occasional professional cleaning).

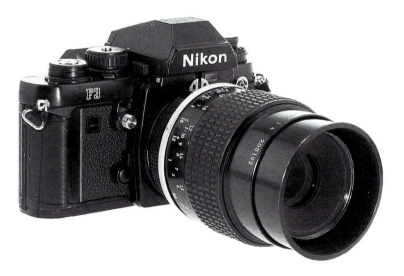

Figure 5–15
Single lens reflex 35-mm camera. In the system that we recommend, a simple camera body that can be operated manually is preferable to a more sophisticated, computerized unit. (Courtesy of Nikon Corporation)

CHAPTER 5   Uniform Photography in Aesthetic Facial Surgery

A critical feature of any camera is that it interface completely with the overall "system" of lenses and other accessories chosen for medical photography.

Lenses

The quality and characteristics of the lens used in medical photography are the most critical link in the photographic system, and *no compromise should be accepted in selection of the best possible lens.*

The standard lens in the typical 35-mm system is usually about 50 mm. If used for patient photography, it creates unpleasant and inaccurate parallax distortion in facial portraits and thus significantly limits its use. Ideally, the "medium" telephoto lenses, particularly those designated "macro" and possessing longer focal lengths, serve best for accurate photographic recording. Medium telephoto lenses (90 to 105 mm) are ideally suited for portrait photography because they minimize facial distortion and allow a comfortable working distance between the patient and photographer while providing a full-frame image (Fig 5–16).

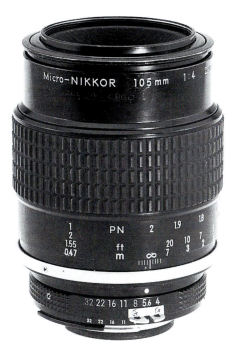

Figure 5–16
The 105-mm Auto Micro-Nikkor remains the preferred medical lens for portrait photography. (Courtesy of Nikon Inc.).

In a medical office setting where space for photographic setup is usually limited, the 105-mm Auto Micro-Nikkor telephoto lens is an ideal choice (see Fig 5–16). Relatively fast lenses (F2.0 or F2.8) are available. For the majority of facial photography, the 105-mm lens may be racked out to its maximum focal length for complete standardization and uniformity of distance and image size. From sitting to sitting, then, all patient photographs will be of exactly the same dimensions (Fig 5–17,A–C).

For close-up views (e.g., scars, lesions, orbit), predetermined distances may be marked on the lens to ensure distance uniformity for each of these specific views.

Motor Drive

Automatic film winders and motor drives (battery operated) are a convenience but not a necessity for accurate medical photography (Fig 5–18). Motor drives are most efficient when employed for the rapid, undelayed recording of photographs in the surgical suite, where time becomes more important. Multiple exposures can be made rapidly at different aperture settings ("bracketing") without removing the photographer's eye from the viewfinder or pausing to advance the film manually.

In addition, motor drives save wear and tear on the film advance lever, a source of potential eventual breakdown in even the best equipment. The surgeon-photographer must simply weigh the cost-benefit-convenience factor of the motor drive in his work against the added expense and inconvenience of battery replacement to power the unit.

CHAPTER 5 Uniform Photography in Aesthetic Facial Surgery

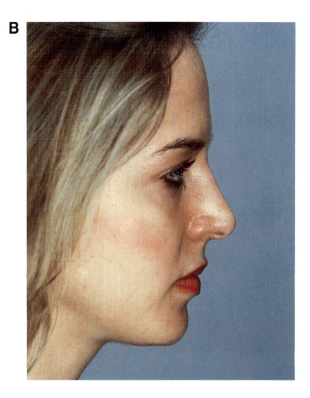

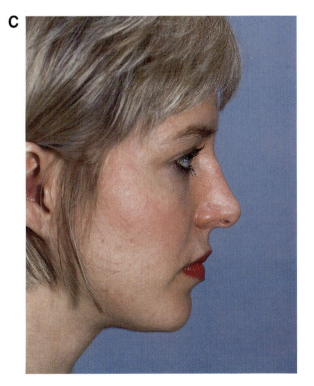

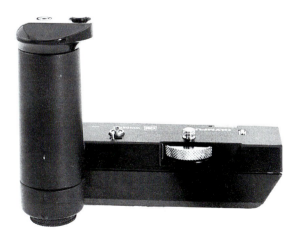

Figure 5–17
A–C, patient photographs recorded at various times with an emphasis on standardization and uniformity.

Figure 5–18
Typical motor drive that may be attached to the camera body for more convenient image recording.

111

Data-back

The standard camera back may be replaced or augmented easily with a device called a data-back (Fig 5–19); selected data are imprinted onto the film each time a frame is exposed (Fig 5–20). The date, time, shutter speed, aperture, and other more personal codes preselected by the photographer can be imprinted. Dates of preoperative and postoperative pictures are particularly useful if the surgeon is heavily involved in teaching. Precise data imprinted on the photograph can be a convenience in storage and retrieval systems, particularly those amenable to microcomputer information storage. Data-backs add significantly to the overall weight of the system and slightly to the bulkiness. Each data-back is ordinarily system specific; each company produces a data-back compatible with its own equipment system.

Film

Among the myriad types of film available for photography, the Kodachromes set the standard for the industry today (Fig 5–21). Both Kodachrome 25 and 64 produce color transparencies of faithful color, extremely fine grain (and therefore sharp images), and stable emulsions, all absolute prerequisites for ultimate quality in medical photography. These laudable characteristics translate into significant advantages for the facial surgeon. If enlargements of the transparency are to be made (for publication or exhibits), the fine grain of the Kodachromes allows significant enlargement without noticeable loss of sharp detail. Color slide transparencies lend themselves better than any other format to storage, retrieval, and cataloging, a significant advantage when a slide library numbers in the tens of thousands. In medical education, the 2 × 2 slide transparency represents the current world standard, and slide projectors (ordinarily the carousel slide projector or its close equivalent) are found in almost every teaching institution in the world.

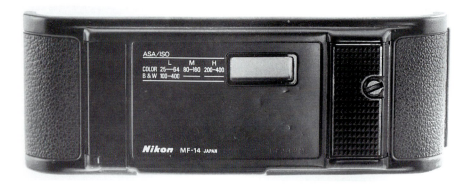

Figure 5–19
Camera data-back utilized for imprinting selected information onto the exposed film. (Courtesy of Nikon Corporation.)

CHAPTER 5   Uniform Photography in Aesthetic Facial Surgery

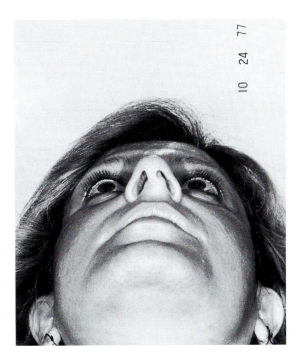

Figure 5–20
Data imprinted on film.

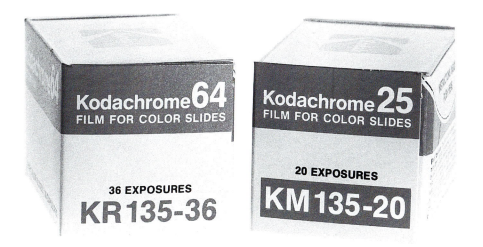

Figure 5–21
The standard of excellence against which all other films are compared remains the versatile Kodachrome 25. For the disciplined office photographic setting, Kodachrome 25 is unequaled in its uniformity, color, sharpness, and archival value. (Courtesy of Eastman-Kodak, Rochester, NY)

Perhaps more faithfully than any photographic film available, the Kodachromes reproduce colors representative of human skin tones. Batches of film developed in Kodak emulsion processing possess longer archival retention of true colors than any other film by far (testing laboratories have assigned an estimate of at least a 50-year stability for Kodachrome emulsions when stored under the proper conditions of relative darkness, low humidity, and stable cool temperatures). This is substantiated by our experience: K-25 slides taken 20 years ago and projected scores of times in relatively hot projectors still retain true and faithful colors. Ektachrome slides conversely fade much earlier when exposed to ambient or projected light.

Finally, color slides are the most economical of all photographs, thus encouraging the photographer to be generous in the number of exposures taken in important shooting situations. Since slides are easily and accurately reproduced (and even enhanced) rapidly and faithfully in modern slide reproduction units, copies can be quickly made for teaching and publishing purposes, thus allowing the original to be properly stored under stable conditions for archival purposes.

A further major advantage of the slide transparency is its use for ready reference in the operating room. Projecting the patient's photographs in the operating room in life size and in full color during surgery provides the ultimate in moment-to-moment comparisons of minute and critical details during the surgical procedure (Fig 5–22).

One significant drawback to regular use of the Kodachromes does exist: development must be carried out in Kodak processing laboratories at various sites throughout the country. Although this requirement ensures a reliable degree of quality control, it is time-consuming and frustrating to a surgeon requiring the results of his exposed photographic rolls as quickly as possible.

Shooting Kodak Ektachrome film allows the development of a usable slide within a few hours, which may be a major advantage when color transparencies are urgently needed and long-term retention of stable colors and hues is not as critical. For this reason we prefer Ektachrome slides only when transparencies are required within a matter of hours and long-term storage and archival retention are unimportant.

An adjunctive system providing a backup capability and an instant printed image is the Polaroid system of cameras and film. It can be quite useful to record two or more instant Polaroid prints during the initial patient consultation (a frontal and lateral view will usually suffice). These photographs are not of the quality and sharpness inherent in the slide transparency, but they can be a valuable visual springboard to facilitate communication between the patient and the surgeon. In addition, they can be filed in the patient's chart for ready evaluation at subsequent visits (Fig 5–23) and ultimately may be presented to the patient sometime in the postoperative period, a courtesy ordinarily greatly appreciated.

Figure 5-22
Patient color slides projected in the operating room during surgery allow moment-to-moment comparison of the patient's upright image in various positions during the surgical procedure. Since many of the details of facial anatomy change during recumbency, these intraoperative comparisons hold significant value for diagnostic and technical decision making.

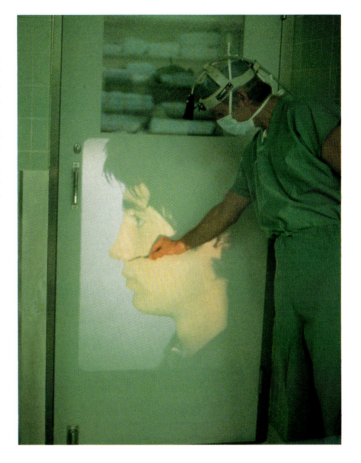

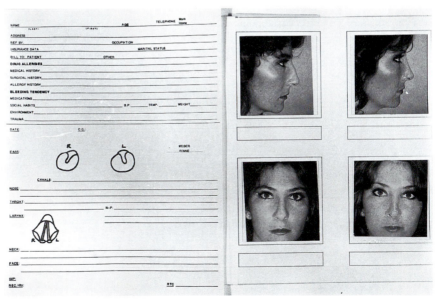

Figure 5-23
Polaroid prints filed in the patient chart for rapid comparisons.

Polaroid prints by themselves are only an adjunct to the more refined slide transparency photographs described and are not acceptable as the only system of photographic recording to be used. In addition, they are relatively expensive.

Relatively instant color Polaroid prints may be produced from 2 × 2 slides obtained with the recommended standardized system. Slide-to-print copy units manufactured by Polaroid (the Polaprinter) and Vivitar are inexpensive and simple to use (Fig 5–24). Such prints are useful for filing and patient review as well as for insurance and legal records.

Electronic Lighting

With the exception of faulty patient positioning, inaccurate lighting represents the most common error in medical photography. A brief review of any current journal covering facial surgery will reflect this inadequacy: photographic prints in overexposed, underexposed, and poorly modeled modes. To some degree this is surprising since with only a minimum of effort lighting of extraordinarily high quality and uniformity can be achieved.

In the past decade one of the major advances in photography has been the development of remarkably powerful, lightweight, and relatively inexpensive electronic flash units. Since the control of light is perhaps the most critical challenge in creating an accurate image, the electronic flash has simplified indoor photography as never before. A spin-off from space age technology, compact flash units are sources of enormous energy controlled by miniaturized microcircuitry. With the possible exception of daylight, no other lighting provides such clean and natural lighting. With these tools at hand, then, superior medical photographs should be simpler than ever to create.

Electronic flash units are an exceptionally good value since even the smallest, least complex units will provide many thousands of flash bursts, a remarkable savings over the conventional use of flash bulbs. Flash units containing "thyristor circuits" prevent surplus energy from the flash unit from reaching the flashtube, thereby conserving the power extended by each individual flash burst and shortening the recycle time for the capacitor to become fully recharged.

In facial surgery in particular, the camera and electronic flash are ordinarily used in two fundamental ways. The first and most frequent use involves the recording of standard and uniform preoperative and postoperative pictures for analysis, record keeping, and medicolegal documentation. Once the proper setup is arranged for these repetitive photographs, the photographer simply needs to follow the exact same protocol from sitting to sitting to ensure that the recorded images are uniform.

The best portrait photographs are consistently made by using dual electronic flash units positioned to either side of the camera and synchronized to fire simultaneously when triggered by the camera shutter release (Fig 5–25). The distance from the camera to each flash unit is again a matter of

Figure 5–24
Polaroid prints may be rapidly created from 35-mm slides by the use of the Polaroid Polaprinter. (Courtesy of Polaroid Corporation)

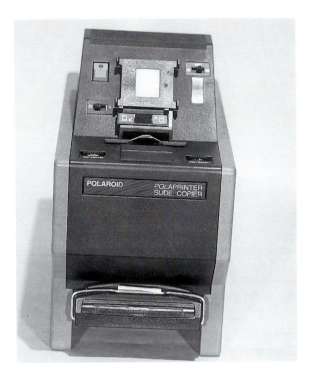

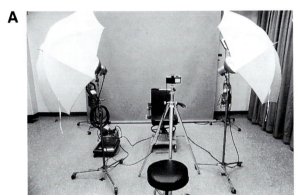

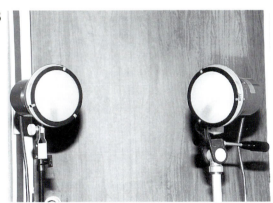

Figure 5–25
A and **B,** dual electronic flash heads positioned at an equal distance from the camera body provide ideal and uniform lighting from sitting to sitting.

personal taste, but in order to achieve uniform facial lighting without casting asymmetrical modeling shadows (an interesting but medically inaccurate effect), the flash heads should be approximately the same distance from the camera and at nearly the same level as the camera. In this manner uniform lighting can be achieved from session to session with the same patient, thus making it easy to compare serial photographs accurately.

Preventing harsh background shadows is accomplished quite simply in the following fashion. First, the patient should be moved sufficiently forward of the background so that harsh shadows are significantly softened. Within the limits of space and comfort, positioning the patient at least 2 ft from the background will accomplish this goal. If diffusing screens or umbrellas are used on the individual flash heads to soften and diffuse the incident light, less severe shadows will result. Although acceptable portrait facial images can be made by using a single electronic flash unit positioned on the camera body itself, this on-camera flash technique produces a characteristically flat, two-dimensional effect, with harsh highlights and washed-out skin tones as typical side effects. In addition, unacceptable and unnecessary shadows are almost always cast on the background by the single on-camera flash.

Optimal patient photography therefore requires the use of studio-grade electronic flash units positioned in some fashion on either side of the camera (Fig 5–26). Our preference and recommendation are for choosing a small studio-type electronic flash setup that occupies little space in the medical office, is capable of powerful bursts of light output allowing smaller aperture settings (and therefore greater potential depth of field), and provides superb modeling capability to capture in great detail the precise form of the human face (Fig 5–27).

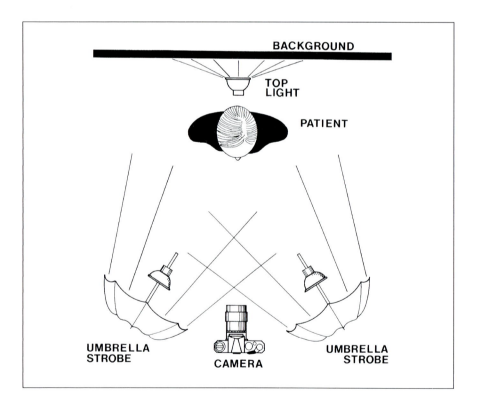

Figure 5–26
Illustration of the photography arrangement recommended and used daily by the senior author.

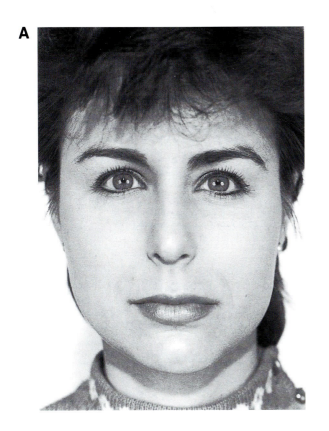 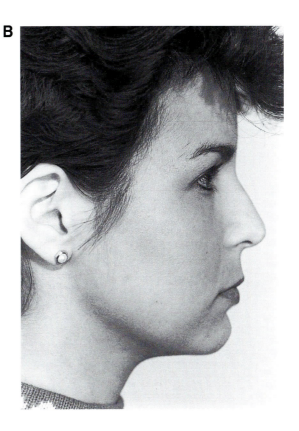

Figure 5-27
A and **B,** these shadow-free photographs of a patient in different head positions demonstrate excellent detailing of the facial anatomy.

In addition, the dual electronic studio flash units, because of their remarkable power output, allow the photographer to use indirect, diffused, or softened light to eliminate bright spots and harsh highlights to produce the very best image.

A recommended arrangement for dual studio flash units is illustrated in Figure 5-26. The two flash units are positioned on either side of the camera at approximately the same distance from the subject. Mounted on lightweight aluminum telescoping stands, the position and height of these units can be easily and quickly adjusted according to the patient's height and individual needs. Connected to the camera body by a power cord, the units fire simultaneously when the shutter is released because they are controlled by a central power pack.

Second, employing an overhead "kicker" or "key" light (see Figs 5-13 and 5-26) positioned on the ceiling and activated by a remote "slave" device will illuminate the background, effectively eliminating any potential shadows and adding a backlighting effect that further improves the picture quality and creates a nearly three-dimensional effect. These remote slave units are inexpensive and are even produced as self-contained screw-in strobe bulbs.

Many studio strobe flash units are provided with a so-called modeling light consisting of a weak continuous light source that is mounted near or within the strobe unit. Modeling lights allow an assessment of the effect that placement of the dual strobe units will have on the ultimate image recorded and, in imperfectly lit rooms, allow improved focusing prior to exposing the image.

Once the dual electronic strobe units have been positioned to personal taste and satisfaction, it is mandatory to perform the simple but critical sample exposure tests. A subject with average skin tones is seated on the rotating stool or chair provided in front of the background and the face and head positioned in the frontal plane. A series of test shots is then recorded with the patient holding a small 3 × 5 card (or tongue blade) on which has been recorded the f-stop for that particular shot (Fig 5–28). Sample shots are made in the lateral and oblique positions as well since one may wish to use slightly different lighting in these positions (this of course implies that the lighting differences will be carried forth for all future photographs of that same patient for complete standardization). Selecting the best exposure from this test series will now be a simple matter for the surgeon, and that preferred setting can henceforth be used to maintain complete uniformity of lighting and exposure from sitting to sitting.

It should be appreciated that all variables have been thus eliminated except for patient positioning, the most commonly inaccurate factor in uniform photography. The photographer must constantly be on guard for minor variations in patient positioning and correct them before the image is exposed.

CHAPTER 5 Uniform Photography in Aesthetic Facial Surgery

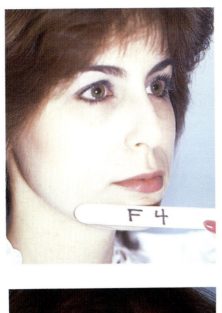
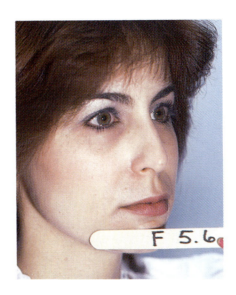
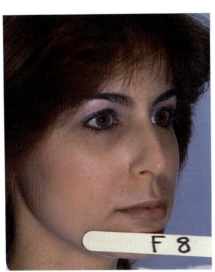
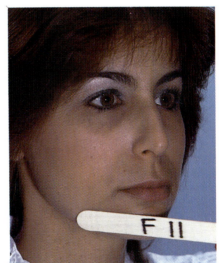
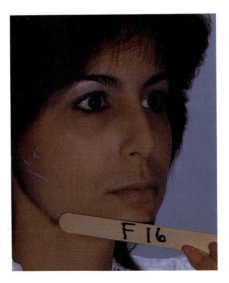

Figure 5–28
A–E, series of patient photographs taken at progressively different f-stops in order to quickly determine the ideal aperture setting for all future studio photography.

Office Photography Suite

For convenience we use a section of one of our large examining rooms as a photography area (Fig 5–29). Dedicating a separate room to photography is preferred by some surgeons. We prefer the convenience of having equipment set up in the principal examination room so that a patient can be photographed without having to move from room to room, thus conserving vital time and streamlining the photographic process. A complete series of preoperative photographs requires only 90 seconds to record.

A few feet from the standard examination chair sits a small stool with a low back. The stool should allow the patient's feet to rest on the ground for comfort as well as posture. Each of the flash heads is positioned 4 ft from the stool at approximately 30 to 45 degrees from the patient. Various objects and paintings are placed strategically throughout the room to facilitate the different required views of the patient during the photography session.

Ideal views recommended for various facial surgery operations are listed in Table 5–1. Of necessity, some departures or additions to these routine views will be required when special or unique findings are necessary to document.

Table 5–1

Recommended Views for Facial Surgery Operations

Blepharoplasty
- Frontal, close-up
- Frontal, eyes open
- Frontal, eyes closed
- Frontal, upward gaze
- Lateral (right and left)

Mentoplasty/submentoplasty
- Frontal, full
- Frontal, close-up
- Lateral (right and left)

Otoplasty/auricular deformities
- Frontal
- Posterior head
- Lateral (right and left), close-up
- Oblique (right and left), close-up

Rhinoplasty
- Frontal
- Lateral (right and left), in repose
- Lateral (right and left), smiling
- Oblique (right and left)
- Base
- Close-up, as required

Rhytidoplasty
- Frontal, in repose
- Frontal, smiling
- Frontal, grimacing (to demonstrate mimetic muscle function)
- Frontal oblique (right and left)
- Lateral (right and left)

CHAPTER 5   Uniform Photography in Aesthetic Facial Surgery

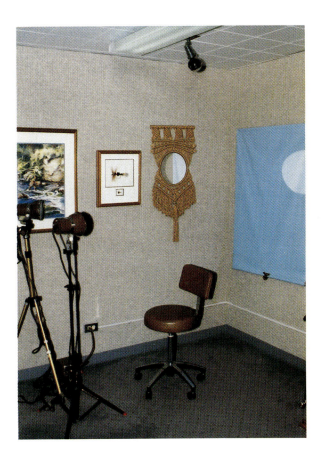

Figure 5–29
The space required for ideal office photography need not be extensive. A corner of the examining room measuring no more than 5 × 6 ft serves admirably for rapid recording of all required patient views. The convenience of transferring the patient only a few feet from the examining chair to the photographic setting represents an additional advantage.

Summary

Although setting up a medical photography suite may seem complicated and expensive, in reality it is neither. Following the recommendations reviewed in this chapter provides a simplified and structured starting point for the reliable and uniform recording of accurate photographs from sitting to sitting. If one adheres rigidly to standards of uniformity and consistent reproducibility, a great body of information can be accurately recorded.

Suggested Reading

- Tardy ME: *Principles of Photography in Facial Plastic Surgery*. New York, Thieme-Stratton, 1992.

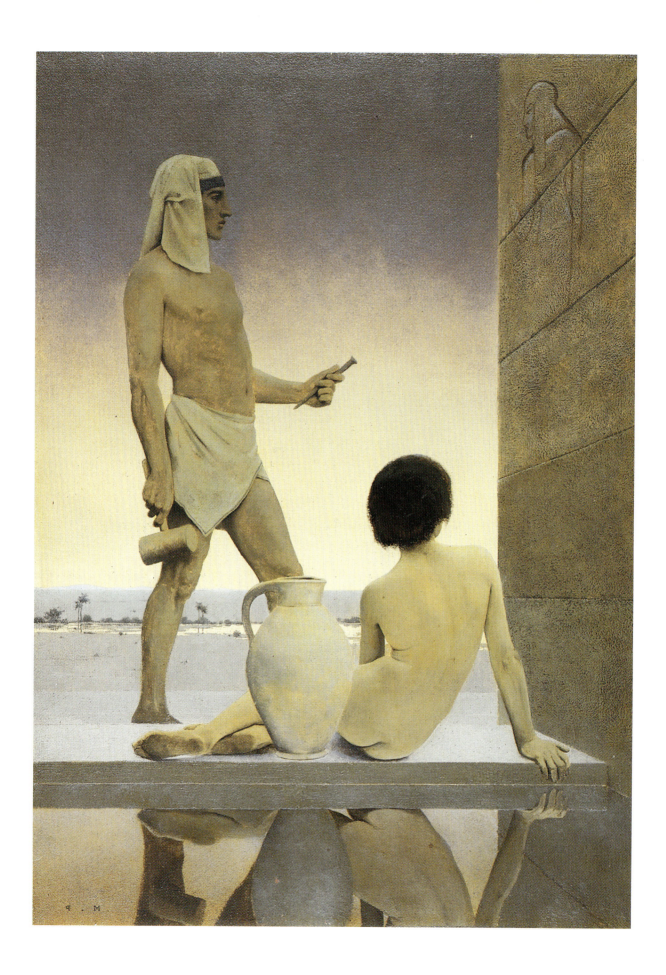

CHAPTER

6

Aesthetics, Analysis, and Judgment

PART I BASIC PRINCIPLES

> *Youth is in man, a mere flash, and full advantage of its opportunities should be taken to improve and enjoy one's body, intellect and spirit. If the latter is not the case, frustration and thus, many other problems will emerge. Man has not yet finished being young, when he is already starting to be old.*
>
> **Mario Gonzalez-Ulloa**

Concepts of Beauty

Universally, those who attempt to specifically define the parameters of beauty encounter frustration. No collection of mathematical lines or angles, preferred by the ancient Greeks, serves infallibly to guide the surgeon seeking a blueprint for his tissue repairs and repositioning. "Proportion" and "harmony" are features regularly cited as a preferable circumstance; however, dramatic exceptions to these universal rules are routinely encountered in strikingly beautiful faces whose unique features display pleasing *disproportion*.

Clearly, true beauty in the final analysis only exists "in the eye of the beholder." More importantly, for facial surgical purposes, the perception of attained personal beauty and positive self-image in the eyes of the operated patient ranks paramount. Therefore cultural and ethnic differences and perceived preferences broaden and make relative only the traditional mathematical parameters for facial beauty (Fig 6–1, A–C). All experienced surgeons have occasionally experienced the profound personal chagrin of encountering the unexplainably displeased patient whose postoperative outcome, in the surgeon's eyes, ranks at the very pinnacle of his concept of beauty. In the absence of some major undetected, occult psychological disturbance, this dichotomy of opinion surely reflects differing individual opinions of what defines facial beauty. Nonetheless, facial surgeons, no matter how technically skilled and facile, must master the concepts of balance, symmetry, proportion, and harmony. Equally important is the facility to modify and rearrange facial features in a subtle or major way while effectively camouflaging incisional scars and producing a non-surgical-appearing outcome. Accurately appreciating, interpreting, and describing what one "sees" in a face is seldom a gift of inheritance but requires rehearsal, study, and refinement. True beauty in any particular medium may not be recognized owing to the undisciplined and unrehearsed senses of

CHAPTER 6   Aesthetics, Analysis and Judgment

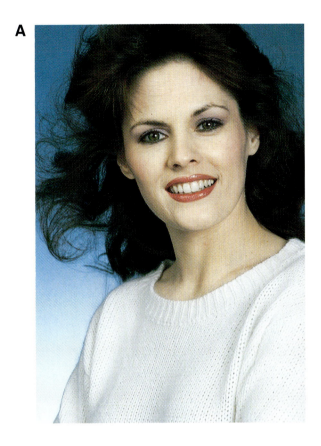
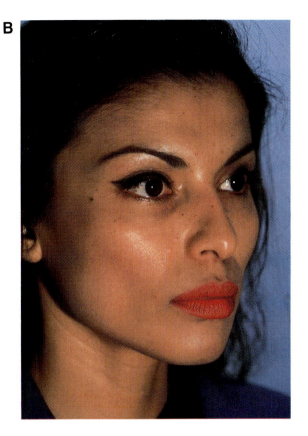
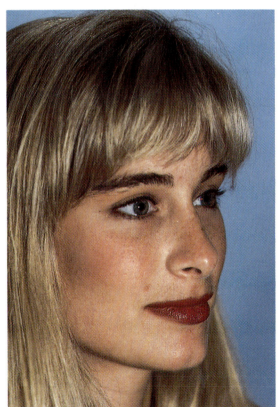

Figure 6–1
A–C, three individuals of widely different ethnic background who despite significantly differing identical facial features share the parameters of harmony and proportion that characterize beauty.

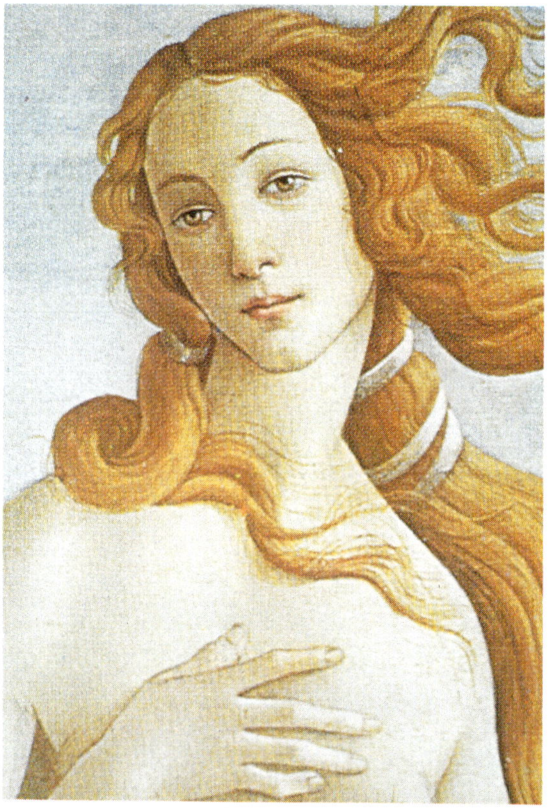

Figure 6–2
Renaissance painting (Botticelli's Venus) revealing characteristics of beauty that are timeless and enduring.

the viewer. Annually one marvels at the early clumsy inability of otherwise highly intelligent and academically credentialed resident surgeons to "see" normal and variant features shown clearly before them, much less discuss them with finesse. Almost without exception, it is equally remarkable to witness their rapid appreciation for and interpretation of the subtleties of facial analysis as repeated and disciplined rehearsal awakens and reveals a developing eye for detail.

Gillies succinctly emphasized this truism:

The majority of failures in plastic surgery are due to errors, the commission of which would lead to failure in any form of surgery. Thus mistakes in diagnosis due to inadequate examination are perhaps the most common cause of indifferent treatment. This element of difficulty and diagnosis may not at first sight be obvious. The word diagnosis in this work is used in its literal sense, mainly to mean a thorough knowledge of the condition present—i.e., the exact loss in terms of anatomic structure.

Thus repair, reconstruction, and aesthetic reorientation of less-than-ideal facial features must not be solely based on free and improvised personal feelings or impressions, but on a surgical art more strictly aligned to the laws of geometry and proportion.

CHAPTER 6 Aesthetics, Analysis, and Judgment

In any learned discussion of the beautiful face, the opinion is frequently expressed that the parameters and societal conceptions of beauty change, or at least evolve, over centuries. To the contrary, any careful examination of portraits prepared by the ancients belies this observation. To be sure, styles change, cultural and ethnic variations exist, and preferences are modified, but the elements of true beauty appear to have persisted nearly unchanged since the earliest recordings of mankind (Fig 6–2).

Thoughtful facial surgeons, in addition to developing the relative uncomplicated skills of technical surgical excellence, must continuously *hone and refine* their analytic and perceptive skills of diagnosis to instantly appreciate the obvious disproportions and disharmonies witnessed in any face while judging the vital influence of the more subtle influences of light, shadow, skin texture, and overall proportional balance upon the intended outcome. They above all else must develop the capability to predict and foresee the visualized final result long before surgical alterations commence. This requires a self-developed sense of the "ideal normal" applied to the human face that is sharpened by experience and applied in concert with a clear and accurate understanding of the individual patient's expectations.

Francis Bacon wrote with particularly sharp insight into the ephemeral notion of beauty:

In beauty, that of favor (feature) is more than that of color; and that of decent and gracious motion more than that of favor (feature). That is the best part of beauty, which a picture cannot express. . . . There is no excellent beauty that hath not some strangeness in the proportion. Man cannot tell whether Apelles or Albert Durer were the more trifler; whereof the one would make a personage by geometrical proportions; the other by taking the best part out of diverse faces to make one excellent. Such personages, I think would please nobody but the painter that made them. Not that I think a painter may make a better face and never was; but he must do it by kind felicity (as a musician that maketh an excellent pair in music) and not by rule. A man shall see faces, but if he examined them part by part, you shall find never good; and yet altogether do well.

Proportions of the Aesthetic Face

Universally accepted guidelines and canons of facial proportions exist (Figs 6–3 to 6–5) but represent only general standards for evaluation and comparison. The unquestioning acceptance of rigid proportions and measurement values as characteristics of an attractive face fails to give proper expression to the variations witnessed in mankind. Thus the art of facial aesthetic surgery requires an understanding of what mathematical characteristics exist in an "ideal normal" face and the artistic talent to create appearance improvements in faces that may depart significantly from accepted norms. The patients pictured in Cases 1 through 8 represent a wide variety of facial characteristics. A detailed analysis of each is instructive in defining favorable and unfavorable features and proportions.

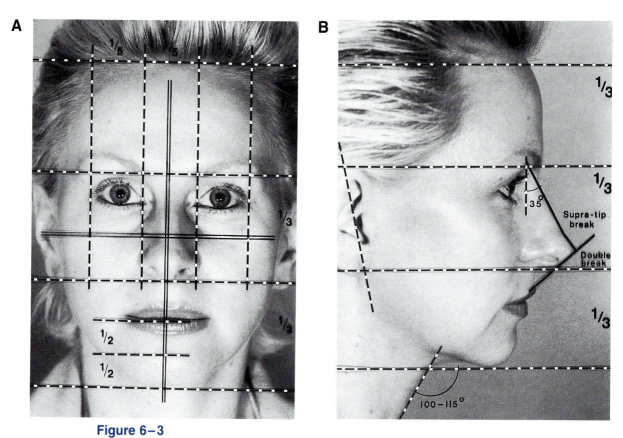

Figure 6–3
A and **B**, recognized and accepted principles of facial proportions and harmony. In any face, balance of aesthetic units creates a pleasing appearance.

CHAPTER 6 Aesthetics, Analysis, and Judgment

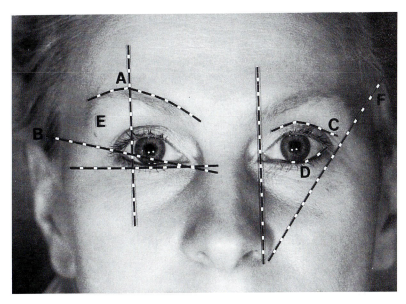

Figure 6-4
In the orbital aesthetic unit, a pleasing appearance is characterized by an arching eyebrow positioned well above the supraorbital ridge *(A)*, a slightly upward angulation to the horizontal axis of the eye *(B)*, a defined upper lid crease *(C)*, a taut lower lid abutting the globe at about the lower edge of the iris *(D)*, and a well-defined supratarsal cleft and infraorbital space free of redundant skin *(E)*.

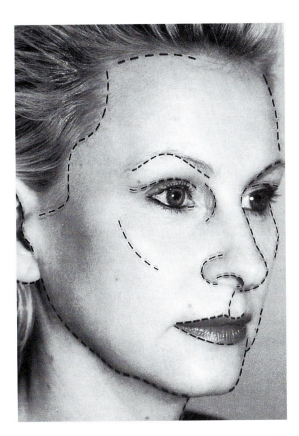

Figure 6-5
Beautiful faces are largely characterized by a collection of gently curved lines defining the dimensions and borders of facial features. Straight lines are seldom observed in ideal faces. Aesthetic surgical procedures should be planned to emulate this principle.

Case 1

56-Year-Old Woman

ANALYSIS

Favorable
- Normal weight for frame, height
- Attractive features—balanced
- Good bone structure
- Ideal skin quality and texture
- No excess facial fat
- Eyes dominate face—attractive
- Little apparent skin damage despite high sun exposure
- Facial symmetry
- Long sweeping jawline
- Elegant long neck
- Little submental fat

Unfavorable
- Etched fine skin lines
- Developing forehead creases
- Crepey eyelid skin
- Deepening perioral radiating lines
- Early platysmal banding
- Slight mandibular asymmetry

Frontal
- Attractive, favorable hair distribution and styling
- Early forehead creases
- Minimal glabellar creasing
- Good brow position above the orbital rim with a favorable brow arch
- Early redundant upper lid skin; a good supratarsal cleft persists
- Aesthetic upward lateral slant to the eyes
- Minimal periorbital creasing
- Slight mandible asymmetry
- Early lower lid creasing, redundancy, fat
- Favorable cheekbone prominence
- Strong, attractive nose—ideal length without droop or elongation
- Slight elongation of the upper lip with etched creases
- Minimal cheek-lip fold formation
- Fine facial skin etching and creases
- Early red lip involution
- Early drool line with a lateral oral depression
- Early jowling with loss of cheek support

Lateral
- Early jowling with loss of cheek support
- Full, sweeping jawline
- Minimal submental fat
- Early submandibular gland ptosis
- Banding with diastasis of the platysmal borders
- Permanent cervical creasing
- Normal hyoid position
- Long columnar neck

Summary
Nearly ideal candidate for surgical rejuvenation procedures.

CHAPTER 6 Aesthetics, Analysis, and Judgment

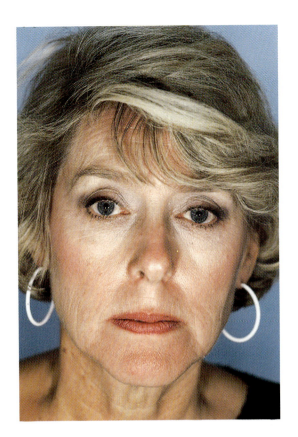
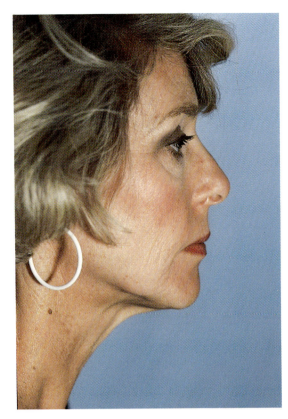
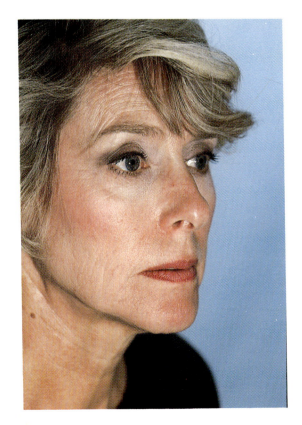

Case 2

50-Year-Old Woman

ANALYSIS

Favorable
- Little skin sun damage
- Attractive face and eyes
- Proper weight for frame, height
- Highly motivated for rejuvenation

Unfavorable
- Delayed request for rejuvenation; some irreversible changes now exist
- Thick skin
- Marked deep facial creases and furrows
- Thin eyebrows
- Asymmetrical upper lid, skin redundancy
- Laxity of the lateral lower lids
- Wide, ill-defined nose
- Nonideal bone structure
- Long upper lip deep furrows
- Deep radiating perioral furrows
- Early chin pad ptosis
- Hanging platysmal bands
- Permanent, deep cervical creases

Frontal
- Deep forehead creases; excess static tension of the frontalis muscles
- Thinning eyebrows with temple/brow ptosis
- Deep glabellar creases
- Asymmetrical upper lids with medial fat herniation
- Lower lid fat herniation
- Deep periocular creasing
- Horizontal nasal root rhytids
- Broad nose: ill-defined
- Long upper lip
- Marked perioral creasing

Oblique
- Thinning temporal hairline
- Temple and brow ptosis
- Redundant upper lid skin, fat, and muscle
- Lower lid herniated fat
- Broad, bifid nasal tip
- Deep perioral and facial rhytids
- Jowling with poor jawline definition
- Hanging platysmal bands

Lateral
- Penciled brow too low
- Upper lid skin hooding
- Lower lid fat: abundant
- Dorsal nasal convexity
- Retraction of the columellar-lateral angle
- Early chin pad ptosis
- Obliteration of the cervicomental angle
- Short columnar neck
- Permanent cervical creasing

Summary
Highly motivated patient who has delayed surgical rejuvenation past the point where it would have been most effective. Procedures undertaken now will create significant improvement but are limited in the s41degree of permanent skin change. This is not an ideal candidate.

CHAPTER 6 Aesthetics, Analysis, and Judgment

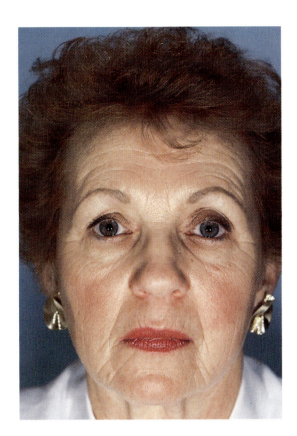
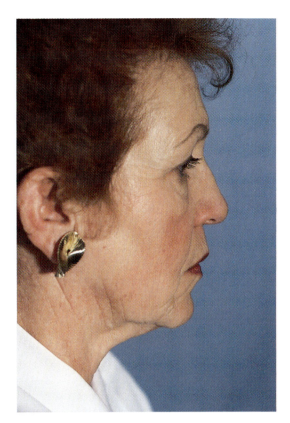
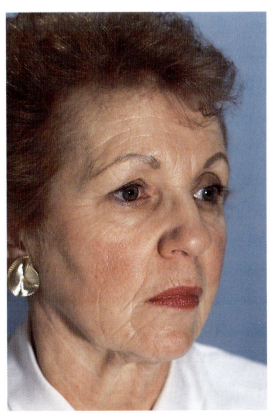

135

PART I   BASIC PRINCIPLES

Case 3

34-Year-Old Woman

ANALYSIS

Favorable
- Young patient—skin elastic but redundant
- Thin with little facial or body fat
- Adequate bone and skeletal structure
- Highly motivated for rejuvenation
- "Sad" look reversible by surgical lifting procedures
- Good hair distribution and styling
- Little submental fat
- Normal submaxillary gland position
- Normal hyoid position

Unfavorable
- Loss of soft-tissue support at a young age (familial)
- Reduced skin tone; flaccidity
- Moderate permanent solar skin damage
- Significant brow ptosis with eyelid hooding
- Slight scleral show
- Prominent cheek-lip folds and nasolabial creasing
- Thin upper lip

Frontal
- High hairline, elongated forehead
- Inferior slant to the lateral portion of the eyebrows; brow ptosis
- Abnormal temporal skin mobility
- Markedly redundant upper lid skin
- Slight scleral show: early lower lid laxity
- Asymmetrical, full, and deep nasolabial folds and creases
- Early elongation of the upper white lip
- Thin upper red lip

Oblique
- Permanent photoaging skin damage
- Eyebrow descended to the level of the bony brow
- Strong, attractive nose
- Early jowl formation
- Early creasing in the lateral canthal area

Lateral
- Advanced temporal/eyebrow ptosis
- Marked eyelid hooding
- Ideal nasal profile
- Prominent cheek-lip fold and "drool" lines coalesce
- Slight retrognathia
- Minimal submental fat
- Long columnar neck with a high hyoid position

Summary
Patient exhibiting, at a young age, a familial tendency toward early aging because of the loss of skin elasticity. Ptotic eyebrows and upper lids create a tired, fatigued appearance, while deep nasolabial creases compound the early-aging appearance.

CHAPTER 6 Aesthetics, Analysis, and Judgment

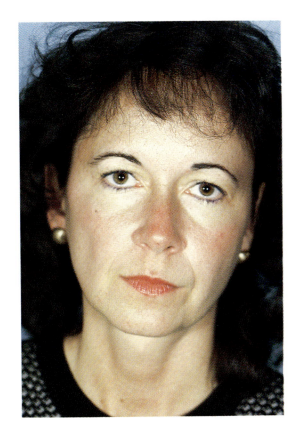
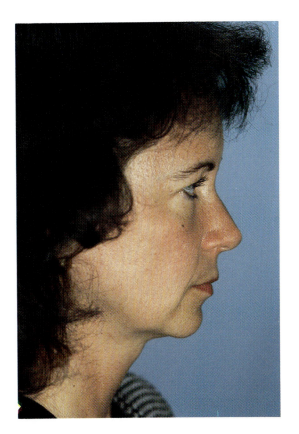
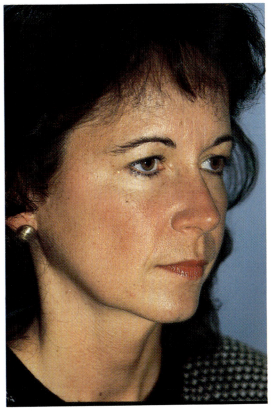

Case 4

62-Year-Old Woman

ANALYSIS

Favorable
- Attractive face and eyes
- Good facial balance and proportions
- Good skeletal and bone structure
- Little photopigmentation despite high sun exposure
- No excess fat
- Good mandibular length

Unfavorable
- Older age group
- Poor skin elasticity
- Significant permanent skin creasing
- Prominent scleral show with inadequate lower lid support and early ectropion
- Deep forehead and glabellar creases
- Forehead, brow, and nasal root ptosis
- Regional facial fat atrophy with hollowing
- Prominent exposed cervical fat pads
- Prominent cheek-lip folds
- Elongated upper lip
- Severe perioral wrinkling and atrophy, involution
- Thin lips with inversion
- Prominent chin
- Severe facial and cervical creasing
- Asymmetrical platysmal banding

Frontal
- Thick, abundant hair
- Forehead creasing
- Glabellar rhytids
- Moderate redundant upper lid skin
- Scleral show with reduced lower lid support
- Lateral canthal rhytids
- Cheek fat atrophy
- Prominent cheek-lip folds and creases
- Marked facial and perioral wrinkling
- Thinning, involuting lips
- Platysmal banding

Oblique
- Temple ptosis with rhytidosis
- Brow ptosis
- Deeply etched permanent creases
- Flat cheekbones
- Prominent jowls
- Deep cervical creases
- Marked brow, temporal ptosis
- Little excess lower lid fat
- Tip-supratip disproportion
- No tip ptosis
- Good upper lip length
- Thinning lips with involution
- Elongated cheek-lip folds
- Mid- and lower-facial fat atrophy
- Redundant cervical skin
- Obliteration of the cervicomental angle
- Ptotic submandibular gland

Summary
Attractive older patient who has delayed the quest for surgical rejuvenation overlong, thus limiting improvement possibilities. Facial fat atrophy creates regional depressions and deep creasing, which are only partially improvable.

CHAPTER 6 Aesthetics, Analysis, and Judgment

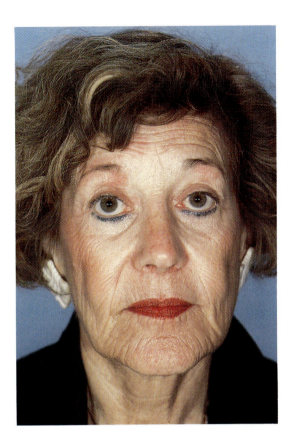
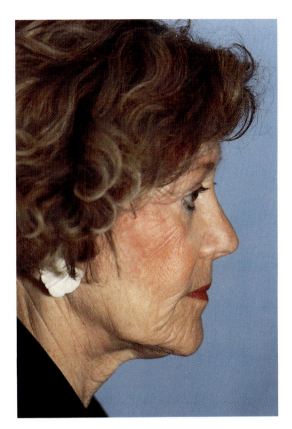
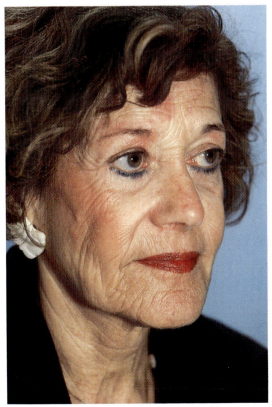

Case 5

42-Year-Old Woman

ANALYSIS

Favorable
- Attractive face and eyes
- Little solar skin damage
- Early aging changes
- Good skin quality

Unfavorable
- Round face without skeletal definition
- Lateral brow ptosis
- Excess facial/cervical fat
- Slightly overweight for height and frame
- Retrognathia
- Poor mandibular cervical definition
- Excess submental fat
- Relatively short columnar neck
- Slight scleral show
- Asymmetrical lower part of the face

Frontal
- Hair frames face well
- Minimal forehead creasing
- Prominent glabellar crease
- Moderate eyebrow ptosis without an arch
- Minimal excess upper lid skin; medial fat
- Slight scleral show
- Herniated lower lid fat
- Prominent midface
- Strong, elegant nasal dorsum
- Full, heavy cheeks and jowls
- Excess lower facial fat
- Early fine lip rhytids
- Submental fat excess
- Deep cervical crease formation

Lateral
- Attractive nose without ptosis
- Heavy ptotic thick cheek and jowl
- Retrognathia, deficient lower third of the face
- Prominent, elongated cheek-lip fold
- Poor mandibular line; excess fat
- Hyoid slightly lower than ideal
- Short columnar neck

Summary
Attractive patient whose rejuvenation surgery would best be postponed until appropriate weight reduction is realized. Particular attention to the lower third of the face and submental area is mandatory, and facial suction lipectomy is vital to complement the cervicofacial lifting procedure.

CHAPTER 6 Aesthetics, Analysis, and Judgment

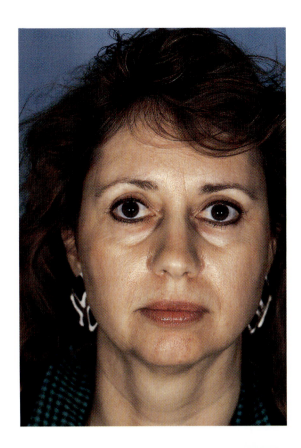
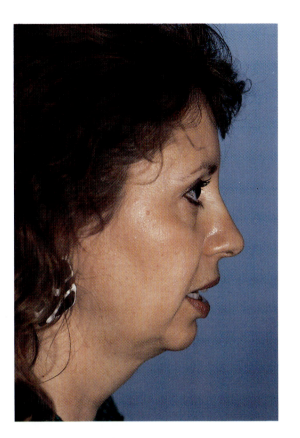
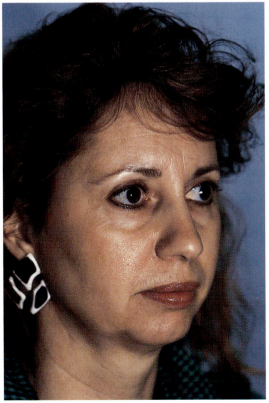

Case 6

57-Year-Old Man

ANALYSIS

Favorable
- Proper weight for frame, height
- Little facial fat
- Good bone structure
- Normal facial proportions

Unfavorable
- Photoaging skin damage
- Permanent skin creasing
- Heavy cheek-lip folds
- Reduced skin elasticity
- Scleral show

Frontal
- Retained youthful hairline
- Photoaging skin damage
- Deep forehead creases
- Brow and temple ptosis
- Minimal excess upper lid skin
- Scleral show; lax lower lid
- Lower lid fat herniation
- Permanent facial rhytids
- Prominent cheek-lip folds
- Thinning lips
- Elongated nasolabial creases

Oblique
- Brow and temple ptosis
- Prominent supraorbital ridge
- Slight scleral show
- Permanent periorbital rhytids
- Strong masculine nose
- Preauricular rhytids
- Fine perioral rhytids
- Cheek and jowl ptosis

Lateral
- Favorable hair and sideburn distribution
- Lower lid fat
- Handsome nose without aging droop
- Dependent cheek and jowl
- Submental fat with platysmal banding
- Loss of cervicomental angle definition
- Favorable mandibular structure

Summary
Male patient with favorable facial proportions and features for rejuvenation.

CHAPTER 6 Aesthetics, Analysis, and Judgment

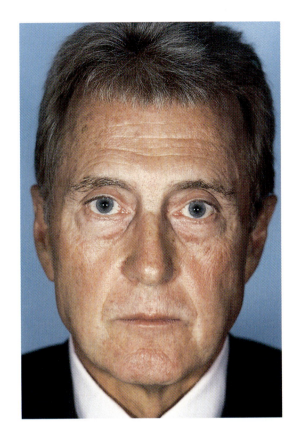
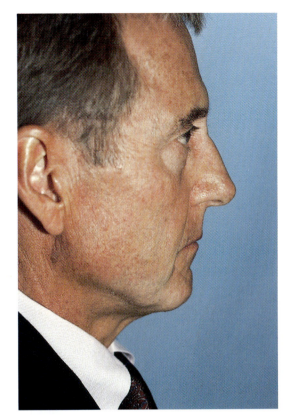
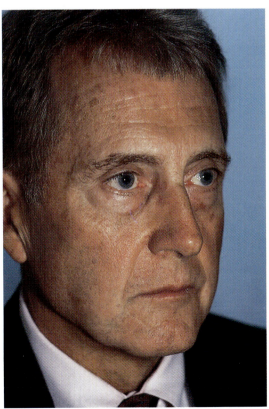

143

Case 7

55-Year-Old Woman

ANALYSIS

Favorable
- Favorable skin quality
- Good bone structure
- Early aging changes
- Attractive face and eyes
- Reasonable facial balance and proportion
- No excess facial or cervical fat
- Subcutaneous good soft-tissue padding
- Minimal forehead crease; no glabellar lines
- No nasal elongation or ptosis

Unfavorable
- Sun-damaged skin with photopigmentation
- Brow asymmetry
- Prominent nose
- Early elongation of the upper lip
- Asymmetry of the cheek-lip creases
- Slight mandibular asymmetry
- Asymmetrical platysmal bands
- Modest retrognathia
- Large (disproportionate) earlobes

Frontal
- Blotchy skin photopigmentation
- Good retained forehead/brow support
- Higher left eyebrow
- Excess upper eyelid skin
- Early fat herniation of the nasal quadrant and upper lids
- Good lower lid support
- Excess lower lid fat
- Increased nasal width
- Asymmetry of the mouth, cheek-lip mandible creases
- Asymmetrical platysmal banding

Oblique
- Good cheekbone structure
- Slight elongation of the upper lip
- Early creasing of the upper lip
- Enlarged, creased earlobes
- Permanent cervical creasing

Lateral
- Upper lid hooding
- Prominent dorsum; supratip prominence, creases; tip-supratip disproportion
- Prominent cheek-lip fold and early "drool" line
- Early jowling
- Obliteration of the cervicomental angle by a hanging platysmal band
- Enlarged earlobe
- Slight ptosis of the submandibular gland
- Modest retrognathia

Summary
Excellent candidate for rejuvenation surgery. Good bone structure provides a positive platform for redraping of soft tissues. Nasal and earlobe reduction would complement the basic rejuvenation procedures.

CHAPTER 6   Aesthetics, Analysis, and Judgment

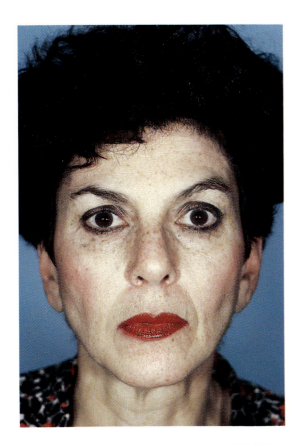
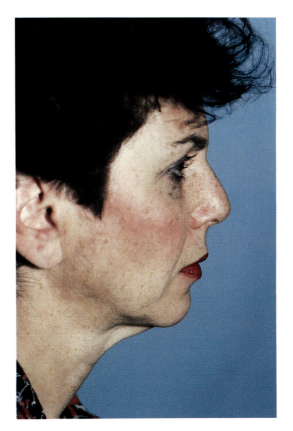
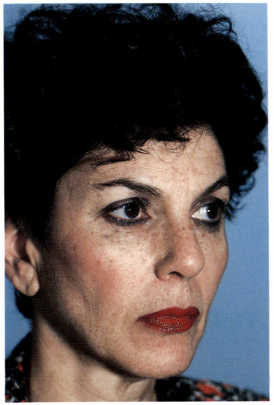

145

Case 8

40-Year-Old Woman

ANALYSIS

Favorable
- Excellent facial proportion with symmetry
- Thin skin—ideal fat cushion
- Good bone structure
- No forehead/brow ptosis
- Excellent brow arch
- Attractive eyes
- Minimal excess eyelid skin
- Moderate lower lid fat
- Proportionate nose, upper lip
- Sweeping jawline
- Minimal submental fat
- Long columnar neck

Unfavorable
- Thin, dry skin
- Multiple pigmented nevi
- Slight nasal asymmetry
- Permanent neck creasing

Frontal
- High hairline; abundant hair
- Good retention of forehead/brow support
- No significant forehead/glabellar creases
- Early, moderate upper lid fat
- Herniated lower lid fat
- Slight nasal tip asymmetry
- Shallow nasolabial creases
- Full mouth; proportionate, attractive

Oblique
- Ideal "double-tuft" temporal hair distribution
- Aesthetic arch of the eyebrow
- No significant upper lid fat
- Good lower lid support and position
- Excellent cheek bone structure
- Strong dorsal nasal profile
- Youthful earlobe
- Early oral commissure "drool" lines
- Early jowling

Lateral
- Multiple facial/cervical nevi
- Slight alar-columellar disproportion
- Strong elegant nose, slightly overlong
- Ideal lip posture
- "Drool" line oral commissure
- Early jowling
- Early blunted cervicomental angle
- Aesthetically long columellar neck

Summary
Favorable skin quality and bone structure with only early aging changes qualify this patient as a near-ideal candidate for facial rejuvenation.

CHAPTER 6 Aesthetics, Analysis, and Judgment

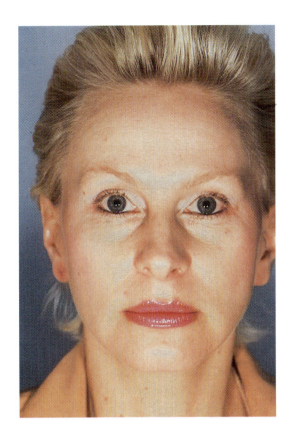
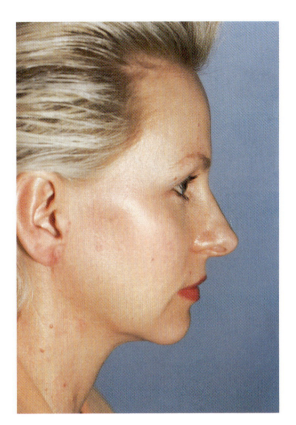
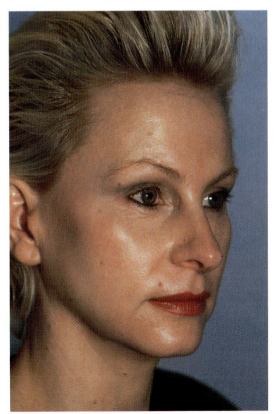

PART I BASIC PRINCIPLES

Preoperative Facial Evaluation

The evaluation of facial features is inaugurated at the moment the surgeon and patient meet. During the brief moments of initial greeting and into the more detailed and specific period of examination, facial proportions, balance, and particularly animation are assessed in ongoing fashion. Much can be learned about patient motivation, expectation, and realism during the casual conversation that takes place during the initial period of making the patient at ease. Highly useful to elicit is the level of knowledge about plastic surgery possessed by the patient, information of value to the surgeon in individually structuring the interview and examination. Of equal interest are what event or decision triggered the visit to inquire about the details of surgery and how the patient was referred. Inquiring about the patient's occupation and interests frequently allays the understandable anxiety and even embarrassment that often accompanies the facial consultation. It is instructive to learn why this particular time was selected to investigate surgical consultation. Of extreme interest is an initial determination, often evident early in the interview, of whether the individual seeking surgery seems well motivated and, in broad terms, "sensible."

Reviewing the medical and surgical history previously recorded by the office staff rather commonly reveals additional medical facts not previously provided since patients are surprisingly careless or circumspect in giving personal and medical details to someone other than the physician. Particular emphasis should be placed on any and all medications routinely taken. The use of aspirin, blood pressure medication, antidepressants, and sleeping medications is vital to ferret out and document. Previous plastic surgical procedures, the circumstances and motivation for their performance, and the patient's level of satisfaction with the outcome can provide vital clues in diagnosis and understanding. Known or suspected allergies or untoward reactions to medications must be specifically delineated and recorded. Thus as the remainder of the medical history is elicited, pathways of communication begin to open between the surgeon and prospective patient that provide clues as to the reasonableness of the surgery request. The ideal circumstance is to develop an atmosphere in which the patient feels free and comfortable to confide in the surgeon without reservation. In reality, all during the interview process two relative strangers proceed to make judgments about each other: the patient about whether he or she can have unqualified confidence in the surgeon consulted, and the surgeon about whether a favorable outcome is likely to be achieved that will result in a satisfied and happy patient. In the simplest terms, each attempts to determine whether he or she "likes" and can develop essential trust in the other.

Gaining some degree of understanding of the patient's depth of knowledge and accuracy of perceptions about plastic surgery often provides a useful guideline for continuing the interview and examination. Patient requests during the initial encounter generally fall into one of two categories: those who request surgical correction of a specific feature area and those who ask the surgeon to provide an overall evaluation of the present

CHAPTER 6   Aesthetics, Analysis, and Judgment

condition of the face and which procedures or combination of procedures might be indicated to effect improvement and rejuvenation. Each surgeon must decide for himself whether it is appropriate to recommend procedures that are not specifically requested. Almost without fail definite stated or unstated clues emerge during the consultation to guide the surgeon's approach. Full and complete facial assessment is always essential and is routinely accomplished.

Infrequent occasions do arise in which it becomes obvious early in the interview process that surgery of any kind is inadvisable. In these circumstances no purpose is served by undertaking the usual complete examination, and tactful disengagement with the patient is advisable.

We begin the examination process with the patient in a comfortable examining chair that may be rotated or elevated as needed to examine the facial features alternately in different lighting. Strong full frontal lighting prevails throughout most of the evaluation, but tangential lighting is useful to demonstrate facial contouring as well as shadows cast by elevated or depressed scars.

With a three-way mirror positioned so that both the patient and surgeon can participate in specific evaluation, the patient is asked to point out exactly the area(s) disliked or to be altered (see Fig 1–3). If concern is expressed about a series of features disliked, it may be instructive to have him rate the complaints in order of importance or concern since defects clearly obvious to the surgeon may provide little concern to the patient. It is better to gain this information early in the evaluation than to risk potential embarrassment later when a feature pleasing to the patient is criticized. Providing a common Q-tip to be used as a pointer is a useful trick to delineate specific points of concern. Once the chief concerns and complaints are fully elicited, the complete facial and neck examination ensues. If a single isolated area or feature has generated the patient's concern, we begin with a formal, detailed evaluation of the specific area first and discuss and demonstrate its significance, variation from the range of normal, and the options and alternatives for improvement. Evaluation of the remaining facial features follows, their condition pointed out, and options suggested for repair *only* if the patient has been judged receptive or eager for information. For the vast majority of individuals this information, offered as educational and informative, is welcomed; however, one must be sensitive to that small group of prospective patients who may find this method off-putting. Patients who request or obviously are eager for an assessment of the range of improvement possibilities for the entire face and neck undergo a complete, feature-by-feature analysis of the face and an explanation of the procedures that may reasonably be expected to result in significant improvement without undue risk.

To ensure completeness, it is usually preferable to begin the evaluation in the upper part of the face and proceed inferiorly. Throughout this process the texture, quality, varying thickness, elasticity, and degree of sun damage to the skin in differing regions are evaluated by inspection and palpation with the thumb and forefinger. Palpation with the most gentle and delicate touch possible reassures patients that the surgeon places high value on technical delicacy. Skin lesions, wrinkling, variable pigmentations, and any scars are pointed out. Particular and strong emphasis is placed upon documenting to the patient facial asymmetries (both in repose and upon animation), which almost always exist to one degree or another.

In the forehead region features of importance include the level and character of the hairline, the degree and symmetry of the horizontal aspect of the forehead, and the precise vertical or oblique glabellar wrinkling (including oblique sleep creases). Hypertonicity of the frontalis muscle, if present, is documented, along with the resultant effect on the eyebrow position (Fig 6–6). Alterations in or recession of the normal hair pattern is demonstrated and the character of the typical "double tuft" of hair in the temporal region pointed out. The shape, symmetry, heaviness, and relationship of the brows to the supraorbital rim should be recorded, along with the effect on upper lid contour when the brows are manually lifted to a normal position.

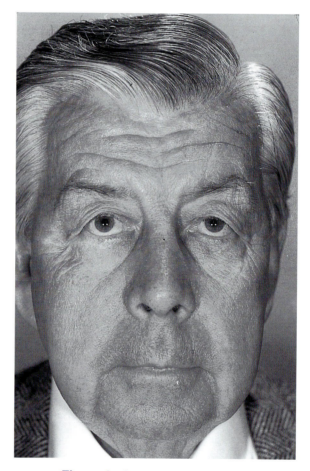

Figure 6–6
Hypertonicity of the frontalis muscle.

CHAPTER 6 Aesthetics, Analysis, and Judgment

The orbital region suffers the earliest impact of the aging process and thus requires especially attentive evaluation, including the degree and character of excessive upper lid skin and fat, lid ptosis, lateral hooding, the degree of horizontal inclination of the eye, and the nature of the upper lid crease. In the lower lid excess skin and fat are documented (both in forward gaze and during upward and lateral globe movements), any untoward scleral show or ectropion observed, and tonicity assessed by pulling the skin away from the globe and observing the character and rate of its return to a normal position against the globe. Weakening of the lower lid support structures with excess horizontal laxity is commonly encountered. Laxity and ptosis of the temporal aesthetic unit is searched for and the effect of temporal lifting upon brow position and the lateral "laugh lines" noted both in repose and while smiling. Vision in each eye is assessed and tests for diminished lacrimation carried out if the history is at all suggestive of dryness or irritation. The presence of fat or fluid in the malar pads is noted.

The mid and lower portions of the face are assessed next, both in repose and in varying degrees of animation. Asymmetries must be carefully noted and drawn to the patient's attention, particularly if they result from an imbalance or weakness in mimetic muscle function. A critical determination of the relative mobility of the facial skin, subcutaneous tissues, and layers of the superficial musculoaponeurotic system (SMAS) is then performed to ascertain how easily these layers glide over the underlying skeleton of the face. Rolling the soft tissues between the fingers provides information about the thickness and amount of subcutaneous fat and skin elasticity. The presence of ptotic malar fat pads, jowls, and prominent cheek-lip folds or creases is usually obvious. Critical to the success of any rejuvenation surgery is the angular and prominent skeletal bone structure—the malar eminences plus the width, length, and symmetry of the mandible. Inequalities of the two sides of the mandible, with variable deviation of the lower part of the face, are regularly encountered. Perioral rhytidosis, lengthening of the upper lip, thinning of the red lip portions, and midface retrusion all accompany the aging process. The influence of dentition on the mouth and lips is checked.

Examination next occurs in the submental region and the effect of the head-up and head-down positions on cervical anatomy noted. Loose and hanging skin and platysma muscle are palpated, stretched, and lifted laterally and upward to determine the potential benefits of lifting and repositioning procedures. The degree and extent of the submental fat accumulation may be judged rather accurately by palpation and ballottement between the thumb and forefinger. Critical to the potential surgical improvement is the relative position of the hyoid-thyroid complex and its influence upon the nature of the cervicomental angle. Columnar neck length is assessed. The patient is asked to forcibly pull the corners of the mouth downward to create dynamic contracture of the platysmal bands and throw them into broad relief for study (Fig 6–7). Excess regional fat depositions in the neck requiring removal by direct excision or suction lipectomy to maximize the ultimate contouring possible with lifting maneuvers are documented. Ptotic submaxillary glands emerging below their normal anatomic sites—behind and above the level of the mandibular border—must be noted.

During this examination, a continued oral interview of the patient ensues to gather information about the patient's reasons for requesting surgery and whether his motivation is high and appropriate. Constantly and progressively, an operative "game plan" is developing in the surgeon's mind, a mental rehearsal of potential operative improvements to be realistically realized on the basis of the individual patient's unique anatomy and facial features.

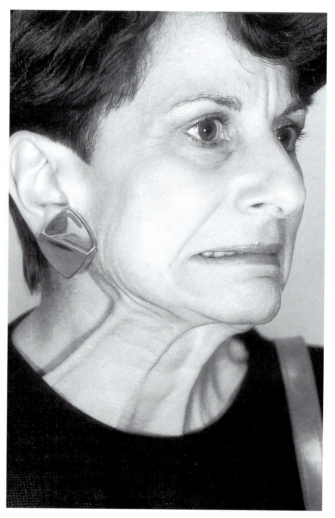

Figure 6–7
Borders of the platysma muscle break through into broad relief by hypercontraction when patient is asked to forcibly pull the corners of the mouth downward.

CHAPTER 6 Aesthetics, Analysis, and Judgment

Suggested Reading

- Farkas LG: *Anthropometry of the Head and Face.* New York, Raven Press, 1994.
- Farkas LG, Kolar JC: Anthropometrics and art in the aesthetics of women's faces. *Clin Plast Surg* 1987; 14:599–616.
- Powell N, Humphreys B: *Proportions of the Aesthetic Face.* New York, Thieme-Stratton, 1984.
- Romm S: *The Changing Face of Beauty.* St Louis, Mosby, 1992.

PART II

FACIAL AESTHETIC AND LIFTING PROCEDURES

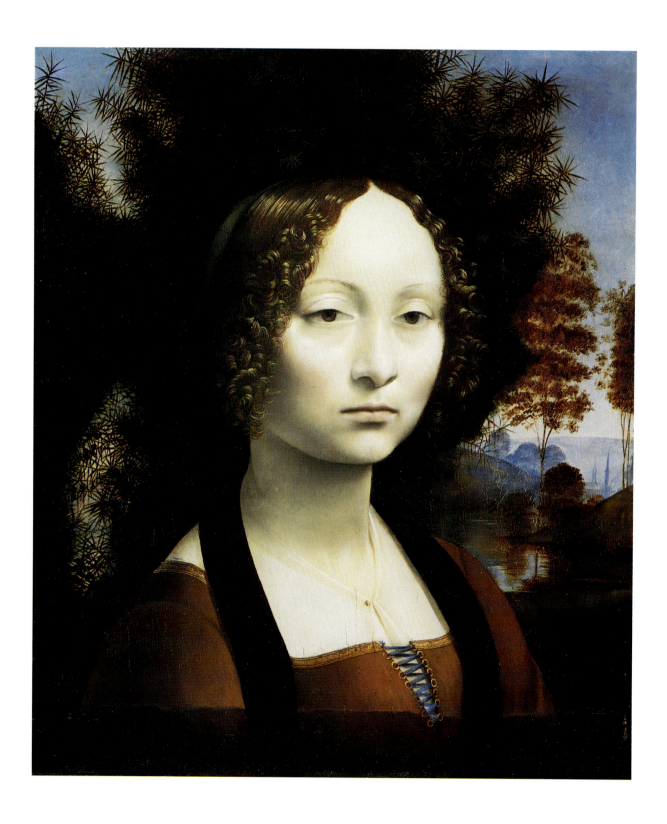

CHAPTER

7

 # Forehead-Lift

> *Forty is the old age of youth;*
> *Fifty the youth of old age.*
>
> **Victor Hugo**

Diagnosis and Candidate Selection

The relentless passage of time combined with gravity inevitably creates forehead and eyebrow drooping and malposition. The aesthetic facial unit comprising the eyelid-orbital region, when flawed by gradual aging, asymmetry, or familial abnormality, cannot always be satisfactorily rejuvenated with eyelid surgery alone. Ptotic eyebrows may compound the problem of redundant upper eyelid skin by crowding the eye and producing an abnormal appearance of both fatigue and premature aging. A temporal quadrant visual deficit may develop, further justifying interventional surgery to restore lost function. If upper lid blepharoplasty alone is used in attempts at correction, the eyebrow is often drawn nearer the lid margin and adequate delineation of the infrabrow cleft obliterated by sacrificing excessive upper lid skin in a misguided attempt to correct this problem. Incorporating one of the brow elevation procedures to enhance the resultant appearance is a preferred approach that preserves sufficient upper lid skin to achieve a pleasant sweeping delineation of the upper lid cleft.

Blepharoplasty alone is less effective in improving and recontouring the lateral orbital rhytids ("crow's-feet" or "laugh lines"), which contribute to the aging appearance and thereby displease patients. Oblique and vertical glabellar frown lines remain unchanged without direct surgical interruption of the involved animation muscles. Some form of adjunctive "lifting" procedure in the upper third of the face is thereby required to augment the improvement achieved by blepharoplasty. Most useful among these are the *brow-lift (browplasty), temporal (temple) lift,* the *midforehead lift,* and the *forehead (coronal and pretrichal) lift.* Specific indications exist for each and will be explored later.

Careful patient selection to ensure effective, satisfactory outcomes assumes major importance in all forms of aesthetic surgery, especially important in orbital region rejuvenation. Patients regularly request eyelid surgery when instead or in addition to eyelid surgery they need forehead-, brow-, and temple-lifting. Educating patients about the most effective procedure(s) often requires superior communication skills and gentle guidance, since few patients are aware that forehead/brow ptosis is responsible for the aging orbital changes apparent. Clearly more of the surgeon's time must be ex-

CHAPTER 7 Forehead-Lift

pended to realize the laudable goals of effective patient understanding and truly informed consent.

Patient selection, particularly from the viewpoint of *motivations* and *expectations*, assumes major importance in the caliber and effectiveness of the final outcome. In aesthetic surgery, pure technical excellence will not always result in a happy, satisfied patient. Useful guidelines to patient selection (and rejection) exist; each individual, however, requires careful and sensitive screening to identify proper candidates.

Although different regions of the face age at different rates, influenced primarily by genetic factors, the upper facial third possesses its own unique fashion of aging (see Fig 1–6). As elasticity progressively declines, the forehead, temple, and glabellar skin descends. Ptotic low-positioned brows develop, crowd the orbital region, and increase the degree of skin redundancy in the upper lid area (Fig 7–1). Fine lines, the result of gravity and repeated orbicularis muscle contraction, appear at the lateral canthus and temple (Fig 7–1). Progressively deep horizontal creases appear in the forehead, the consequence of repetitive frontalis muscle contraction and hypertonicity (Fig 7–2) (their absence in a paralyzed forehead validates this observation). Synergistic actions of the corrugator and procerus muscles produce vertical, oblique, and horizontal creases in the glabella and nasal root (Fig 7–3).

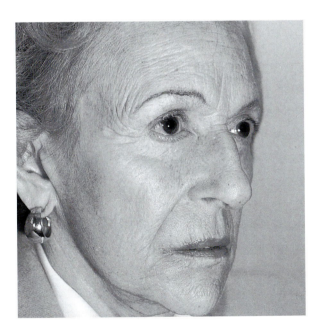

Figure 7–1
Developing aging characteristics of the forehead, temple, brow, and upper lid. Forehead rhytids develop, the brow descends to or below the level of the orbital rim, the temporal area relaxes and drifts caudally, and upper lid redundancy becomes apparent—often to a profound degree.

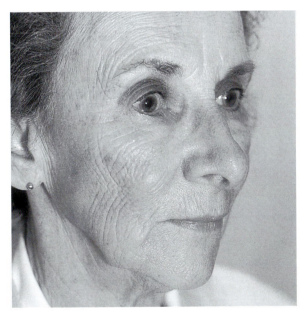

Figure 7–2
Deeply etched rhytids caused by a combination of aging, animation, and excessive sun exposure produce a near-checkerboard pattern in the lateral canthal and temple regions.

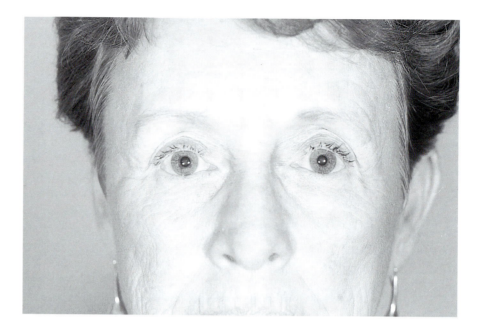

Figure 7–3
Vertical, oblique, and horizontal rhytids in the glabella and nasal root produced by synergistic actions of the corrugator and procerus muscles.

Forehead-lifting procedures may be effectively combined with methods to rejuvenate the middle and lower facial thirds (facelift and necklift). Since the various regions of the face may age at different rates, forehead/brow-lifting is also commonly accomplished as an isolated procedure or as a preliminary step to blepharoplasty.

With rare exceptions, the brow elevation procedure should be carried out *prior to* upper lid blepharoplasty, thereby facilitating judgment as to the precise amount of upper lid skin excised and thus preventing an over-aggressive elevation of the brow–upper lid complex with consequent difficulty in normal upper lid closure.

Three factors bearing heavily on the surgeon's choice of sequence and combinations of operations are (1) the relative position of the brows, (2) the mobility of the scalp and forehead layers, and (3) the sex of the patient. The male brow classically is heavier in hair content, occupies a more inferior (caudal) position, and is less laterally arched than the female brow, which commonly occupies a transversely horizontal position (Fig 7–4). This effect, although occasionally objectionable in a female, is not usually displeasing in a male. In contrast, the preferred female brow (many variations obviously exist) arches higher laterally than medially, ideally assuming its highest point at about the junction of the middle and outer thirds (Fig 7–5). The female brow typically thins as it courses laterally, and this diminishes the ease of potential scar camouflage in the hair-skin junction. Therefore a critical evaluation prior to technique selection is assessment of the eyebrow position, attitude, and shape with the patient sitting and in

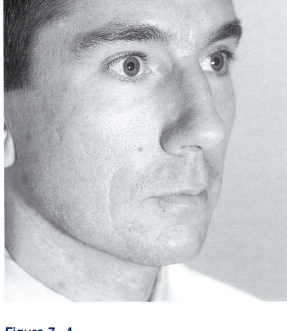

Figure 7–4
Normal position of the male brow, resting at or just above the supraorbital rim. Little brow arch exists.

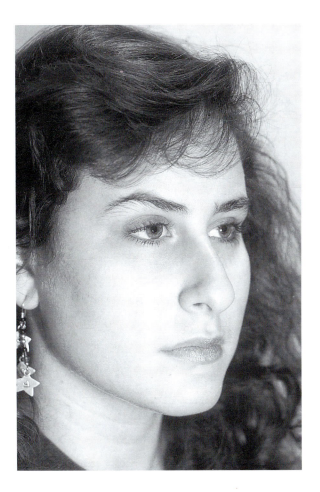

Figure 7–5
Favorable and attractive position and shape of an arching female brow.

repose. By manually elevating the brow and forehead with the patient gazing straight ahead, a tentative judgment can be made about the favorable effect of brow elevation on the aesthetic unit of the eye and orbit (Fig 7–6). Individuals with ptotic brows commonly attempt to unconsciously elevate the brow and cause excessive forehead animation. This facial posture is ordinarily an unconscious habit and gives rise to a "surprised" facial expression as the drooping brow is temporarily elevated (Fig 7–7). Preoperative estimates of the benefits of surgical brow elevation will be much more accurate if all animation is consciously eliminated and the brow position is judged with the patient in complete facial repose. By having the patient close the eyes and open them slowly after allowing the facial muscles to relax, the true brow position in repose may be determined. The individual anatomic situation will then dictate the choice of which of the brow elevation procedures would most favorably complement the planned blepharoplasty operation (Table 7–1).

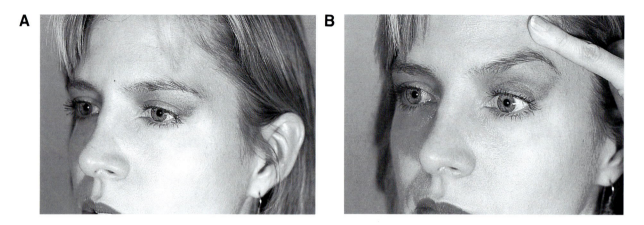

Figure 7–6
A, aging, ptotic brow. **B,** manual elevation of the brow to assess mobility and the effect of a brow or forehead elevation procedure on orbital and eyelid appearance.

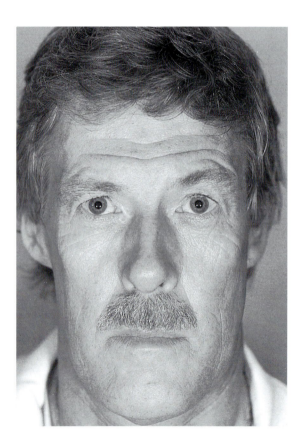

Figure 7–7
Hypertonicity of frontalis muscle.

Table 7–1

Forehead- and Brow-Lifting Procedures

Procedure	Indications and Advantages	Contraindications and Disadvantages
Coronal forehead-lift	■ Ideal and immediate scar camouflage ■ Treats all aspects of the aging forehead and brow	■ Limited use in males ■ Elevates hairline ■ Vertically lengthens the upper ⅓ of face ■ Elongated scar ■ Possible prolonged hypoesthesia of the scalp ■ Less fine tuning of the brow position
Pretrichal forehead-lift	■ High hairline ■ No vertical forehead lengthening ■ Preserves the hairline ■ Treats all aspects of the aging forehead and brows ■ Immediate scar camouflage (with hair) ■ Improved "fine tuning" of the brow position	■ Possible visible (exposed) scar ■ Possible prolonged hypoesthesia of the scalp
Mid forehead-lift	■ Prominent horizontal crease ■ Preserves the hairline ■ Improved "fine tuning" of the brow position ■ Corrects brow asymmetry	■ Possible visible (exposed) scar ■ Avoid in oily, thick skin
Mid forehead/brow-lift	■ Prominent horizontal crease ■ Improved "fine tuning" of the brow position ■ Corrects brow asymmetry	■ Possible visible (exposed) scar ■ Treats brows only ■ Avoid in oily, thick skin
Direct brow-lift	■ Accurate brow elevation ■ Preserves forehead/scalp sensation ■ Patients with abundant brow hair preferred ■ Immediate scar camouflage (with hair) ■ Corrects brow asymmetry	■ Possible visible (exposed) scar ■ Treats brows only
Temporal-lift	■ Ideal and immediate camouflage ■ Improves brow position and temple laxity	■ Not useful for midforehead glabellar creases ■ No effect on medial aspects of the brow

Surgical Goals

The goals associated with rejuvenation surgery of the brow and upper portion of the face are straightforward and include the following:

- Elevation of ptotic eyebrows
- Reduction of redundant upper lid skin
- Elevation of the forehead
- Modification of forehead rhytids
- Reduction of glabellar rhytids
- Elevation of the temporal aesthetic unit
- Reduction of lateral canthal "crow's-feet" rhytids
- Correction of eyebrow asymmetry

The coronal forehead-lift, properly performed, results primarily in long-lasting cephalic elevation of ptotic eyebrow position. Overaggressive brow elevation must be assiduously avoided to prevent an abnormal surprised look on the final facial appearance.

Attenuation of the mimetic activity of the procerus and corrugator muscles by surgical division or removal reduces glabellar rhytid appearance and forestalls further worsening of these objectionable lines, but cannot be expected to completely eliminate creases permanently etched in the glabellar skin. Elevation of the glabellar and nasal root skin improves redundancy in this area and ameliorates transverse nasal creases in the nasal radix.

Transverse forehead rhytids can be expected to undergo improvement in direct relationship to their depth and length of existence. Following coronal forehead-lifting with attenuation or removal of segments of the frontalis muscle, transverse creases generally undergo a degree of smoothing and reduction in crease depth; seldom, except in younger surgical candidates, do they undergo total elimination.

Finally, the forehead-lift results in a variable degree of reduction in upper eyelid and temporal unit skin excess and redundancy and thus reduced direct skin excision during blepharoplasty. Accordingly, during rejuvenation procedures aimed at improving the appearance of the aging orbital area, blepharoplasty should always be accomplished *after* forehead-, temporal-, or eyebrow-lifting.

With proper technique, the effectiveness and longevity of upper facial lifting procedures is highly satisfactory, regularly outlasting improvement gained by lower facial lifting procedures.

Since very little swelling or edema ordinarily results following upper facial lifting procedures, patients commonly return to normal activities only a few days following surgery. Bruising and ecchymosis are uncommon, and since incision stitches and staples are hidden in the hair-bearing skin, the procedure(s) are camouflaged immediately.

Since forehead-lifting performed through a coronal incision above the hairline necessarily produces a higher frontal hairline, only patients whose facial appearance will not be unfavorably influenced by a vertically enlarged forehead should undergo the procedure. An acceptable alternative

CHAPTER 7   Forehead-Lift

that preserves the existing hairline utilizes pretrichal incision at the hairline margin.

If forehead lifting is contemplated for patients who have undergone previous blepharoplasty, caution should accompany significant raising of the eyebrow and upper lid skin position lest permanent lagophthalmos result.

Surgical Techniques

Specific Anatomic Considerations

Although apparently a more extensive procedure, the forehead-lift is in reality not complicated as long as a healthy respect for normal anatomy is maintained. The relevant topographic anatomy in forehead-lifting is portrayed in Figures 7–8 to 7–16. Anatomic structures to which specific attention should be paid include the frontal and temporal hairlines; the frontalis, corrugator, and procerus muscles; the supratrochlear and supraorbital nerve and vessels; the frontal branch of the facial nerve; and the subgaleal tissue plane. The following anatomic factors should be also be evaluated:

- Forehead height relative to the facial proportions
- Hairline: frontal and temporal
- Abundance of frontal and brow hair
- Skin quality, texture, sebaceous quality, and thickness
- Skin elasticity and mobility
- Scalp (galeal) mobility
- Degree and depth of forehead wrinkling
- Eyebrow position and mobility
- Eyebrow anatomy and symmetry
- Degree of dermatochalasis
- Lateral canthal hooding
- Temporal rhytidosis

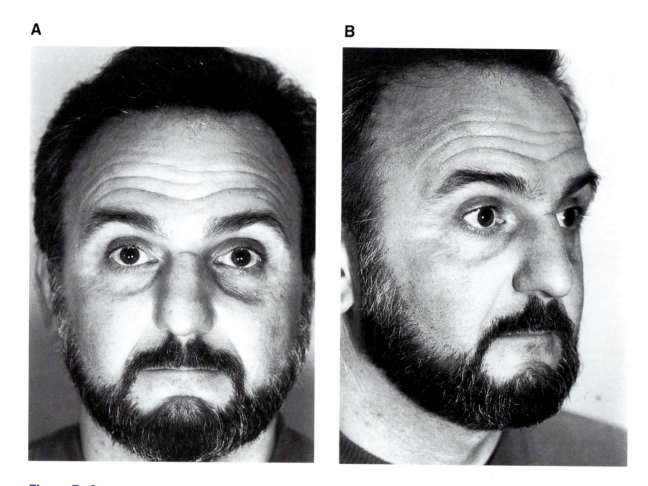

Figure 7–8
A and **B,** hypertonicity of the frontalis muscle produces deep horizontal forehead rhytids, often with the appearance of a surprised expression.

CHAPTER 7 Forehead-Lift

Anesthesia

Coronal forehead-lifting is carried out under intravenous analgesia supplemented by local anesthesia and, along with browplasty and temporal-lift, can also be performed on an outpatient basis on well-motivated patients. General anesthesia, if preferred by the patient, is equally satisfactory. If local anesthesia is chosen, infiltration to block the supraorbital and supratrochlear nerves at the upper level of the eyebrows, augmented by infiltration along the intended line of incision in the hairline, is sufficient to create excellent local anesthesia. (It is imperative to appreciate that infiltration near the facial nerve frontal branch may result in a temporary partial or complete frontal paralysis for a short period.) One percent lidocaine with 1:100,000 epinephrine, freshly mixed, is sufficient to provide local anesthesia.

Preferred and Alternative Techniques

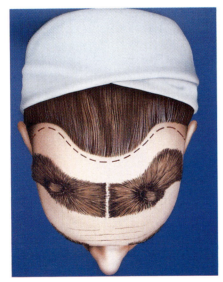
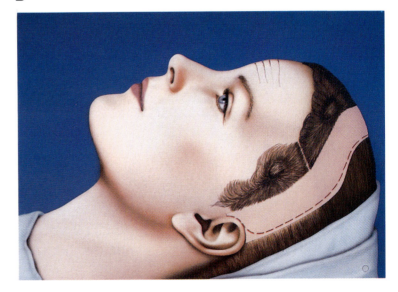

Figure 7–9

A, and **B,** the incision is sited and marked in a coronal fashion and placed far enough posterocephalically behind the frontal hairline that an excision of 1 to 2 cm of scalp anterior to the incision will place the resultant scar 2 to 4 cm behind the hairline. Hair is left intact and not shaved as depicted here. The exact site and geometry of the incision will be dictated by the shape of the frontal hairline and the individual mobility of the scalp and forehead soft tissues. The lateral wings of the incision may extend to the supra-auricular temple or, for maximal temple-lifting, beyond the tragus of each ear in a sinuous fashion from the temple into the junction of the auricle with the face. Scar camouflage is thereby facilitated. If a high forehead exists, the incision may be modified centrally by curving its midline aspect into the junction of the widow's peak and forehead.

Beveling the coronal incision protects residual hair follicles. Advancing the incision in short segments will allow continuous control of incisional bleeding by pressure, pinpoint cautery, and Rainey clips. Since the anterior edge of the incision will ultimately be excised, hot cautery to control bleeding has no deleterious effect.

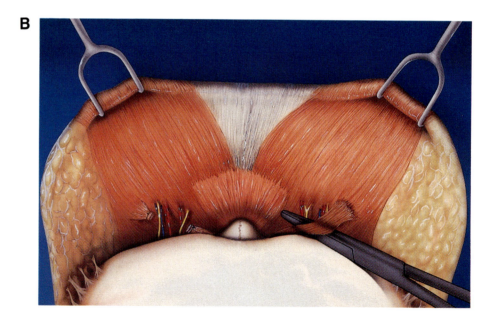

Figure 7–10

A, and **B,** as the supraperiosteal subgaleal plane is entered, the dissection may now proceed rapidly and bloodlessly with sharp and blunt dissection and is carried in this manner down to the level of the supraorbital ridges. The periosteum is left intact to this point in the procedure. The Shaw hemostatic scalpel possesses great value in maintaining profound hemostasis while allowing rapid dissection in the subgaleal plane. Here the corrugator muscles are shown being dissected away from vital neuromuscular bundles. With blunt dissection, the extent of the corrugator muscles is delineated and isolated from the supraorbital neurovascular bundle, which is religiously protected.

CHAPTER 7 Forehead-Lift

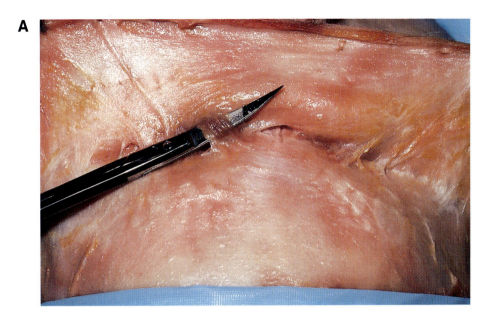

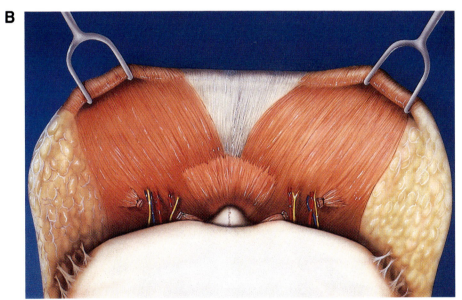

Figure 7-11
A, and **B,** the corrugator muscles are separated from their bony origin, cross-clamped, and 1 to 1.5 cm of muscle excised.

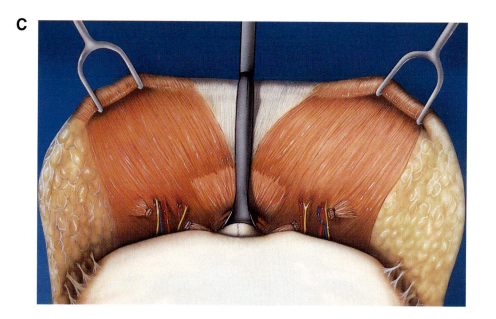

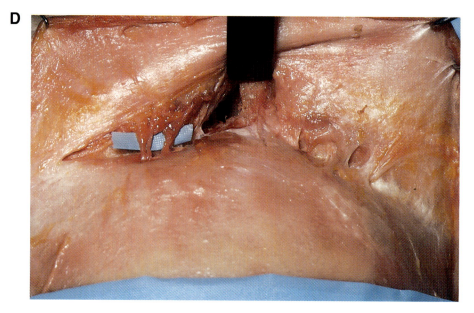

Figure 7–11 (cont.)
C, and **D,** if desired at this point, the procerus muscle may be partially excised and elevation of the dorsal nasal skin accomplished as an additional benefit (**C** and **D**).

CHAPTER 7 Forehead-Lift

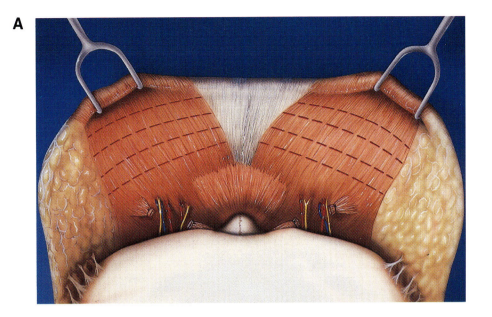

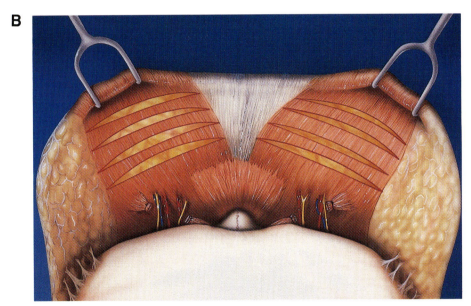

Figure 7–12
A–C, the previously marked transverse skin creases on the forehead are then visually related to the undersurface of the forehead flap. Transverse strips of the frontalis and subcutaneous tissue (1.0 to 2.0 cm) are excised by sharp dissection and care taken to preserve intact muscle at the region of the neurovascular bundles. This important resection releases the "rubber band" tension effect of the frontalis muscle on the wrinkled, ptotic forehead and is the principal factor in allowing a prolonged reduction of forehead creases.

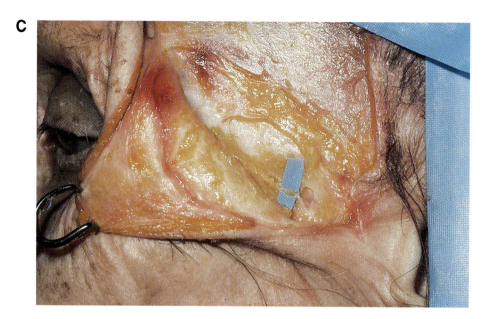

Figure 7–12 (cont.)
C, laterally, any interruption or excision of frontalis muscle should be located at least 3 cm above the orbital rim in order to protect the frontal branch of the facial nerve **(C).**

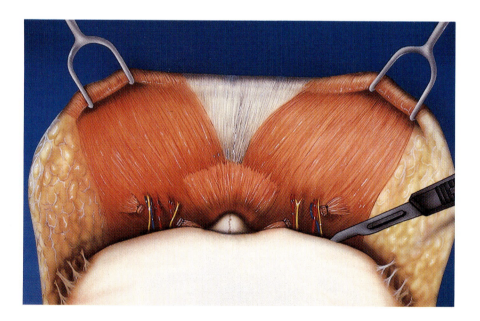

Figure 7–13
Increased elevation improvement is gained by incising the periosteum at the supraorbital rim with the Shaw scalpel and releasing the periosteum and orbital skin for added upward elevation by dissection with the Joseph periosteal elevator.

CHAPTER 7   Forehead-Lift

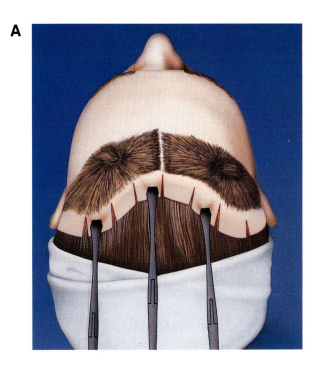 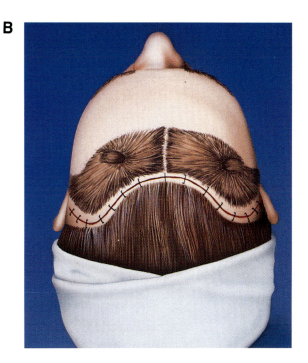

Figure 7–14
A, and **B,** after absolute and meticulous hemostasis is secured, the flap is advanced and redundant skin excised in segments, with an immediate improvement in appearance noted. Incisional closure is relatively rapid with 4-0 polydioxanine dermal sutures complemented by surgical skin clips in the scalp. Commonly, no drains are required.

Before excising portions of the flap, the scalp posterior to the coronal incision should be pushed forward to determine its mobility and elasticity, factors influencing the amount of flap excised.

The coronal forehead lift can be expected to produce a relatively long-lasting elevation of the entire forehead and brow. Transverse forehead creases and wrinkles are considerably improved but should not be expected to disappear entirely, and normal animation is preserved. Congenitally low brows assume a more normal cephalic position after a forehead-lift, as do brows rendered ptotic by the aging process. Brow elevation thus exerts a salutary effect on redundant upper eyelid skin and allows a more conservative and accurate skin resection during upper lid blepharoplasty. Clearly, deep vertical rhytids are best treated by muscle excision through the forehead-lift.

Pretrichal Forehead-Lift
An alternative approach to forehead- and brow-lifting is the pretrichal forehead-lift, accomplished by siting the coronal incision at the junction of the hairline and cephalic forehead. Although the resultant scar is theoretically not as well camouflaged as that resulting from a coronal forehead-lift, scars located at the junction of two major facial landmarks ordinarily

heal in an inconspicuous manner if meticulously repaired (particularly if reverse beveling through hair follicles at the hairline is utilized), and appropriate hairstyling can be utilized to completely camouflage the surgical scar. In patients with an increased vertical proportion to the forehead and a high hairline, this approach is useful since it avoids further elevation of the hairline with a consequent increase in vertical forehead height.

Surgical Technique

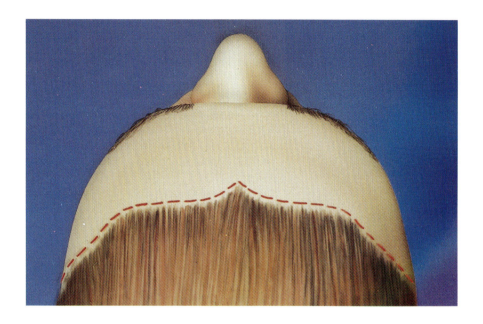

Figure 7–15
The incision proceeds in a curvilinear fashion, following and parallel to the hairs of the frontal hairline, and can on occasion be irregularized with Zs or steps to create an uneven scar and aid in eventual scar camouflage.

The subgaleal plane is entered, and the procedure then ensues in essentially the same manner as that accomplished during the coronal forehead-lift procedure (see Figures 7–10 to 7–14).

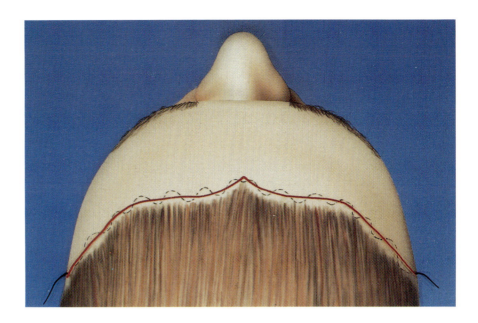

Figure 7–16
Meticulous incision closure with dermal-to-dermal interrupted 4-0 PDS sutures followed by a running locked epithelial suture of 6-0 Prolene is necessary for ideal scar healing.

On occasion, reverse beveling of the hairline incision and division of some of the hairline hair follicles are useful in that a portion of the frontal hairline hairs will regrow through the incision, thus creating improved scar camouflage.

Midforehead-lift

Specific anatomic criteria must be met before the midforehead-lift technique is contemplated; only a select few individuals are thus good candidates for this approach. A typical candidate must possess prominent transverse forehead creases into which the incision and ultimate scar may be camouflaged (Fig 7–17). Thinner nonsebaceous skin is preferred over thick, oily, textured skin in order to promote better camouflage. Patients with high or progressively receding hairlines may benefit from this approach since the overall vertical height of the upper third of the face will be slightly reduced after surgery, thereby improving overall facial proportions.

Because the incision lies closer to the ptotic brows, more exact repositioning of the desired elevation of brow posture is usually possible.

The midforehead-lift differs substantially from the coronal and pretrichal forehead-lift in that the plane of elevation of the flap is created *subcutaneously* rather than subgaleally.

Surgical Technique

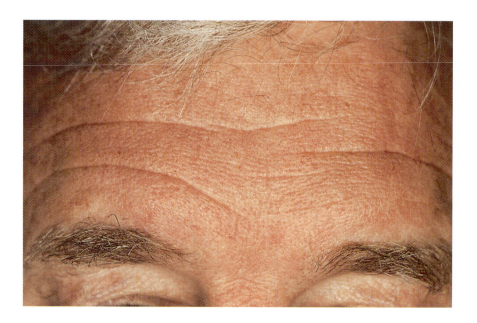

Figure 7–17
Ideal deep and asymmetrical creases of a male forehead for camouflage of midforehead-lift incisions.

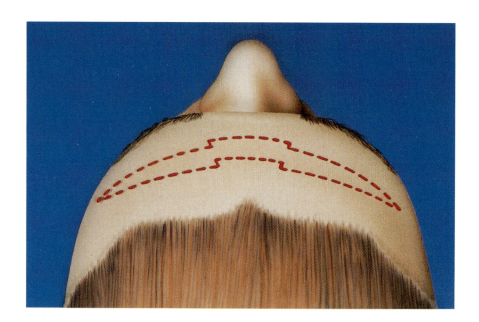

Figure 7–18
A high, completely transverse forehead skin crease is selected for incision siting. The incision is limited to the *subcutaneous plane,* initially avoiding penetration of the galea. Irregularization of the transverse incision during closure is useful in certain patients to optimize scar camouflage.

CHAPTER 7 Forehead-Lift

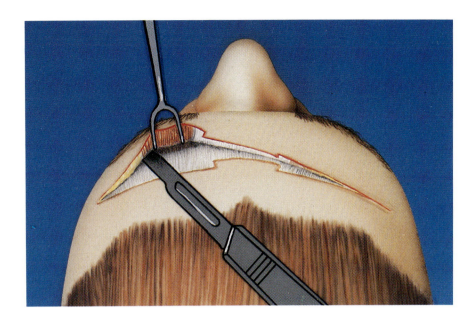

Figure 7-19
With blunt and sharp dissection using the Shaw hemostatic scalpel, elevation of the inferior subcutaneous flap ensues down to the level of the brow and root of the nose.

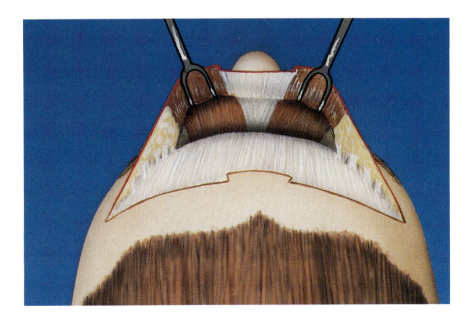

Figure 7-20
This broad exposure maximizes visualization of the corrugator and procerus muscles, which are treated in the same fashion as in the coronal and pretrichal forehead-lifts.

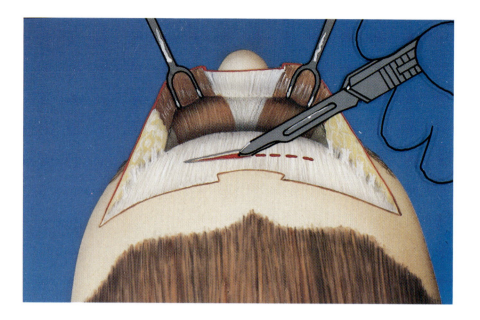

Figure 7–21
To isolate and resect or attenuate these muscles, a transverse galeal incision is created 3 cm above the nasal root and enters the subgaleal plane. This incision must not extend beyond the supraorbital nerves in order to preserve sensory innervation to the forehead. Meticulous hemostasis is paramount but usually easily ensured with the hemostatic scalpel.

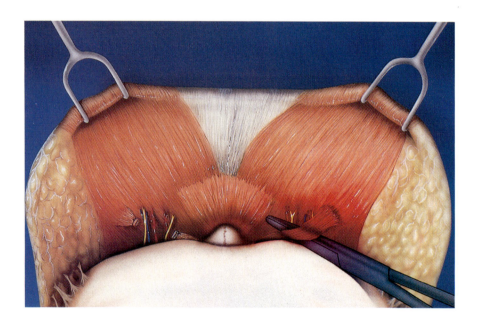

Figure 7–22
Excision of the overactive corrugator and procerus muscles at the glabella is now easily accomplished under direct vision in a manner similar to that described during coronal forehead-lifting.

CHAPTER 7 Forehead-Lift

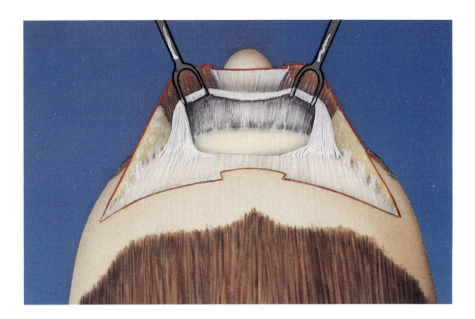

Figure 7–23
Cephalic subcutaneous elevation of the incision edge superior to the incision ensues for 1½ to 2 cm to allow skin edge eversion for closure; selected incisions of the paired frontalis muscles are carried out to release overlying deep creases.

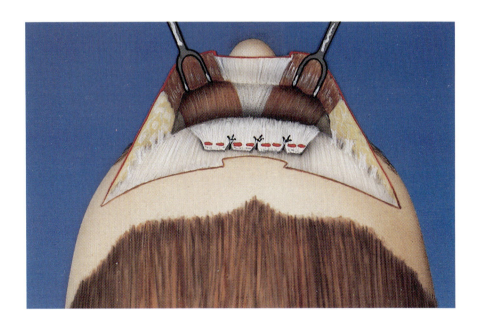

Figure 7–24
Before skin closure, the transverse galeal incision undergoes closure, after excision of any excess tissue, with 4-0 PDS sutures.

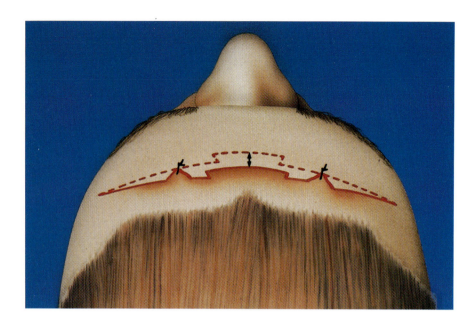

Figure 7–25
By retracting the inferior flap upward, the amount of redundant skin created by the preferred degree of brow elevation may be accurately estimated and excised. The degree of skin excision medially and laterally may be tailored to effect a desirable unequal elevation of asymmetrical brows.

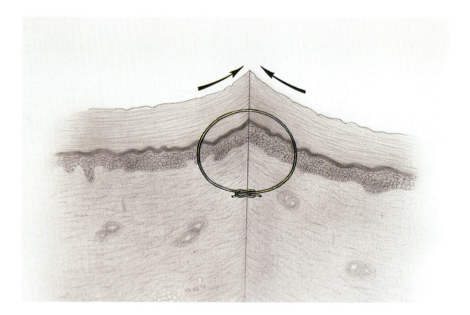

Figure 7–26
Exacting and meticulous dermal and epidermal suture closure is vital to the success of these techniques. Multiple buried, everting dermal sutures of 5-0 PDS approximate the dermis and prevent even the slightest tension in the everted skin edges.

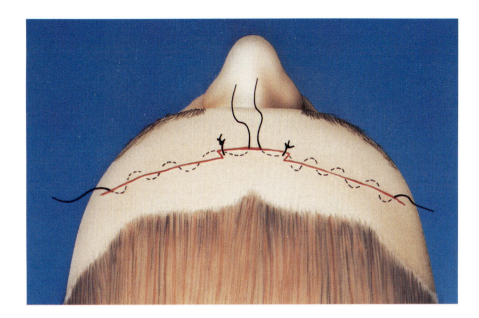

Figure 7-27
Incision closure follows with a 6-0 running Prolene suture, which is removed in 4 to 5 days and replaced with antitension skin strips. If the anatomic criteria listed above are followed in patient selection, a highly acceptable level of scar camouflage may be expected with ultimate healing.

Midforehead Browplasty

Men with ptotic brows and prominent midforehead or suprabrow skin creases are potential candidates for this technique in which the forehead incisions do not cross the midline and interconnect, further maximizing scar camouflage. Incisions sited in creases at different levels on either side further enhance scar camouflage. Improved brow posture may be accurately and effectively realized with this more limited approach, but deep glabellar and horizontal forehead rhytids are better approached by the other forehead-lifting procedures.

This procedure is thus quite limited in the treatment of forehead creases by myotomy but is highly effective in "fine-tuning" the ultimate brow position and shape in preparation for blepharoplasty, particularly in patients with asymmetrical brow lines. In addition, a significant degree of lateral canthal hooding and temple ptosis improvement results with proper incision placement since the incision generally courses more lateral than that of a direct brow-lift. At all times the "danger zone" of the region of the frontal facial nerve branch in the temple must be respected (see Fig 7-12,C) and excessive dissection, cautery, and traumatic stretching and manipulation avoided during flap retraction.

Surgical Technique

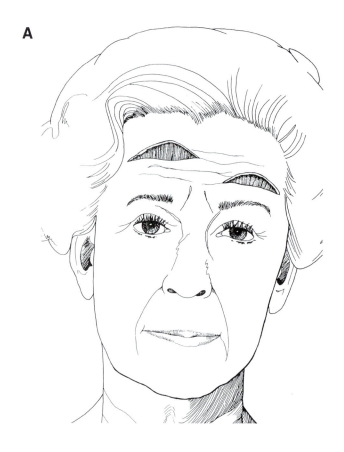

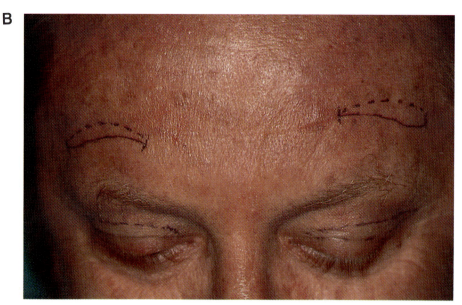

Figure 7–28
A and **B,** prominent creases lying above the lateral aspects of the brows are selected for incision siting, often selecting the second highest crease encountered. If possible, selecting creases at different levels above each brow results in superior scar camouflage potential.

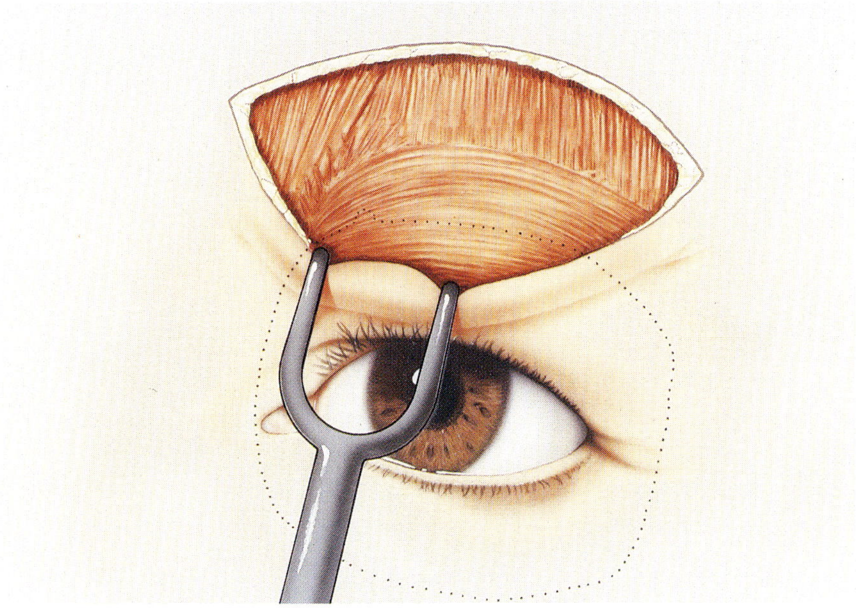

CHAPTER 7 Forehead-Lift

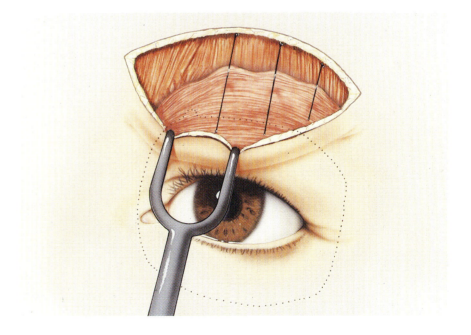

Figure 7–29
The incision enters the *subcutaneous plane;* the inferior flap is dissected to the level of the brow or just below while remaining superficial to muscle. If hypertrophied orbicularis muscle exists, selective transverse myectomy ensues.

Figure 7–30
In selected patients the muscle and dermis of the brow are suspended to the periosteum superolaterally with three or four 5-0 nylon sutures, but this additional maneuver is not always found necessary to produce lasting brow elevation.

PART II   FACIAL AESTHETIC AND LIFTING PROCEDURES

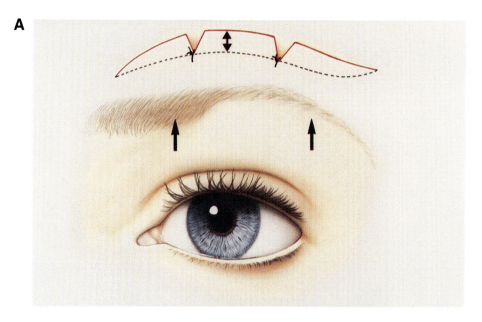

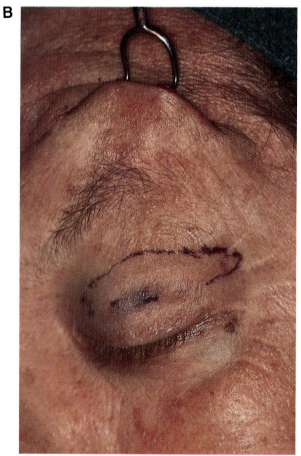

Figure 7–31
A and **B,** as the brow is retracted to the desired new cephalic position, excessive skin of the inferior flap becomes apparent and is excised.

CHAPTER 7 Forehead-Lift

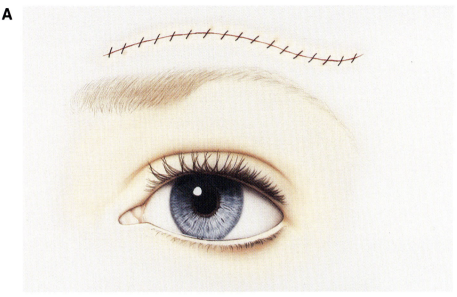

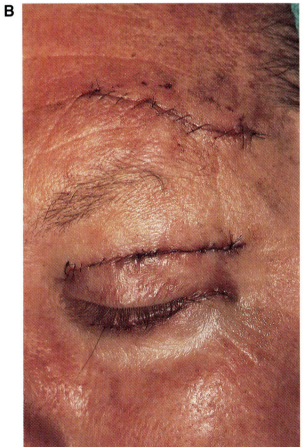

Figure 7–32
A and **B**, meticulous dermis opposition with multiple buried interrupted 5-0 PDS sutures closes the wound firmly and is followed by an everting, running 6-0 Prolene skin closure.

Postoperative Care Principles

Incisions are dressed with NeoDecadron ophthalmic ointment, Adaptic gauze, and a light, circumferential, nonpressure dressing of Kerlex gauze rolls.

At 24 hours the initial dressing is replaced for an additional day; thereafter no dressings are required. Shampooing with gentle cleaning of the hair occurs at 48 hours, when the hair may be blow-dried on a cool setting.

At 10 to 12 days we remove all staples and any external sutures. Full activities may be resumed at this time.

Results and Outcomes

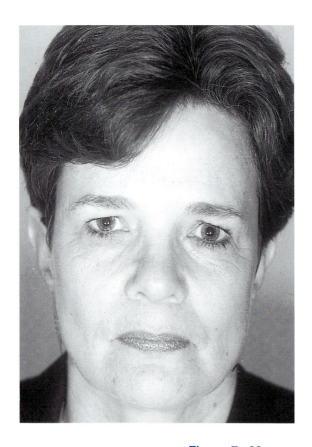 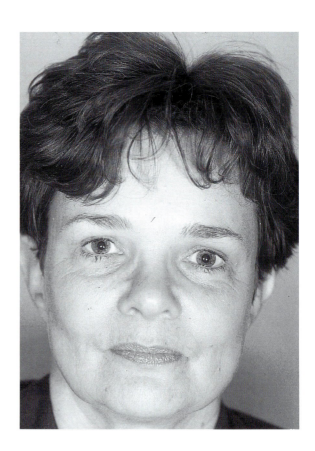

Figure 7–33
Middle-aged patient with forehead and brow ptosis compounded by deep-set eyes and prominent supraorbital bony rims. A tired and aged appearance results. Following a coronal forehead-lift combined with blepharoplasty, the patient's expression is markedly improved.

CHAPTER 7   Forehead-Lift

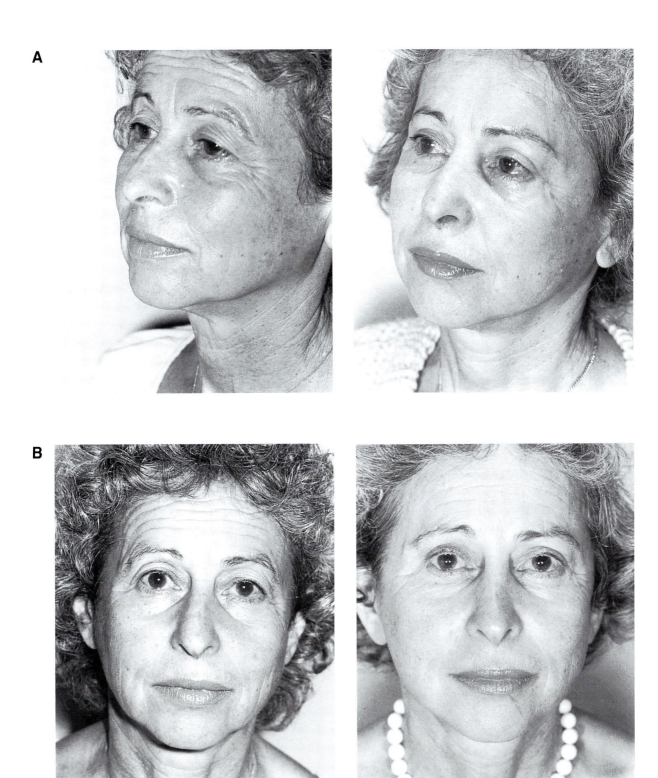

Figure 7–34
A and **B,** improved result from a coronal forehead lift and blepharoplasty in a patient with deep rhytids, hypertonic frontalis activity, a ptotic brow and temple, and upper and lower lid skin redundancy. The oblique view documents significant improvement in the temporal, lateral canthal, and eyelid regions.

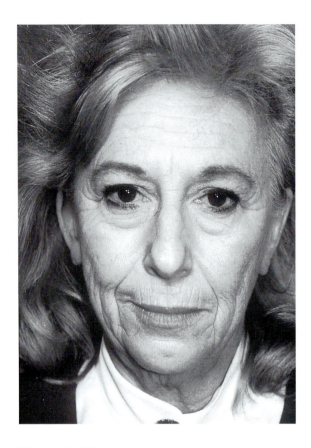 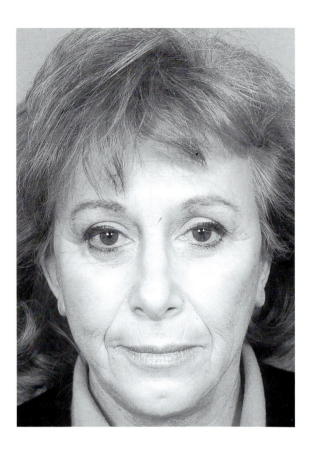

Figure 7–35
Improvement in forehead and glabellar rhytidosis with a coronal forehead-lift combined with blepharoplasty.

CHAPTER 7   Forehead-Lift

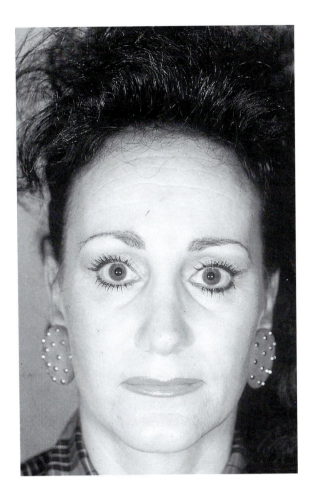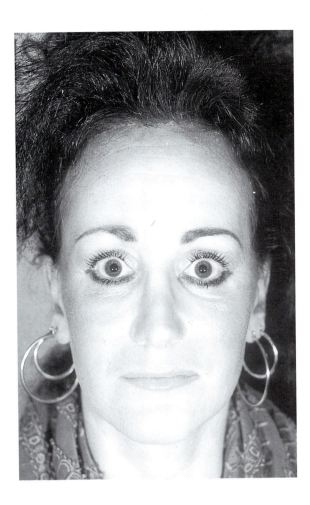

Figure 7–36
Pretrichal forehead lift accomplished in a patient with a high forehead aesthetic unit. Glabellar creases are eliminated, forehead rhytids are reduced, but forehead vertical height has not been altered. Scar camouflage at the hairline has been maximized by irregularizing the incision closure.

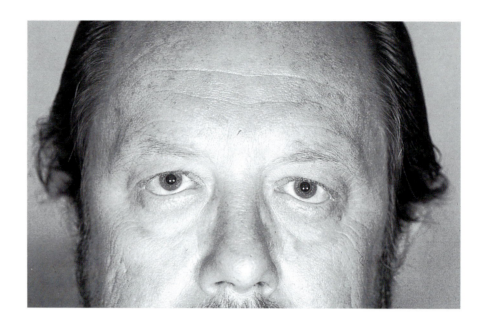

Figure 7–37
Midforehead browplasty in a male patient.

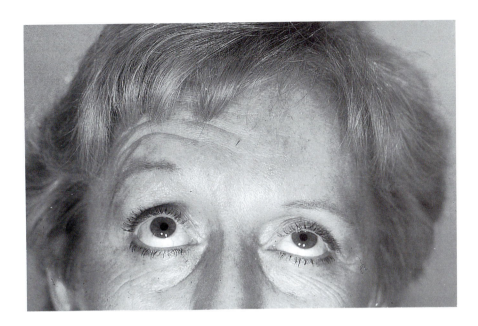

Figure 7–38
Unilateral forehead paralysis several months after a coronal forehead-lift performed elsewhere.

Sequelae and Complications

Few untoward sequelae result from forehead-lifting. Because of the coronal incision, *numbness of the scalp* posterior to the incision persists for several weeks. Minor but annoying paresthesia and dysesthesia occasionally accompany eventual full return to sensation. Possible complications of forehead/brow-lifting include the following:

- Hematoma
- Flap necrosis
- Infection
- Alopecia
- Seventh-nerve paresis
- Scalp hypoesthesia
- Scalp paresthesia
- Neuralgia
- Incision pruritis
- Widened or depressed scar
- Scar depigmentation
- Brow asymmetry
- Elevated hairline
- Abnormal soft-tissue contours

The forehead lacks animation for several days postoperatively; this temporary condition is soon less profound than before because of frontalis muscle attenuation. Permanent unilateral forehead paralysis is rare (Fig 7–38).

No serious complications have been experienced by the authors. Slight *spreading of the scalp scar* is generally totally prevented by employing permanent subcutaneous buried dermal sutures and by avoiding excessive flap closure tension.

Alopecia resulting from excessive flap tension or damage of hair follicles by too-superficial undermining or thermal cautery is essentially totally preventable.

Postoperative *hematomas* demand exploration and bleeding control if encountered in the early postoperative period since flap necrosis can occur if hemostasis is not immediately secured. At a later time, hematoma extraction with small liposuction cannulas may hasten the resolution process.

Lagophthalmos (a greater potential in patients who have experienced previous blepharoplasty) may be avoided by conservative lifting surgery characterized by frequent positioning checks of the eyebrow and temporal unit position during the procedure.

Infection, although a distinct possibility when elevation of any large flap occurs, appears to be rare.

Suggested Reading

- Becker FF, Johnson CM, Smith O: Surgical treatment of the upper third of the aging face, in Papel I, (eds): St Louis, Mosby–Year Book, pp 147–157.
- Brennan GH: *Aesthetic Facial Surgery.* New York, Raven Press, 1991.
- Brennan GH: *The forehead lift.* Otolaryngol Clin North Am 1980; 13:209.
- Castanares S: Forehead wrinkles, glabellar frown and ptosis of the eyebrows. *Plast Reconstr Surg* 1964; 34–406.
- Gleason MC: *Brow lifting through a temporal scalp approach. Plast Reconstr Surg* 1973; 52:141–144.
- Kaye BL: The forehead lift. *Plast Reconstr Surg* 1977; 60:161–170.
- Pitanguy I: Indications for and treatment of frontal and glabellar wrinkles in an analysis of 3,404 consecutive cases of rhytidectomy. *Plast Reconstr Surg* 1981; 67:157–166.
- Rafaty FM: Elimination of glabellar frown lines. Arch Otolaryngol 1981; 107:428–430.
- Spira M: Blepharoplasty. *Clin Plast Surg* 1978; 5:121–137.
- Stegman SJ, Tromovitch TA: Implantation of collagen for depressed scars. *Dermatol Surg Oncol* 1980; 6:450–453.
- Tardy ME: *Surgical Anatomy of the Nose.* New York, Raven Press, 1990.
- Tardy ME, Parras G, Schwartz M: *Aesthetic surgery of the face. Dermatol Clin North Am* 1991; 9:169–187.
- Tardy ME, Thomas R, Fitzpatrick ME: *Facial Rejuvenation Surgery.* Memphis, Tenn, Richards Medical, 1981.
- Webster RC, Fanous N, Smith RC: Blepharoplasty: When to combine it with brow, temple, or coronal lift. *J Otolaryngol* 1979; 8:339–343.

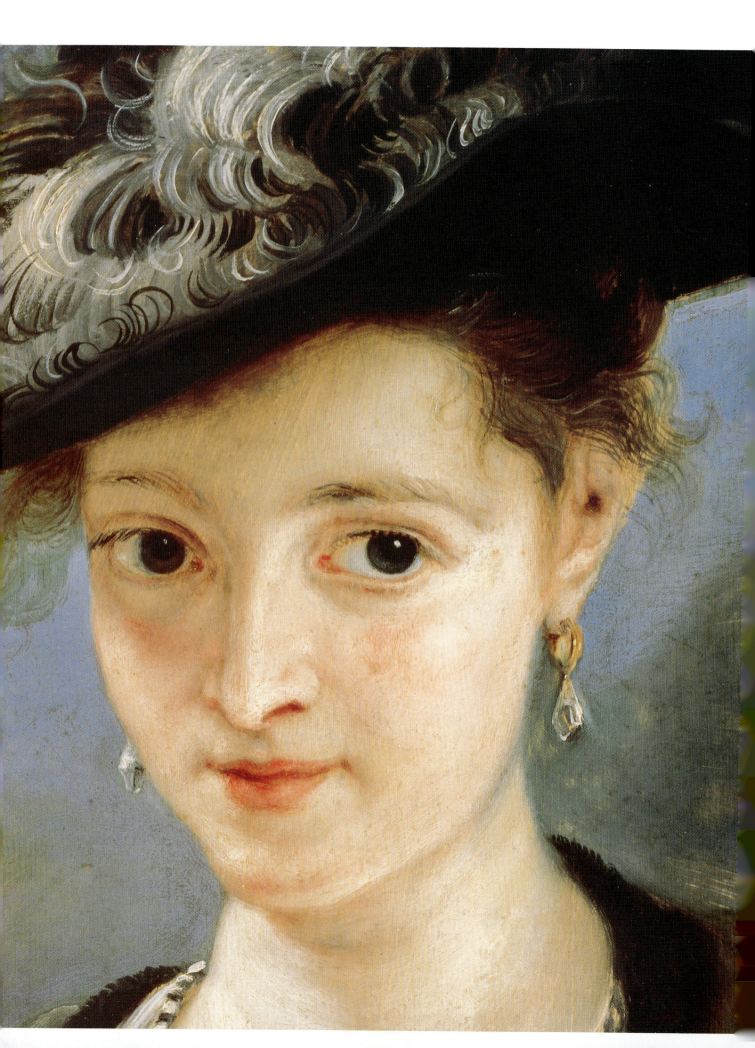

CHAPTER

8

 Temporal Lift

> *As we grow old, . . . the beauty steals inward.*
>
> **Ralph Waldo Emerson**

In selected patients a lifting force can be applied to the lid-brow-lateral canthal aesthetic complex by carrying out an isolated lifting procedure of the temporal (temple) aesthetic unit (Fig 8–1). The patient with early brow and lateral eyelid ptosis and rhytids is an ideal candidate for this approach (Fig 8–2). Its advantages include (1) brow elevation through an incision hidden within the hair, thereby eliminating any visible scar above the brow; (2) selective elevation of the lateral part of the brow and temple; and (3) reduction of the degree of upper lid skin excision contemplated

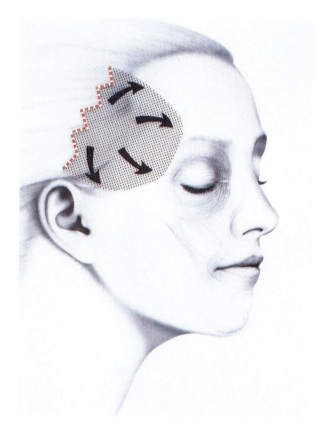

Figure 8–1
Temporal region potentially improved by a temporal lift. The extent of usual undermining is depicted in the *shaded area*.

for blepharoplasty. This operation commonly accompanies blepharoplasty and facelift procedures, with only a few minutes and minimal morbidity added to the overall operation. Local infiltration anesthesia renders the region numb.

The only major structure at risk in this region is the frontal branch of the facial nerve (see Fig 7–12,C), which lies caudal and superficial to the dissection field.

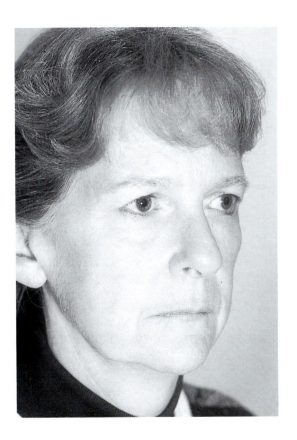

Figure 8–2
This patient with temporal region descent and brow ptosis is a suitable candidate for a temporal lift. Blepharoplasty commonly accompanies the temporal lift to fully rejuvenate the orbital region.

PART II   FACIAL AESTHETIC AND LIFTING PROCEDURES

Surgical Technique

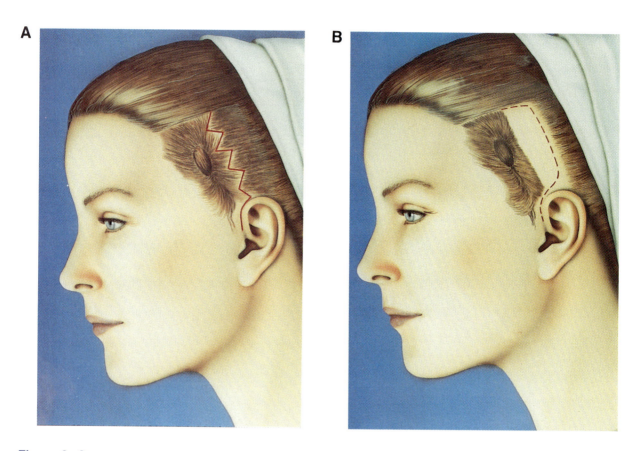

Figure 8-3
A and **B,** the incision, irregularized to provide maximum camouflage, is marked approximately 2½ to 4 cm inside the temporal hairline and carried deep to the level of the hair follicles and up to but not beyond the tissue plane limited by the deep temporal fascia (the scalp hair is not shaved as shown here for ease of illustration). The precise geometrics of the incision will vary with and be guided by the individual frontolateral hairline. The typical "double-tuft" configuration of temple hair in the female must be preserved.

CHAPTER 8 Temporal Lift

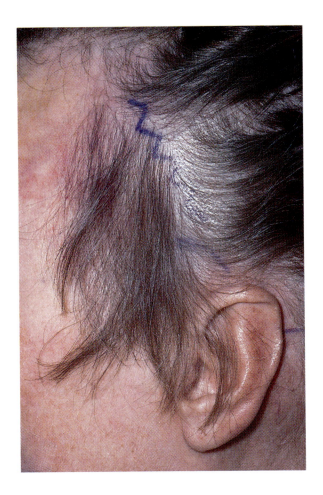

Figure 8–4
Geometrically irregularizing the incision adds additional camouflage to the final scar site.

199

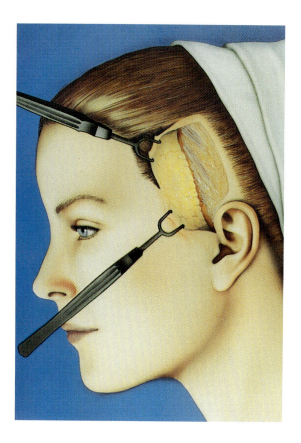

Figure 8–5
With more blunt than sharp dissection, the temporal flap is undermined toward the eye and lateral canthus to just below the level of the brow and ptotic or creased lateral canthal skin. Since the frontal branch of the facial nerve occupies a very superficial position here, dissection progresses safely and bluntly under direct vision aided by good fiber-optic headlighting. The frontal branch is probably more at risk from stretching and/or cautery injury than from careful dissection.

CHAPTER 8 Temporal Lift

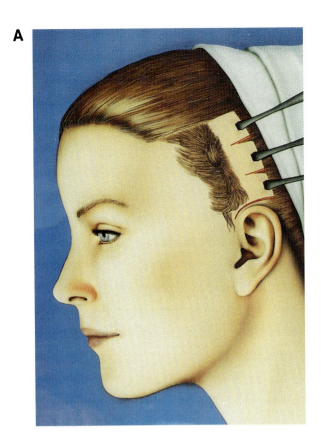
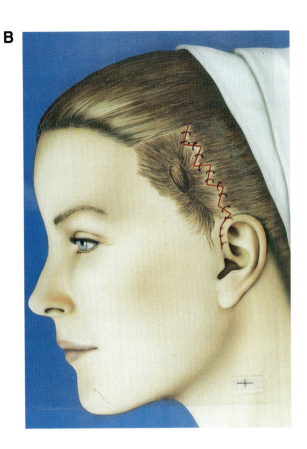

Figure 8–6
A and **B**, the temporal skin unit is then advanced and rotated slightly, the excess trimmed, and an irregularized enclosure made in the hairline with buried dermal sutures of 4–0 PDS (under tension) and stainless steel skin clips in the hair-bearing skin (no tension).

This approach, which in reality is the temporal extension of the traditional rhytidoplasty operation, is effective in immediate brow and temple elevation. In doing so the temporal hairline may be slightly elevated. This fact may be objectionable to individual patients and therefore must be discussed in detail with the patient preoperatively. Like most forms of aesthetic surgery characterized by lifting and rotation forces, a compromise must be reached to provide aesthetic improvement without creating an unnatural appearance or unwanted complications.

Results and Outcomes

Patients treated with temporal lift procedures are demonstrated in Figures 8–7 through 8–11.

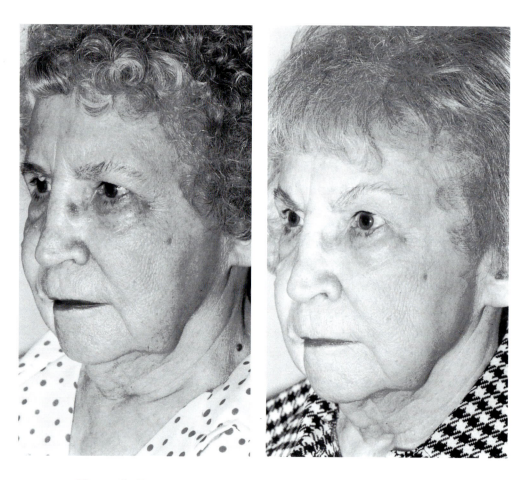

Figure 8–7
Isolated temporal lift performed in a elderly patient to improve a temporal field visual deficit created by extreme temporal, brow, and upper lid skin ptosis. Note significant elevation of the temple and brow. Blepharoplasty was not performed.

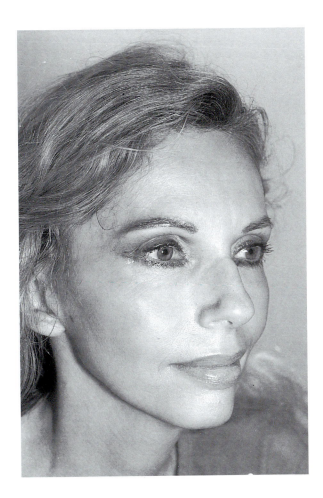 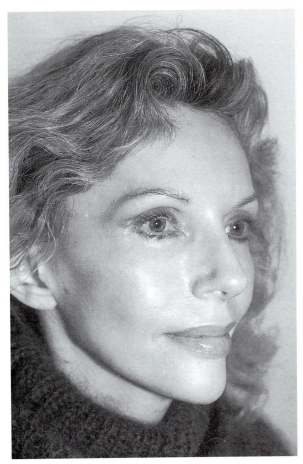

Figure 8-8
Improved brow and temporal region appearance following a temporal lift and blepharoplasty. The effect is subtle but definite. Rhinoplasty adds further refinement to the appearance.

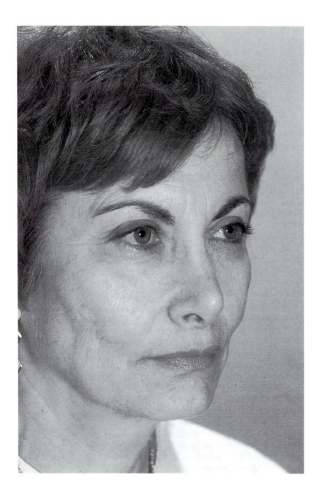 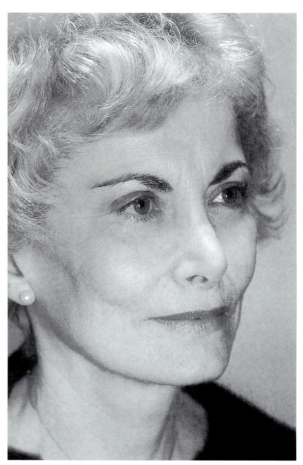

Figure 8-9
Temporal lift combined with blepharoplasty and a facelift. Very little upper lid skin requires removal when a temporal lift precedes blepharoplasty. Note the improvement in the lateral suprabrow rhytids.

CHAPTER 8 Temporal Lift

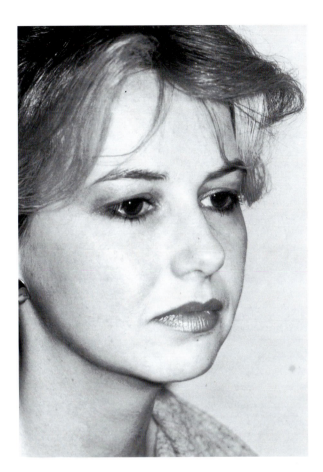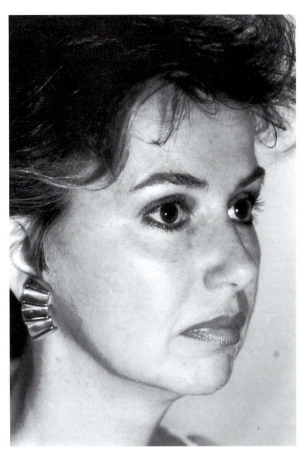

Figure 8–10
Improved, more youthful appearance resulting from a temporal lift and blepharoplasty.

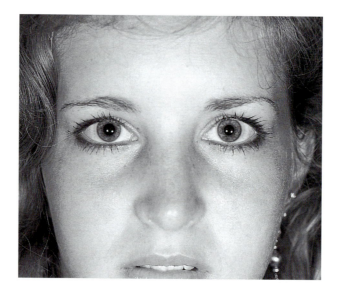
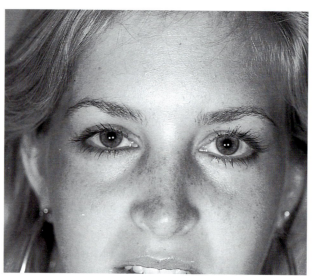

Figure 8–11
Congenital right brow ptosis with consequent eyelid asymmetry in a young patient. An improved result is shown 5 years following a right temporal lift combined with rhinoplasty. Note the improved symmetry and more defined right upper lid crease.

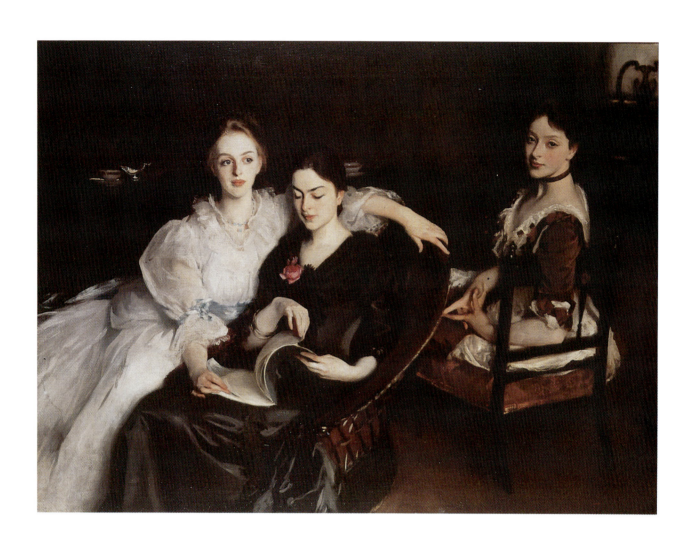

CHAPTER 9

 # Brow-Lift

PART II FACIAL AESTHETIC AND LIFTING PROCEDURES

The eyebrows form but a small part of the face, and yet they darken the whole of life by the scorn they express.

Demetrius

The choice of the most appropriate forehead- and brow-lifting procedure rests upon a combination of anatomic and appearance factors weighed carefully and discussed with the patient before surgery. The *browlift,* the simplest and most direct approach, has significant advantages. The anticipated improvement can be rather accurately demonstrated to the patient preoperatively in a three-way mirror; quite accurate reproduction of this desired position is surgically possible. If asymmetries in brow position exist (Fig 9–1) (often compounded by unequal frontalis muscle action during animation), asymmetrical corrections to restore symmetry are less difficult to achieve with this direct approach by accurate measurement. The brow-lift, depending on the geometric pattern of the excision, may allow selective favorable brow elevation in its nasal, middle, or temporal extent, the brow position being sculpted according to a preplanned scheme. Surgical trauma is minimal, as is the recovery and healing process; the improvement in appearance is immediately apparent.

If indicated and desirable, a direct approach to interruption of the offensive action of the corrugator and procerus muscles from the medial aspect of the brow incision is facilitated, a necessary prerequisite to minimizing glabellar and nasal root rhytids. "Fine tuning" of the final brow position is easily accomplished in browplasty, no vital motor nerves are at risk in the surgical field, postoperative edema is ordinarily quite minimal, and the intended result is immediately apparent to the patient and surgeon alike, a pleasant dividend. If the incision is placed *just inside* the cephalic-most line of brow hairs and carefully repaired with eversion techniques, scar camouflage is generally quite satisfactory. A thin application of brow pencil makeup can render the healing scar inconspicuous until nature provides normal scar maturation and obscurity. *Patients must, however, be willing to accept a lifelong scar at the brow-forehead interface.* In men

CHAPTER 9 Brow—Lift

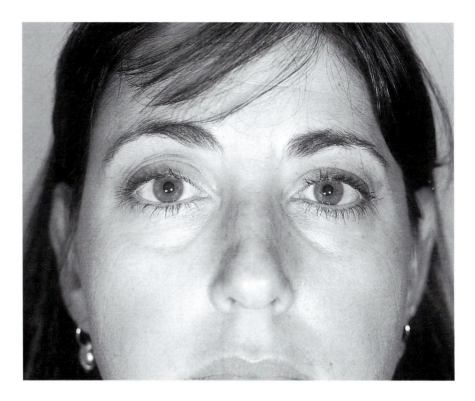

Figure 9–1
Asymmetrical eyebrows, lids, and orbital region, extremely common findings.

with full eyebrows, the healing incision becomes almost immediately hidden by eyebrow hairs brushed upward to conceal the healing incision. Furthermore, repeat brow-lift operations may be carried out, if ever required, through the same incision. In selected individuals with deep lateral midforehead creases, a midforehead brow-lift through an incision placed in the depths of the appropriate crease can be considered as an alternative.

The brow-lift operation has significant limitations that will influence the surgeon's choice of procedure. Rhytids ("laugh lines," "crow's-feet") adjacent to the lateral canthus are improved to only a limited extent by direct browplasty approaches, and then only when the incisions are carried lateral to the hair-bearing brow. Undermining in this area is necessary for even a limited improvement effect, thereby exposing the facial nerve frontal branch to risk.

Surgical Technique

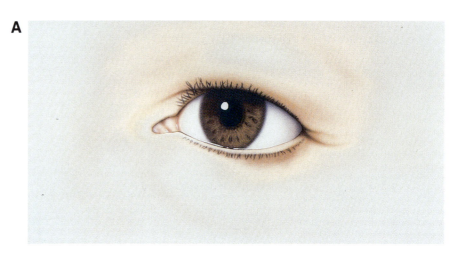

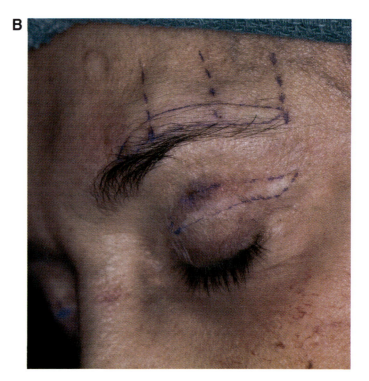

Figure 9-2
Once the decision for the brow-lift is made by developing a diagnostic distinction between isolated brow ptosis **(A),** temporal ptosis and redundancy, and ptosis of the entire upper portion of the face (forehead, temple, and brow), preoperative skin markings delineate the site and geometry of planned excision **(B).** The patient is evaluated and marked while sitting upright *in response* to eliminate spurious brow elevation induced by voluntary or involuntary frontalis action, a common circumstance. If manual elevation of the brow improves the upper orbital space and pleasantly delineates the upper lid cleft, browpexy is judged to be helpful.

CHAPTER 9   Brow—Lift

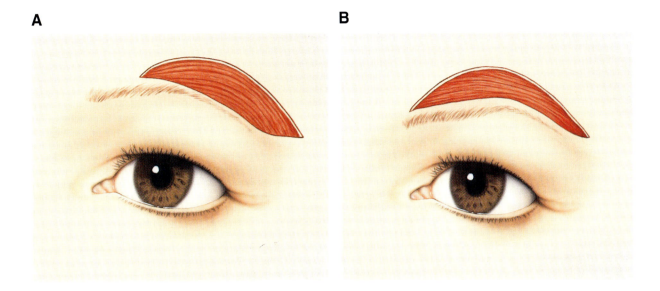

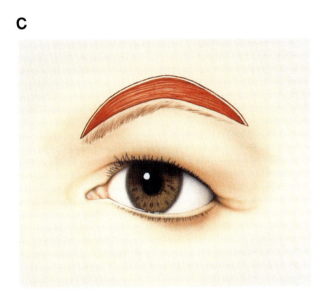

Figure 9–3
A–C, after taking into account the commonly encountered brow position asymmetries, fusiform patterns are outlined above the brow on the forehead skin and the intended final scar placed *just within* the highest row of brow hairs. Brow-lift procedures are best carried out under local infiltration anesthesia, but incisional and excisional judgments must be finalized and marked *before* any infiltration distortion, however slight.

Various geometric fusiform excisional options are available, depending upon the individual's aging characteristics as well as the patient's sex and appearance preference. It can be helpful to create a pattern from x-ray film or other sterile material in order to ensure bilaterally symmetrical marking and excision.

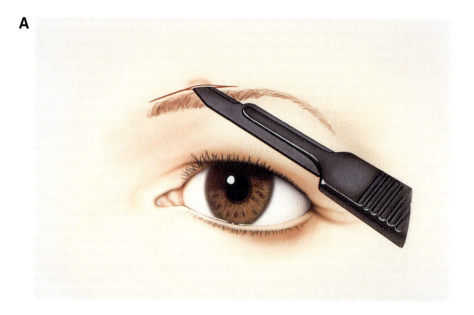

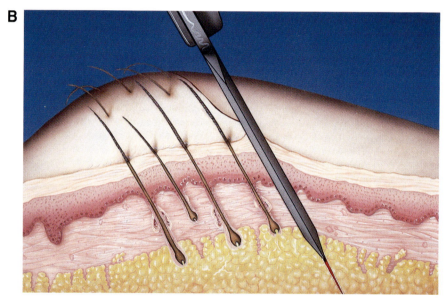

Figure 9-4
A and **B,** after delaying 10 to 15 minutes to enhance vasoconstriction, the initial lowermost incision is created by beveling the scalpel blade to cut *parallel* to the shaft of the upper hair follicles, *just inside* the uppermost row of hairs. Failure to observe this nuance can lead to hair loss and/or a visible scar lying slightly cephalic to the intended brow-forehead interface.

CHAPTER 9   Brow—Lift

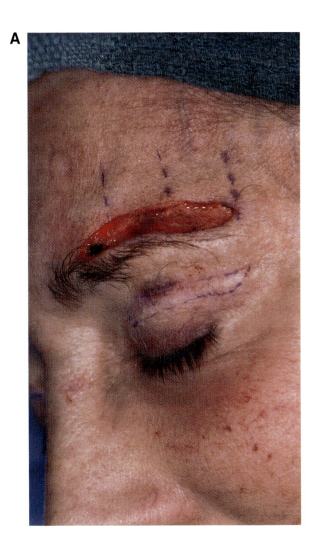
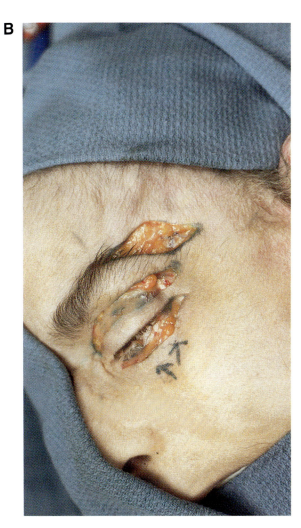

Figure 9–5
A and **B**, following completion of the more cephalic incision, removal of the circumcised segment of skin and subcutaneous tissue is achieved by sharp knife dissection; the skin edges are undermined only sufficiently to allow an eversion of the wound edges on closure. If the lateral canthus rhytids are to be improved, *superficial* separation of the skin from the underlying tissue laterally is necessary to free the redundant skin from the effect of underlying muscle action. It is generally imprudent to carry any portion of the incision medial to the nasal (medial) extent of the brow. Meticulous hemostasis is ensured with pinpoint disposable cautery units. Excision of orbicularis muscle is ordinarily unnecessary.

PART II   FACIAL AESTHETIC ND LIFTING PROCEDURES

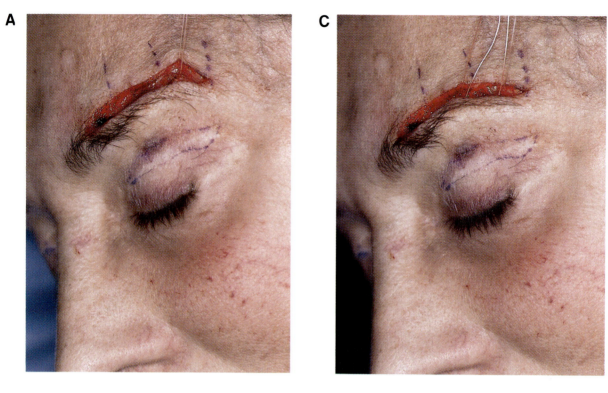

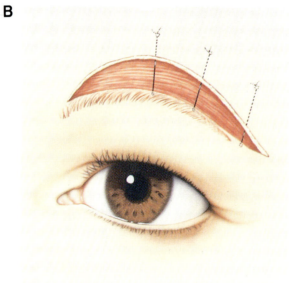

Figure 9-6
A-C, 4.0 Tevdek sutures are placed in the inferior orbicularis fibers to suspend the brow cephalically at the desired location by completing the suture in the galea cephalically.

CHAPTER 9   Brow—Lift

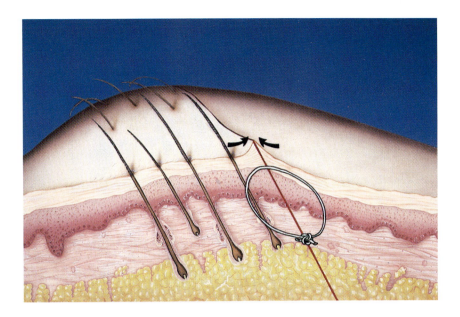

Figure 9-7
Closure is initiated by advancing both muscle and dermis and suturing the dermis with buried everting sutures of 4-0 polydioxanine.

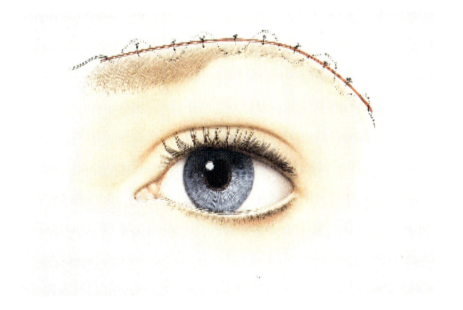

Figure 9-8
Further hypereversion of the closed skin edge with 7-0 nylon sutures ensures a favorable fine-line nondepressed scar.

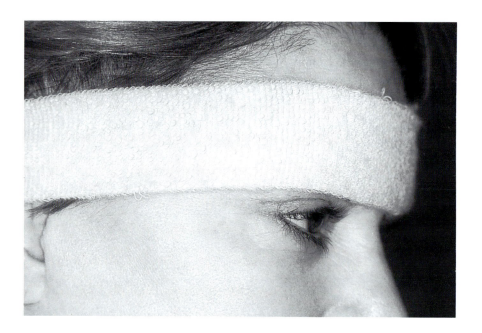

Figure 9–9
The wounds are dressed with a thin application of NeoDecadron ophthalmic ointment. Adaptic gauze and a lightly compressing circumferential dressing are applied for 36 to 48 hours to diminish edema. Minimal swelling and ecchymosis are the rule if tissue handling has been gentle and hemostasis fastidious.

The above procedure accomplishes an isolated long-lasting cephalic repositioning of the ptotic brow and improved delineation of the infrabrow cleft and, if combined with blepharoplasty, should always precede the lid operation in order to avoid creating a permanent lagophthalmos secondary to excessive eyelid skin removal. A brow-lift effectively reduces the degree of lateral orbital skin requiring removal and thus allows the final scar to stop short of the lateral orbital margin.

Glabellar creases (rhytids) may be modified through the brow-lift approach by carrying the dissection into the midforehead to free the skin from the underlying muscles. Insertions of the corrugators are delineated and elevated with a sharp periosteal elevator and the muscle bellies divided or partially resected to attenuate their crease-producing action. The synergistic action of the procerus is similarly eliminated by isolating this superficial muscle with dissecting forceps and dividing or even avulsing its cephalic portion. Improvement in the glabellar rhytids may be expected, but total elimination of eventual glabellar creases is problematic at best. Excessively deep glabellar creases will almost always require the addition of surgical crease resection and scar camouflage closure techniques in addition to the above muscle attenuation techniques.

Light dermabrasion of the glabellar rhytids will often complement the final effect; injectable collagen (Zyderm II) placed in the dermis will efface superficial but not deep glabellar creases. Either of these adjunctive modalities may be carried out at the time of direct brow-lift and muscle resection.

CHAPTER 9 Brow—Lift

Results and Outcomes

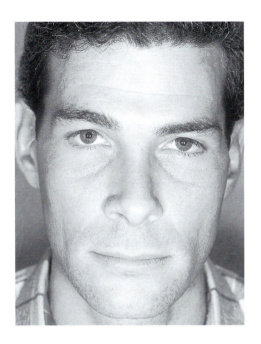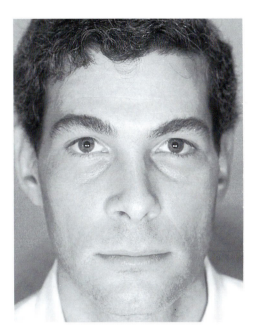

Figure 9–10
Bilateral direct brow-lift to correct congenitally ptotic eyebrows. The outcome provides an immediate improvement in appearance.

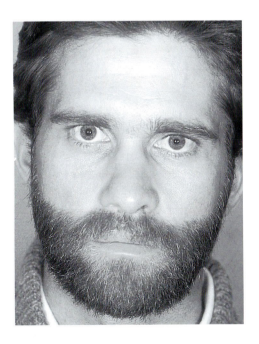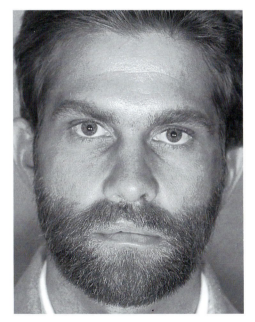

Figure 9–11
Brow-lift carried out in a young man concerned about his "sinister" appearance resulting from a low brow position.

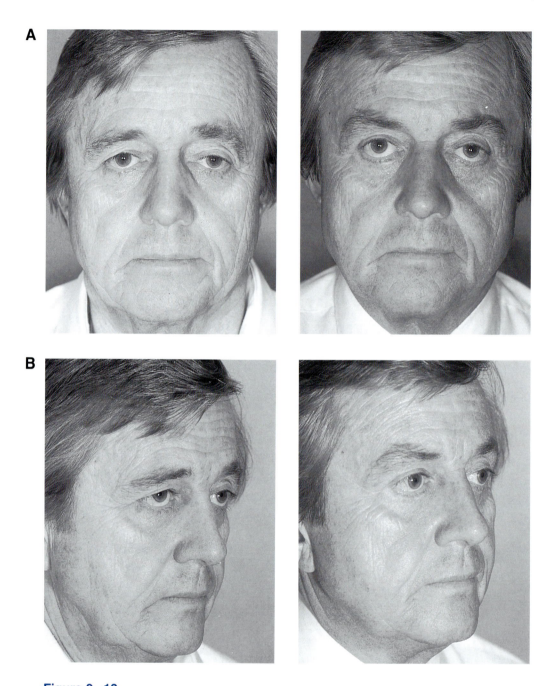

Figure 9–12
A and **B,** aging male who complains of a fatigued appearance despite excellent general health and conditioning. Severely ptotic brows and a hooded eyelid appearance create the expression of sadness. A brow-lift combined with upper lid blepharoplasty restores a much more rested and pleasant facial expression.

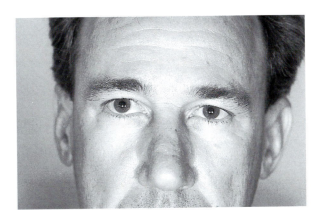 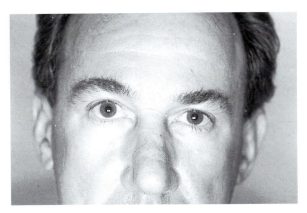

Figure 9–13
Improved orbital expression and appearance following a brow-lift.

Summary and Conclusions

Not all patients concerned about the progressive aging signs about the orbit and eyelids can be satisfactorily improved by standard blepharoplasty procedures alone. If brow and forehead ptosis complicate the aging eyelid appearance, one of three supplemental operations may be employed that are designed to elevate the ptotic brow to a more natural position. Precise placement of the brows is possible by the direct brow-lift approach if the patient and surgeon are willing to accept a suprabrow scar, however inconspicuous. Elevation of the brow and redundant lateral canthal and temple skin and rhytids is favorably accomplished with a temporal-lift and camouflaging the incision in the temporal scalp. The most definitive operation involves the coronal approach to elevation of the entire forehead, brows (both medially and laterally), and temporal skin. When transverse forehead creases, deep glabellar rhytids, and medial brow ptosis complicate the aging condition of redundant eyelid skin and lateral brow ptosis, the forehead-lift assumes the position of the procedure of choice.

In each instance, selection of the appropriate brow-lifting procedure depends upon a *precise diagnosis* of the particular brow-forehead anatomy and its impact upon the aging eye. With few exceptions, the indicated brow elevation operation should *precede* the removal of eyelid skin to avoid over-aggressive blepharoplasty skin sacrifice.

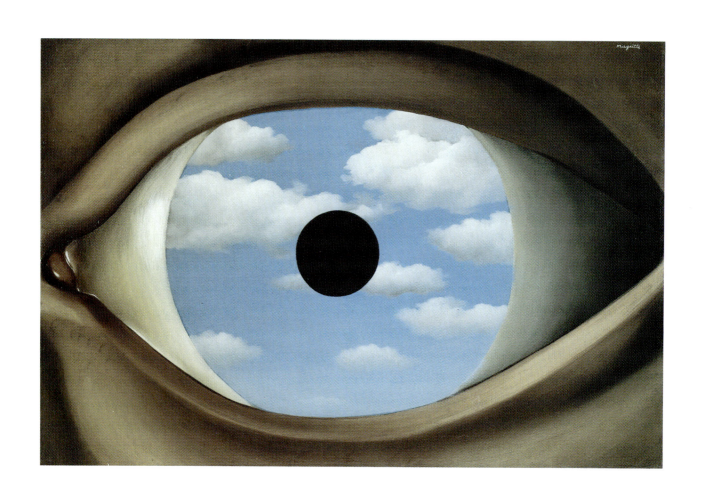

CHAPTER 10

      Aesthetic Blepharoplasty

PART II FACIAL AESTHETIC AND LIFTING PROCEDURES

*The Eye altering
alters all.*

William Blake

Rejuvenation surgery of the eyelids rivals rhinoplasty in its necessity for precision in judgment and delicacy in surgical technique. Surgical errors or healing asymmetries of as little as 1 mm may compromise an otherwise gratifying result. Thus an exacting knowledge of the intricate eyelid and orbital anatomy, coupled with a vital understanding of the principles and dynamics of eyelid healing, is essential for the blepharoplasty surgeon. Furthermore, a clear understanding and conceptualization of the possibilities as well as the limitations of safe eyelid surgery are required of the surgeon and the patient. Attempts to surgically produce a more dramatic result than anatomically feasible invariably leads to disappointment and, occasionally, to complications. Since secondary or revisional blepharoplasty is generally more difficult and potentially more complicated, virtue exists in ensuring an excellent result from primary surgery. If properly executed in carefully selected patients, rejuvenative eyelid surgery results in safe, natural, and long-lasting improvement with ideal camouflage of required surgical incisions. As with rhinoplasty surgery, *there is no single technique that produces a gratifying outcome in every patient,* so a precise diagnosis of the abnormal anatomy is essential to selecting the appropriate technique for repair. Orbital and eyelid asymmetry constitutes the rule rather than the exception; blepharoplasty infrequently produces perfect postoperative symmetry, a fact essential to educate patients about before any procedure is contemplated.

Commonly, evidence of facial aging first makes its appearance in the orbital area (Fig 10–1, A and B) and is characterized by redundant and excessive skin, fat, and muscle in the upper and lower eyelids. In addition, relaxation and stretching of the tarsal plate and tendons may rob the eyelid area of its youthful appearance. Lower lid fat pseudoherniation is seen as early as the late teenage years in certain ethnic populations and as an inherited family trait (Fig 10–2).

Ptosis of the eyebrow and temporal aesthetic unit compounds the aging appearance and requires, in appropriately selected patients, lifting and repositioning procedures *prior* to direct blepharoplasty operations. Significant forehead and brow ptosis may suggest *direct browplasty* or *coronal forehead-lifting* to achieve optimal results with or instead of blepharoplasty repair.

CHAPTER 10 Aesthetic Blepharoplasty

Figure 10–1
A and **B**, the fatigued, saddened, aging appearance of this older male was produced by gravitational and aging changes in the orbital region. Brow ptosis is particularly severe and compounds the upper lid skin redundancy. Relaxation and horizontal excess of the lower lids are apparent.

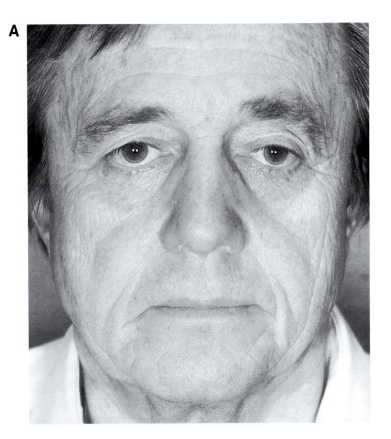

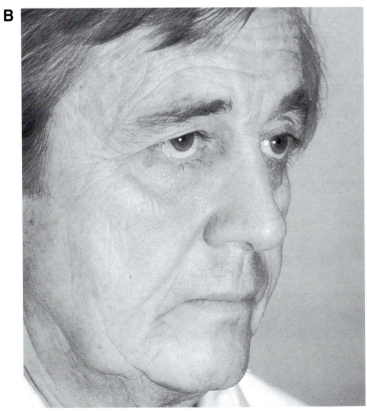

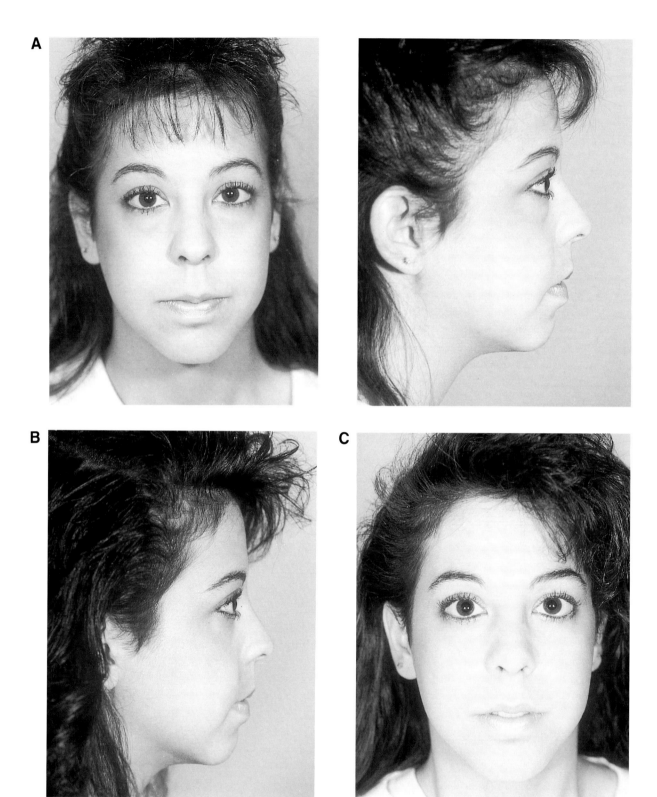

CHAPTER 10 Aesthetic Blepharoplasty

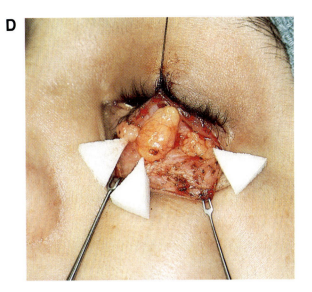

Figure 10–2
A–D, herniated orbital fat in young preadolescent patient, the consequence of a familial congenital tendency. Significant psychological stress resulted from peer group teasing, which disappeared following lower lid fat removal. No lower lid skin was excised. **A**, preoperative. **B**, one week after lower lid blepharoplasty. **C**, six months postoperative. **D**, abundant herniated fat.

Since the human eye and adnexa represent the central point of visual contact and interaction between individuals, the blepharoplasty surgeon has a unique opportunity to ensure that this contact becomes more meaningful.

Diagnosis and Preoperative Evaluation

Critical to the successful outcome of blepharoplasty procedures is a clear and exact determination of the patient's wishes and expectations from rejuvenation surgery. A three-way mirror becomes vital for the accurate exchange of information and views between the patient and surgeon (Fig 10–3). The surgeon must ensure, as accurately as possible, that the patient requesting reparative surgery is psychologically sound and mature with *realistic expectations about appearance outcome*. The patient must be willing to accept the limitations of irreversible aging characteristics such as deep lateral canthal wrinkling, excessively crepe-like skin, and orbital hyperpigmentation. Eyelid and facial asymmetries, present but not appreciated by the majority of individuals, must be pointed out and documented.

Discussions with patients are initiated by general questions regarding health history, followed by detailed inquiries into any past or potential

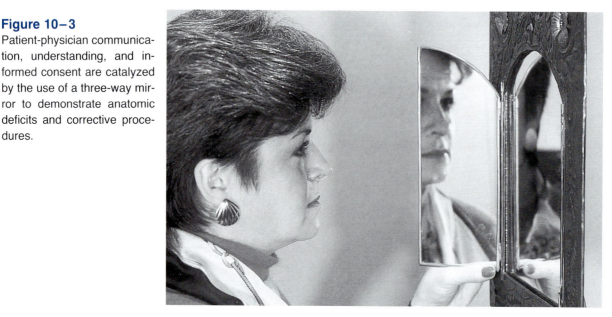

Figure 10–3
Patient-physician communication, understanding, and informed consent are catalyzed by the use of a three-way mirror to demonstrate anatomic deficits and corrective procedures.

ophthalmologic problems. It is vital to document specific medical and pharmacologic allergies and sensitivities. Any history of the regular use of medications that might influence a patient's clotting capabilities (aspirin and similar compounds), reduce basal tear secretion, or have a bearing on the choice of anesthesia during surgery is painstakingly elicited.

A detailed examination of the eye and the orbital adnexa follows. A complete eye examination consultation is firmly recommended for (1) all prospective patients older than age 40 years and (2) all patients with any history or physical finding suggestive of optic abnormality. Consultation with an ophthalmologist *knowledgeable about blepharoplasty* will provide valuable presurgical information relative to unilateral and binocular vision, both corrected and uncorrected, any visual field impairment, corneal sensitivity, extraocular muscle activity, basal tear secretion, and the condition of the lens and retina.

Corneal sensation may be assessed by using a wisp of cotton to stimulate the peripheral cornea. An absent or diminished response demands further neurologic investigation and may contraindicate blepharoplasty surgery. Basic visual acuity and extraocular muscle motion may be assessed easily during the initial consultation. In patients under 40 years of age, routine use of the Schirmer tear test has not been helpful in detecting candidates at risk for the "dry eye syndrome" following surgery; it is carried out only in patients with a history suggesting diminished tear secretion. The latter condition does not uniformly contraindicate blepharoplasty, but surely provides a warning flag that conservative surgery is essential.

With the patient observing in a three-way mirror, a series of vital assessments are next performed. Precisely what features the patient dislikes and wishes to have corrected are discussed in detail. *Ocular asymmetries* and any *unilateral eyelid ptosis* (a common finding) must be pointed out (Figs 10–4 and 10–5). A determination of the degree of excess upper lid skin

CHAPTER 10　　Aesthetic Blepharoplasty

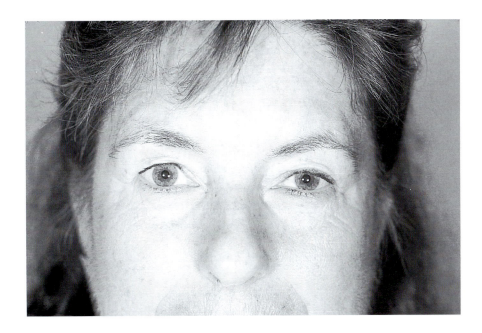

Figure 10–4
Ocular and eyelid asymmetry is exceedingly common among patients who desire blepharoplasty.

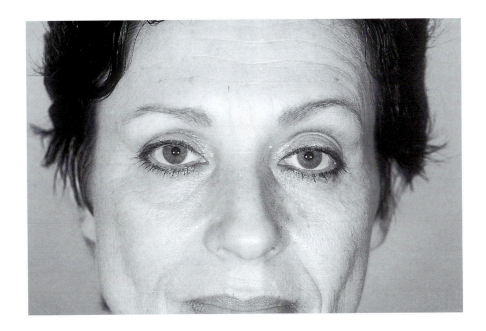

Figure 10–5
Unilateral lid ptosis of varying degrees is a frequent finding in patients seeking blepharoplasty.

along with the level of the eyebrow in facial repose suggests whether or not surgical elevation of the brow, temple, or forehead should precede blepharoplasty to achieve the optimal desired improvement in appearance. Patients often have difficulty in realizing how repositioning the brow results in optimal eyelid appearance; manually elevating the brow provides a reassuring reflected image of eyelid improvement (Fig 10–6, A and B).

With the patient gazing straight ahead, any degree of "scleral show" present in the preoperative state is documented (Fig 10–7). Gently pulling the lower lid away from the globe with the thumb and assessing its return to opposition to the globe are helpful in determining lower lid laxity. If the lid retains sufficient elasticity to "snap back" quickly to its normal position, a lid tightening or horizontal shortening procedure is usually not necessary. Weak lower lids that flow slowly back to the globe after finger retraction (Fig 10–8, A and B) may require reconstruction by some form of horizontal lid shortening procedure, such as lateral canthoplasty or canthopexy, or may require full-thickness excision of a pentagonal segment of the lower lid structure followed by meticulous suture repair in layers.

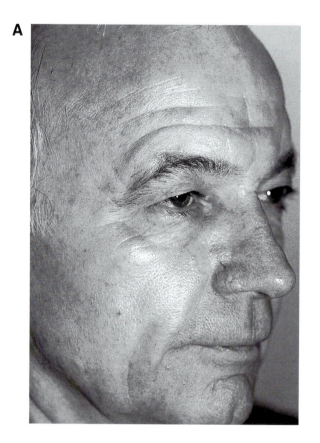
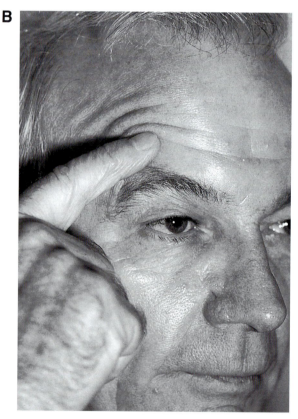

Figure 10–6

A, brow ptosis in an aging male. The brow has descended below the level of the supraorbital bony ridge to crowd the upper eyelid skin. **B,** manual elevation of the eyebrow provides an approximation of the improvement in appearance provided by a brow elevation procedure.

Figure 10–7
Significant scleral show in a patient seeking blepharoplasty.

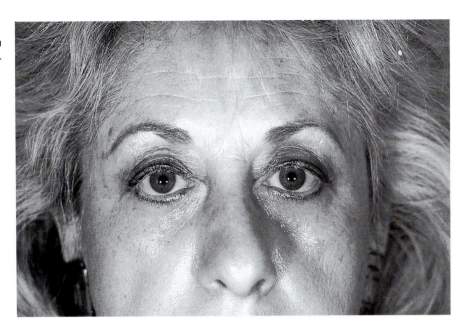

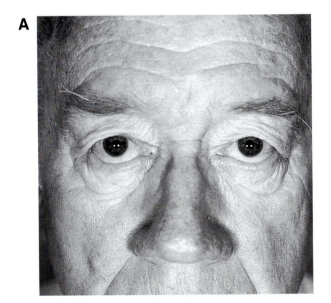
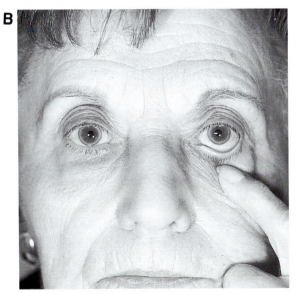

Figure 10–8
A, lax lower lid with marked scleral show and lid eversion. **B**, gross assessment of the elasticity and integrity of the lower lid may be assessed with the "snap test." If a delay in return of the lower lid to its normal position in contact with the globe exists, there is probably a need for a horizontal lid tightening and shortening procedure.

PART II FACIAL AESTHETIC AND LIFTING PROCEDURES

Accurate photographs in the direct frontal view with the eyes closed and with the eyes gazing upward and in the lateral view are taken for appropriate preoperative analysis, archival records, and medicolegal documentation (Fig 10–9,A–E). These standardized photographs are *reviewed with patients preoperatively* to develop to the fullest degree a mutual understanding of the range of reasonable expectations and anatomic limitations.

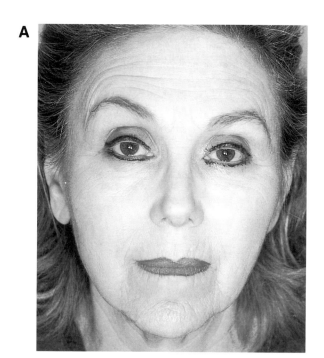

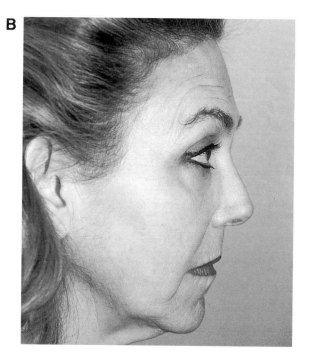

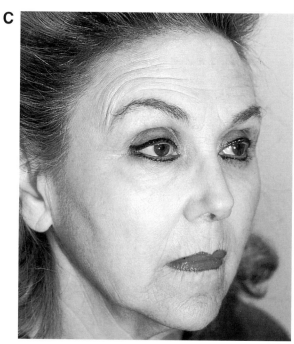

CHAPTER 10 Aesthetic Blepharoplasty

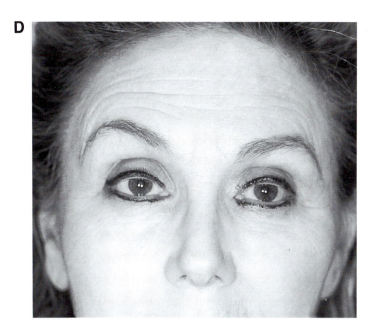

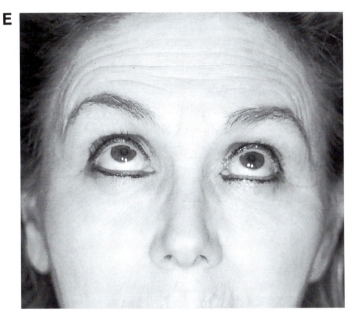

Figure 10-9
Minimum preoperative photographic views essential for blepharoplasty.

Surgical Goals and Planned Outcome

Realistic surgical expectations of blepharoplasty surgery include excision of redundant upper and lower eyelid skin, removal of redundant fat and muscle, and if indicated, horizontal tightening of the lower eyelid supporting structures. In the upper eyelid a clean pretarsal expanse of firmer skin

233

should be apparent, with significant reduction of excess eyelid fullness. A slight lid crease is not undesirable. The lateral brow tissues should be naturally elevated and not encroaching inferolaterally upon the upper lid. The lateral extent of the upper lid incisional scar courses obliquely upward and stops short of the lateral bony rim in most individuals.

In the lower eyelid, firming of redundant, stretched skin along with removal of unsightly fat pseudoherniation benefits the majority of patients. A conservative vertical lid shortening thus results. When lower lid support is poor, a *horizontal shortening* procedure of the lower lid margin and tarsal plate may be mandatory. Protuberant fat should be removed from all compartments down to or below the level of the orbital rim to allow flat redraping of lower lid skin. Any excess bulging orbicularis muscle, apparent upon smiling or in repose, requires horizontal excision. These surgical goals should be accomplished without changing the basic shape and appearance of the eye (Fig 10–10) while camouflaging all incisions in near-perfect fashion. After satisfactory healing, no evidence of the surgical procedure should be apparent to the casual observer, with a completely natural and more youthful appearance being restored (Fig 10–11, A and B). Since every eyelid is anatomically different and unique, the operation will differ slightly from patient to patient.

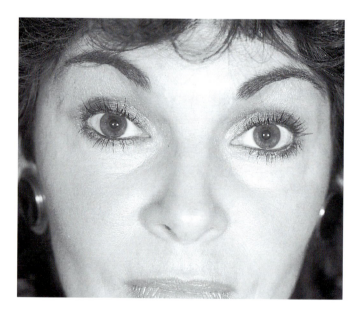

Figure 10–10
Attractive eye appearance in a midlife patient. A gentle, laterally upward slant from the medial canthus to the lateral canthus accentuates a pleasant appearance.

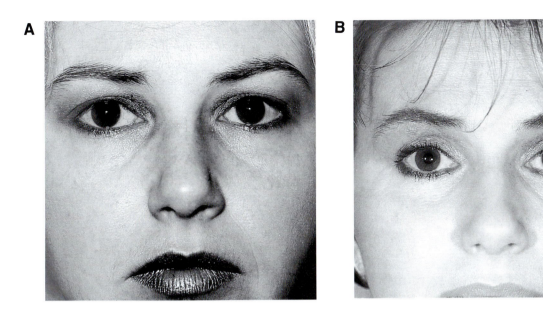

Figure 10–11
Significant and natural eyelid appearance improvement 18 months following blepharoplasty. Note the improved pretarsal cleft development in the upper lid.

Because of the delicacy of the vital structures encountered in the orbital region during blepharoplasty, significant additional safety ensues when measures are taken to *ensure total and complete control of hemostasis* throughout. Delicate dissection techniques with *small sharp scissors* and *disposable battery-operated or bipolar cautery units* regularly result in a near-bloodless operation with the additional benefit of minimal to no postoperative ecchymosis or swelling (Fig 10–12, A and B).

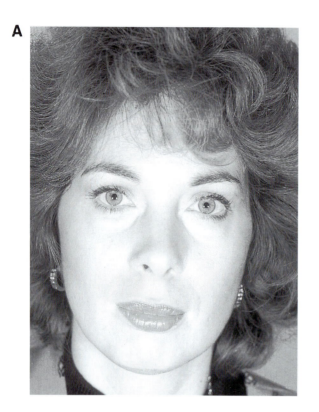
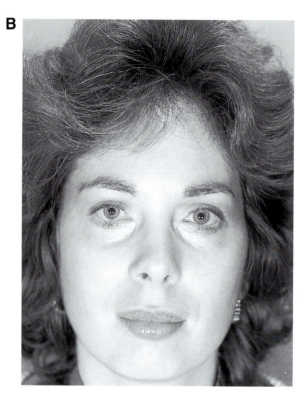
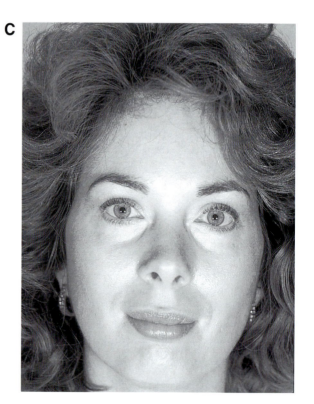

Figure 10–12
Meticulous hemostasis during blepharoplasty commonly produces minimal or no ecchymosis postoperatively, a highly desirable early outcome. **A,** preoperative. **B,** one week after lower lid blepharoplasty. **C,** six months postoperative.

CHAPTER 10   Aesthetic Blepharoplasty

Surgical Techniques

Specific Anatomic Considerations

The complex anatomic structures and their relationship to one another are illustrated and described in Figures 10–13 through 10–20. An exact knowledge of orbital and periorbital anatomy is an absolute prerequisite for performing blepharoplasty.

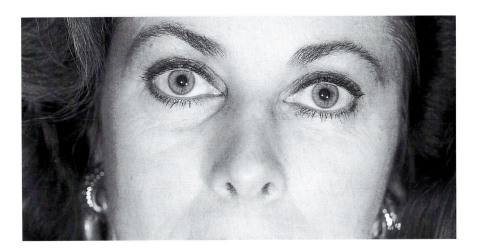

Figure 10–13
A normal, attractive feminine orbital appearance. The eye shape is favorable, the brow position is ideal, and a definitive lid crease exists.

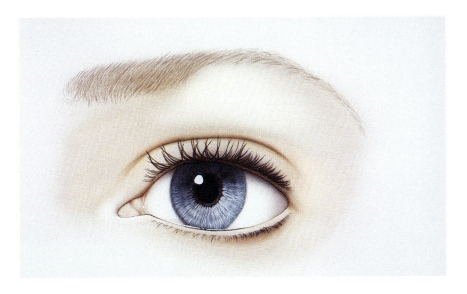

Figure 10–14
Normal surface anatomy of the eye and orbital region.

237

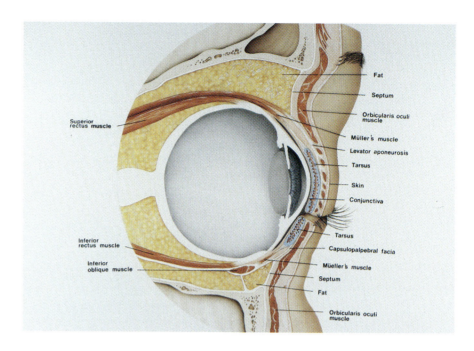

Figure 10–15
Normal anatomy of the eye and eyelids.

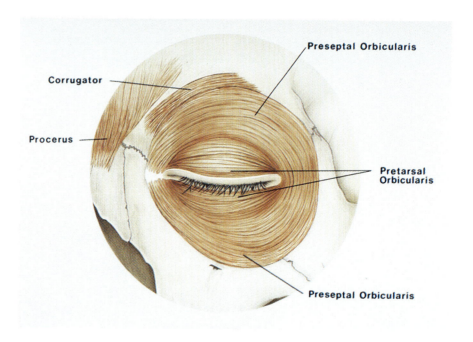

Figure 10–16
The periorbital muscles have an impact on eyelid and orbital skin movement, creating rhytidosis.

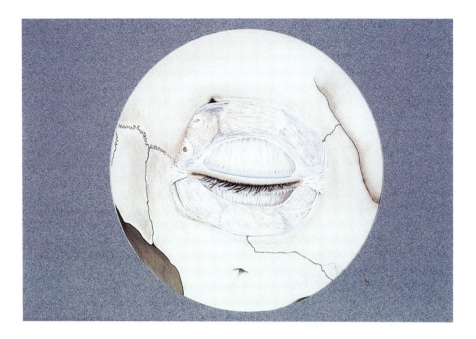

Figure 10–17
Orbital septum relationship to the orbital structures.

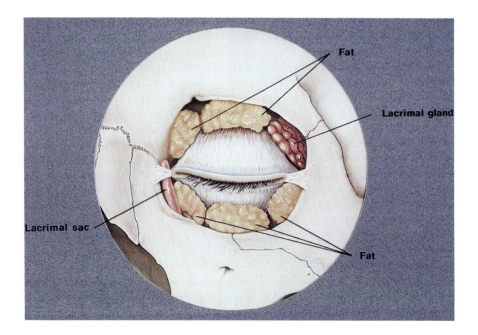

Figure 10–18
Typical fat pads of the upper and lower eyelids. In older patients fat is often not distinctly compartmentalized, but is more confluent and diffuse.

PART II FACIAL AESTHETIC AND LIFTING PROCEDURES

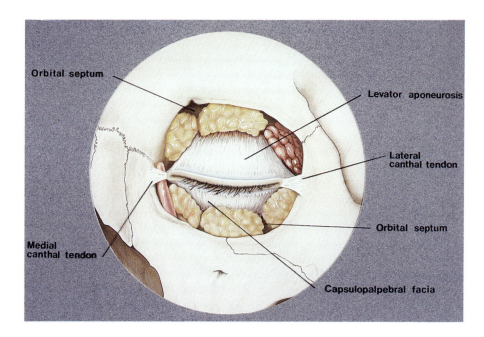

Figure 10-19
View of typical fat pads, canthal tendons, and the capsulopalpebral ligament.

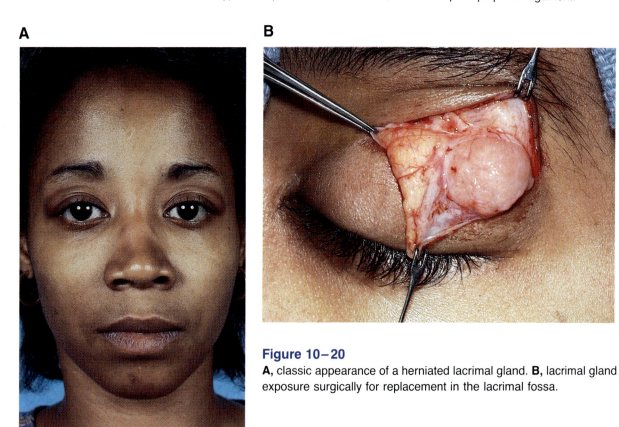

Figure 10-20
A, classic appearance of a herniated lacrimal gland. **B,** lacrimal gland exposure surgically for replacement in the lacrimal fossa.

CHAPTER 10 Aesthetic Blepharoplasty

Anesthesia

The following steps are important in preparing for the operative procedure:

1. The patient is positioned in a slightly head-elevated position on the operating table and cushioned by a soft air or foam mattress.
2. Any residual eyelid makeup or mascara is completely removed and the lids and lashes cleansed with a nonirritating surgical detergent with cotton applicators (eye makeup can be flammable and potentially lead to ignition during cautery maneuvers).
3. Prior to instituting local and intravenous anesthesia, the exact patterns of incision and excision are marked with a fine surgical marking pen aided by a right-angle forceps grasping the redundant skin and muscle (Fig 10–21). *This incision siting is accurate only if accomplished with the patient sitting.* Instructing the patient to move the eyes in the cardinal positions of gaze will aid in confirming the positions of redundant fat in the lower eyelid (Fig 10–22). Animation exposes excessive lower lid muscle hypertrophy for planned excision (Fig 10–23).
4. After patient relaxation 0.5 mL 1% lidocaine with 1:50,000 epinephrine solution, freshly mixed, is injected into each upper and lower lid in the immediate subcutaneous plane (Fig 10–24, A and B). A significant effort is made to avoid distortion of the lid tissues in order to lend more precision to the surgical excision. Use of a 1-mL tuberculin syringe armed with a no. 30, 1-in. needle facilitates this injection and is helpful in avoiding annoying ecchymosis during the injection sequence.
5. Ten to 15 minutes now elapses while intense vasoconstriction ensues and the local and intravenous anesthesia renders the patient relaxed, pain free, and comfortable. This short period further allows the surgeon an opportunity to scrub, study the preoperative color photographs projected in the operating room, and mentally rehearse the planned surgical events once again.

Intravenous analgesia with a potent narcotic and phenothiazine, provided cautiously and incrementally by a competent, sympathetic anesthesiologist and supplemented by an injectable local anesthetic, ensures the maximal safety for blepharoplasty procedures. Intravenous analgesia lends comfort, relaxation, and remarkable amnesia for surgical events while maintaining the patient in a state compatible with voluntary eye and facial movements requested by the surgeon in order to judge the extent and nature of the blepharoplasty. Although some minimal eyelid procedures are certainly possible with only local infiltration anesthesia, inadvertent eyelid movements (well controlled or nonexistent during intravenous analgesia) may render the operation less safe and technically more complicated. General endotracheal anesthesia remains unnecessary and imposes additional risks and surgical disadvantages.

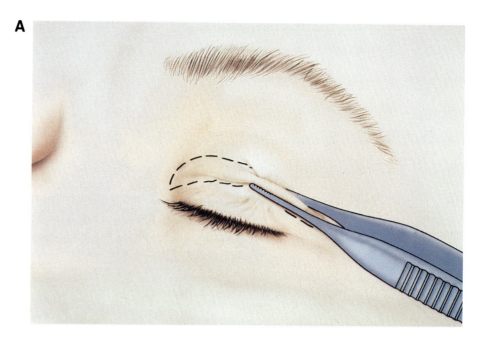
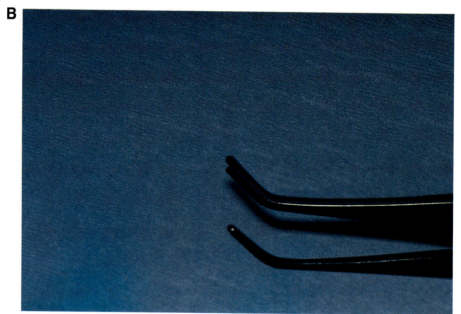

Figure 10–21
A significantly accurate approximation of the extent of redundancy of the upper eyelid skin may be achieved with delicate forceps prior to infiltration of local anesthetic.

CHAPTER 10   Aesthetic Blepharoplasty

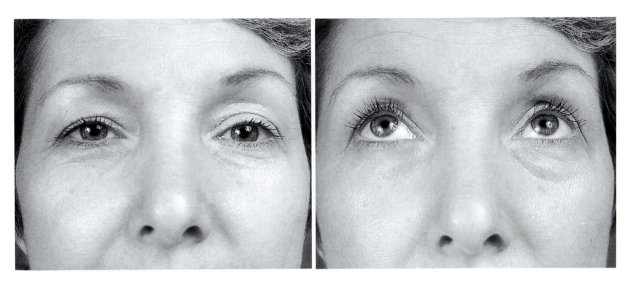

Figure 10–22
Upward gaze facilitates identifying the location and extent of protuberant fat pads. Notice the patient's eyelid asymmetry.

Figure 10–23
Certain patients show abnormal horizontal ridging or "hypertrophy" of the subciliary orbicularis when smiling. If objectionable, this ridging may be safely excised during blepharoplasty.

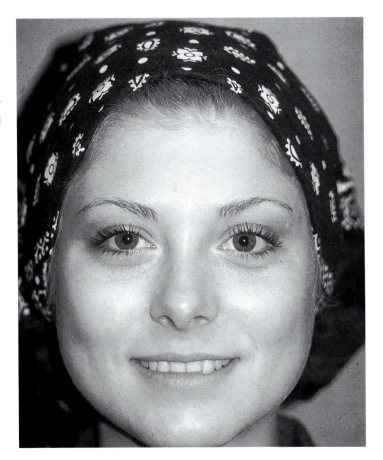

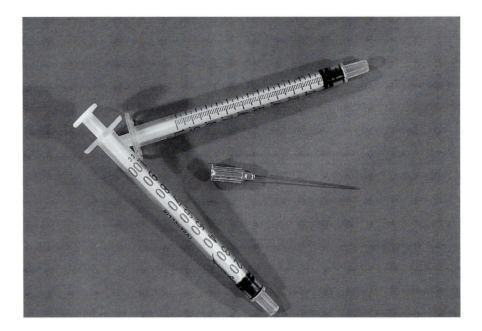

Figure 10–24
A and **B,** a 1-cc tuberculin syringe provides greater precision when injecting eyelid tissue and prevents inadvertent tissue distortion from overinjection.

A seemingly small but critical adjunct to the patient's anesthetic well-being derives from the anesthesiologist or nurse holding the patient's hand during the procedure. Patients regularly comment upon the reassurance provided by this simple gesture during the unfamiliar anesthetic state.

Upon completion of the procedure, an intravenous narcotic antagonist (naloxone [Narcan] or levallorphan [Lorfan]) hastens the patient's recovery and return to an alert state. Essentially no pain should occur following blepharoplasty.

Incisions and Approaches

Preferred incisions in the upper lid vary according to the anatomy encountered and the degree of skin redundancy. The inferior incision is regularly sited approximately 10 mm above the lash line and should be symmetrically placed on each eyelid (Fig 10–25). Medially the incision courses much nearer to the lash line. The cephalic lid incision site is determined by the degree of skin redundancy, the ultimate effect to be accomplished, and the position of the brow in relation to the excess eyelid skin; natural asymmetry may cause this portion of the incision to be sited differently from side to side to restore symmetry. Medially, profound skin redundancy may necessitate M-plasty to achieve smoothness (Fig 10–26, A and B); the incision must *never* be carried into or across the nasal concavity to avoid a visible, bowstring scar. Laterally, the incision heals best in the majority of

CHAPTER 10 Aesthetic Blepharoplasty

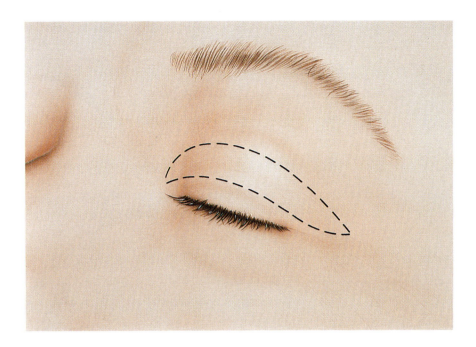

Figure 10–25
The inferior margin of the upper eyelid incision generally falls 9 to 11 mm above the lid margin.

patients when it sweeps upward toward the brow (Fig 10–27) and stops short of the orbital rim margin. If it is necessary to carry the incision further, it should fall in a relaxed skin tension line and be meticulously closed in this region of thicker skin.

The preferred incision to gain access to the lower lid, whether a skin-muscle or skin flap procedure is planned, differs little. Placed 1½ to 2 mm beneath the lash line, medially it stops short of the inferior punctum to take advantage of the ideal camouflage provided by the lower lid lashes (Fig 10–28). Laterally we prefer to limit the incision extent to just at or slightly beyond the lateral canthus.

If skin redundancy demands a longer incision, it is extended horizontally into a skin crease or is swept slightly cephalically to parallel the upper lid incision (Fig 10–29).

A bridge of undissected skin of 5 to 8 mm should be left undisturbed between the upper and lower lid incisions (Fig 10–30). Incisions that course obliquely downward are best avoided for optimum scar camouflage.

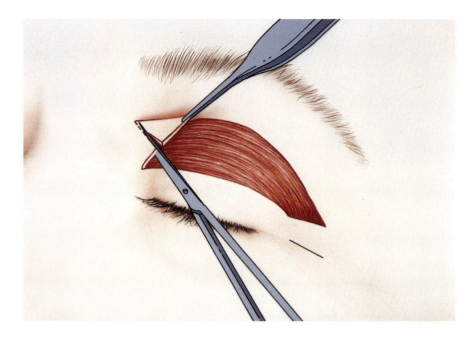

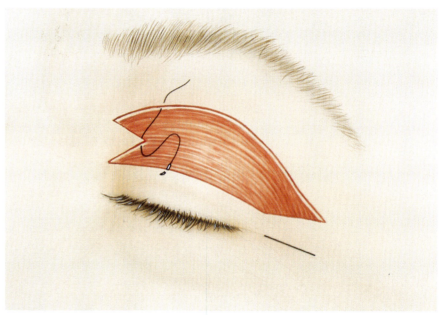

Figure 10-26
Redundant skin medially is best removed by using an M-plasty configuration to avoid carrying the primary incision into the thicker skin and contour concavity of the inner canthus hollow.

CHAPTER 10 Aesthetic Blepharoplasty

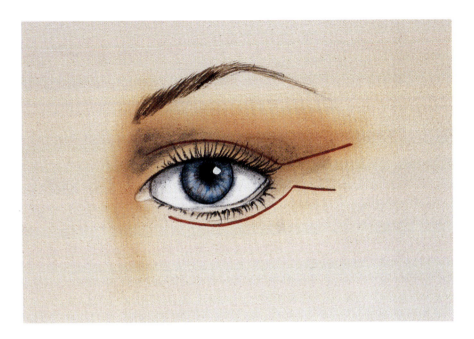

Figure 10-27
The lateral extent of the upper lid incision varies according to the individual anatomy encountered, but in general the incision is best carried obliquely upward for maximum camouflage.

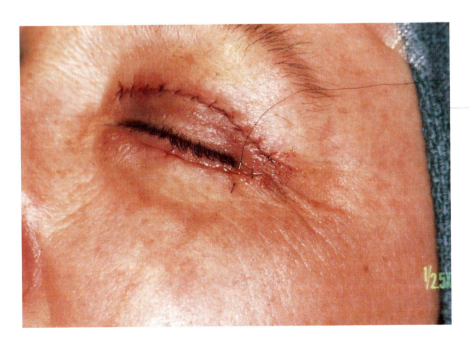

Figure 10-28
Typical lower lid incision 1½ mm below the lash line.

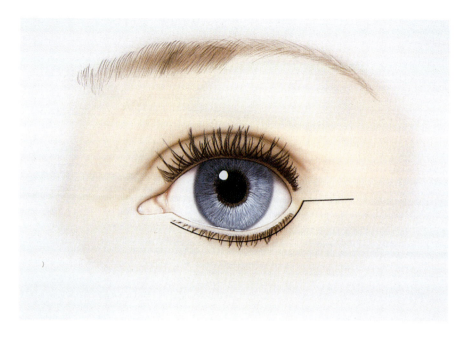

Figure 10–29
Extended lower lid incision into the lateral rhytid for camouflage. This extension is best created directly horizontally or slightly cephalically, never abruptly downward.

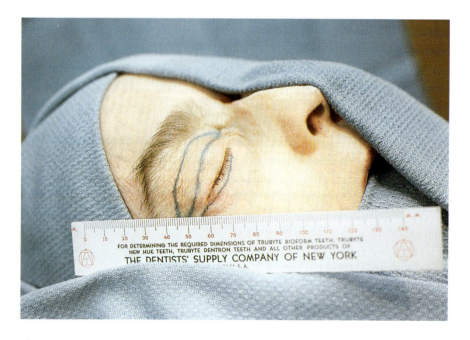

Figure 10–30
For ideal healing and scar camouflage, at least a 5- to 8-mm bridge of nondisturbed skin should exist in the lateral canthal region between the upper and lower lid incisions.

CHAPTER 10   Aesthetic Blepharoplasty

Preferred and Alternative Techniques

Although no two blepharoplasty procedures are ever exactly alike, fundamental similarities exist in our preferred techniques. Strong emphasis is placed on conservative but effective procedures, reduction of surgical trauma to a minimum, and *absolute hemostasis* with each surgical step.

Upper Lid

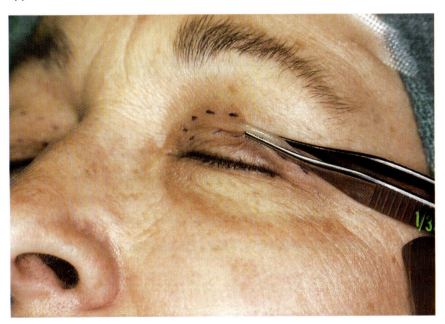

Figure 10–31
With the aid of angled forceps, the planned extent of excision of redundant upper eyelid skin is estimated by bunching the excess tissue between the blades of the forceps. The preoperative skin markings are thus again validated. The ideal amount of excision will result in a very temporary slight amount (1 to 2 mm) of intraoperative lagophthalmos that subsides as the local anesthetic solution is dissipated. Ordinarily a compromise must be struck between excising the amount of skin calculated to provide the best postsurgical appearance while avoiding bringing the eyebrow and the eyelid margin too close together.

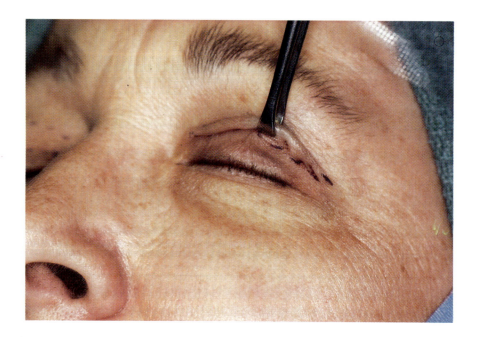

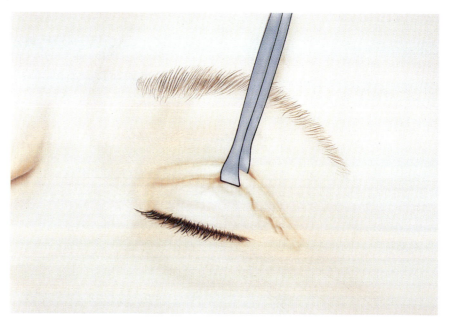

Figure 10–32
The redundant upper lid skin is serially clamped and crushed in the serrated teeth of an Allis forceps along the preoperative skin markings laterally to medially. This helpful maneuver pinches the skin edges together, temporarily crushes the small vessels supplying the thin eyelid skin, adds a further safety check regarding the proper extent of skin excision, and allows total or near-bloodless excision of the upper lid skin with sharp scissors.

CHAPTER 10 Aesthetic Blepharoplasty

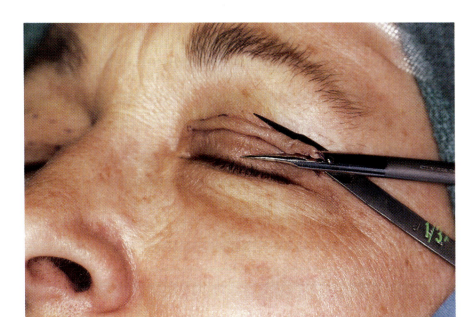

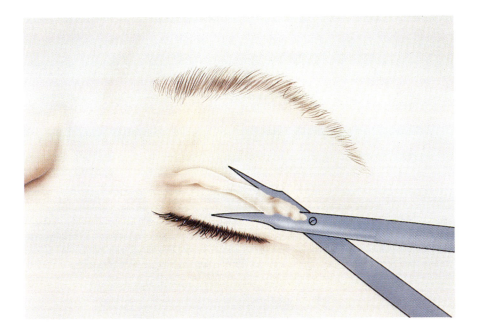

Figure 10–33
Stabilizing the pinched skin roll with delicate toothed forceps and sharp tenotomy scissors facilitates skin removal and ordinarily results in no bleeding along the pre-marked deep edge of the crushed skin roll. Thus all crushed skin is removed and fresh sharp wound margins left for repair. Particularly in very aged skin, a slight amount of intimately attached orbicularis muscle may be included in the excised skin roll.

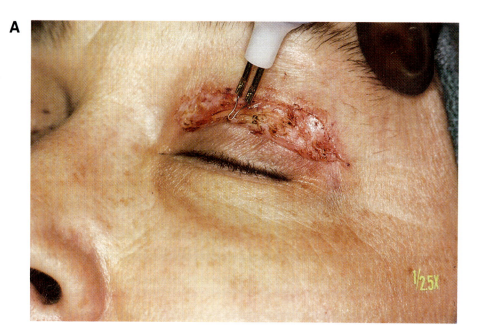

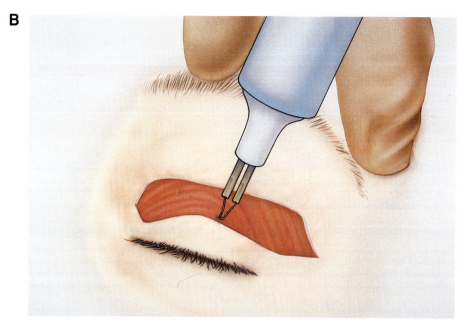

Figure 10–34
A, the entire brow is next elevated by the assistant with two widely spread fingers to open the wound bed; the assistant simultaneously retracts the inferior margin of the eyelid with a moist nasal tampon. **B,** all vessel arcades exposed near the skin edges are cauterized with a bipolar or Concept disposable cautery, along with any vessels noted in the wound itself.

CHAPTER 10   Aesthetic Blepharoplasty

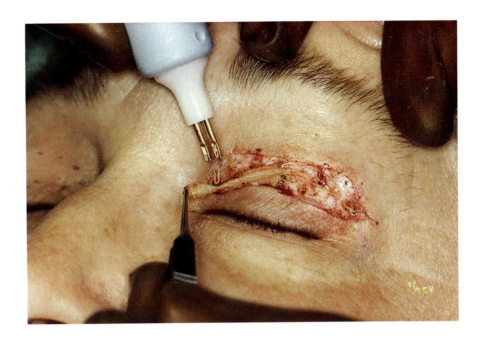

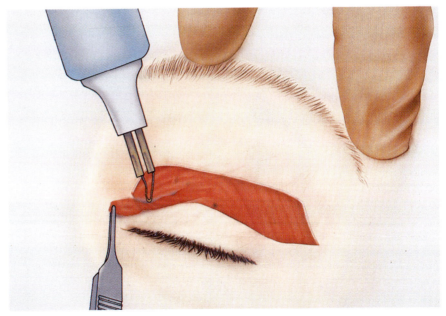

Figure 10–35
If redundant orbicularis muscle exists, a horizontal strip 5 to 8 mm wide is excised laterally to medially with the Concept cautery, which allows delicate removal with no bleeding. This maneuver exposes the preaponeurotic fat for evaluation and possible excision and results in a more clearly defined supratarsal skin crease following eyelid healing; this avoids the need, in the majority of patients, for routine tarsal fixation procedures.

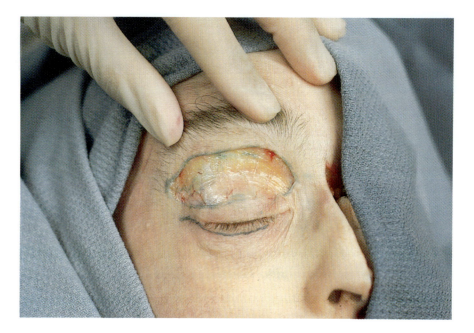

Figure 10–36
Should the upper lid fat be judged excessive and contributing to unaesthetic lid fullness, the orbital septum (and overlying muscle if it exists) is tented up with fine forceps and opened with the Concept cautery. Moistened cotton-tipped applicators then tease and dissect the fat away from its investing delicate fascial bands and allow it to protrude in order to estimate the degree of redundancy.

Figure 10–37
Ordinarily fat removal is required only from the central and nasal portion of the upper lid. Upper lid fat excision should be conservative to avoid creating a hollow-eyed appearance.

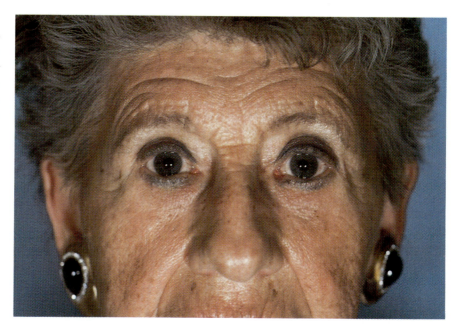

Figure 10-38

Laterally or temporally, a ptotic lacrimal gland can be mistaken for redundant fat because of its investment with fatty tissues. With gentle blunt dissection, however, the reddish brown character of the gland is not difficult to identify.

If doubt exists, a pinpoint cautery test differentiates the tissue accurately—heat applied to fat creates a sizzle, boil, and partial evaporation, while pinpoint cautery to lacrimal gland tissue creates only charring (see also Fig 10-20,B).

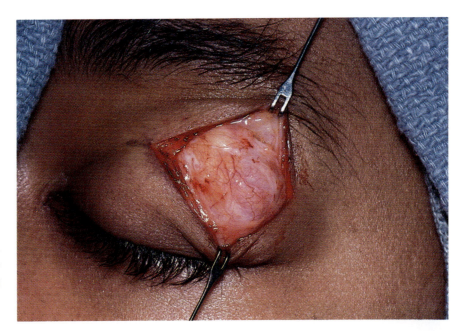

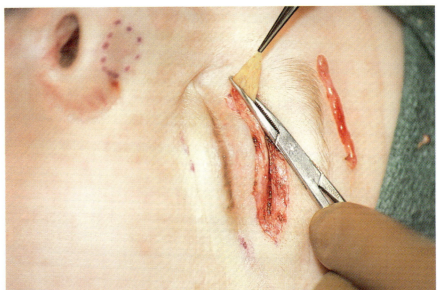

Figure 10-39

With care taken to avoid penetrating any small vessels supplying fat, the base of each fat pad is infiltrated with 0.1 to 0.2 mL plain lidocaine via a no. 30 needle. After cross-clamping the fat pad pedicle, the excess is resected with scissors and a generous cuff of fat preserved for careful cautery coagulation. Cauterization of the pedicle stump seals any open vessels. *Small toothed forceps then stabilize the pedicle while the hemostat is removed to prevent any sudden retraction of a bleeding pedicle into the orbit. This safety measure persists while the pedicle cuff is again cauterized to ensure absolute hemostasis.*

Occasionally in heavy-lidded individuals, an excess of subcutaneous tissue and muscle is encountered temporally over the orbital rim margin. To impart increased definition to the upper lid appearance, this excess tissue may be excised with the disposable cautery when indicated.

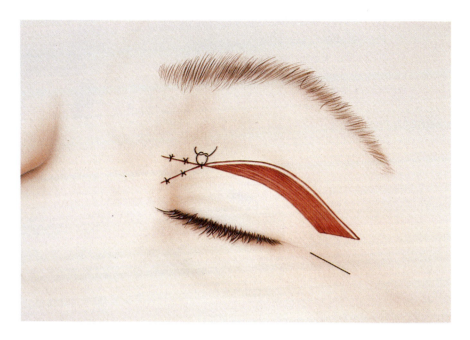

Figure 10–40
A moment is now taken to inspect the upper lid wound for any irregularities or departures from routine anatomy. If excess crepe-like skin exists nasally above the inner canthus, an M-plasty skin excision facilitates a smooth skin appearance without advancing the incision nasally into or through the concavity of the nose-lid confluence. A similar maneuver laterally may prevent extending an elongated incision temporally into the thick skin of the temple. Gentle pressure on the globe reveals any further fat protrusion or excess; additional removal follows if necessary.

Figure 10–41
Finally, the orbicularis fibers within the upper lid are further tightened by multiple pinpoint cautery maneuvers to induce favorable healing fibrosis.

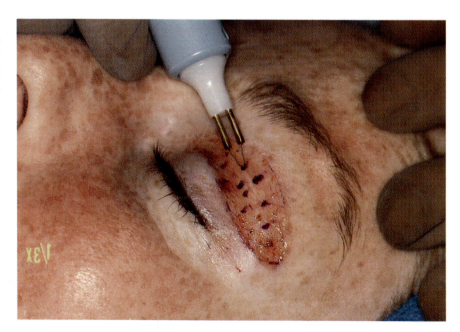

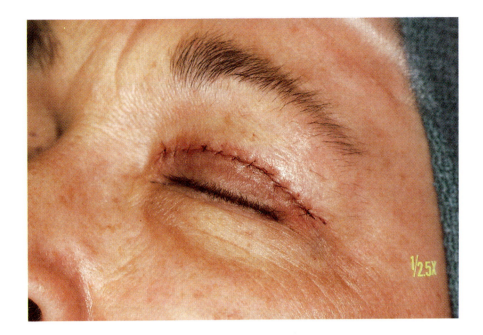
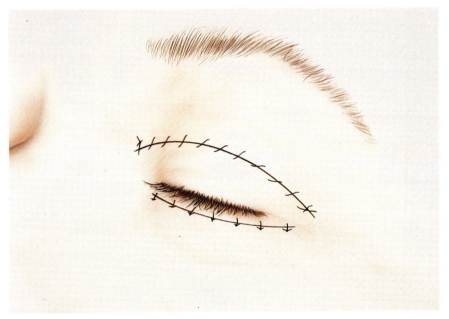

Figure 10–42
Wound closure completes upper lid surgery with a running 7–0 Novafil black suture. This fine suture swagged on a delicate reverse cutting needle driven by the Castroviejo needle holder facilitates atraumatic repair, causes little or no tissue irritation and milia formation, and may be maintained in place for 7 to 10 days before removal without detriment to healing or the development of visible suture tracks. A continuous running intradermal or subcuticular monofilament nylon suture closure is also satisfactory but occasionally produces annoying bleeding and immediate ecchymosis as the needle penetrates dermal vessels generally avoided with a cutaneous repair.

Our routine sequence in four-lid blepharoplasty is initiated by left upper lid blepharoplasty (without final closure), followed by left lower lid blepharoplasty with suture closure. The surgeon switches sides, and after right upper lid blepharoplasty, both upper lids are sutured simultaneously by the surgeon and assistant to facilitate a more rapid operation. Right lower lid blepharoplasty then completes the procedure.

PART II FACIAL AESTHETIC AND LIFTING PROCEDURES

Lower Lid

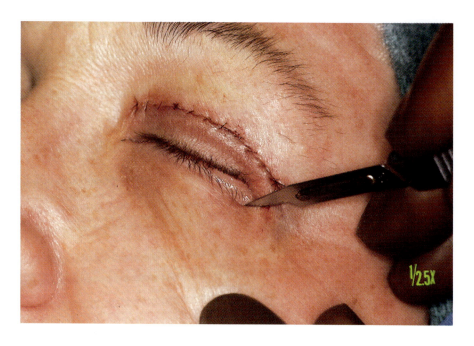

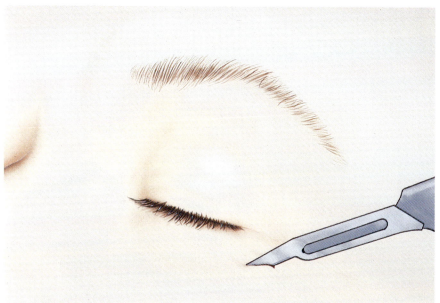

Figure 10–43
In the majority of patients, we prefer the skin-muscle flap approach to fully expose the anatomic elements of the lower lid in need of correction. A stab incision directly to the bony rim, ideally and safely created with a diminutive 15 C Bard-Parker blade, initiates the procedure. Sited 1 to 1.5 mm below the ciliary margin at the lateral canthus, the incision is not extended laterally or superiorly into the lateral lines of expression unless necessary for adequate flap repositioning and tailoring.

CHAPTER 10 Aesthetic Blepharoplasty

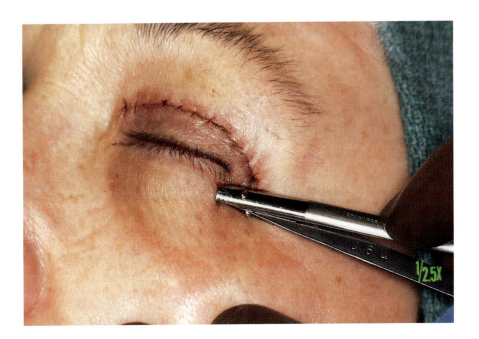

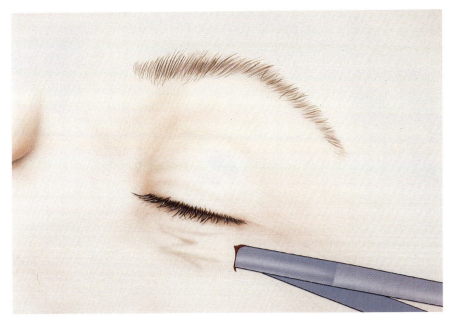

Figure 10–44
The submuscular plane is entered and dissected medially with delicate canthotomy scissors to gently spread the tissues and define the favorable tissue plane between muscle and the orbital septum.

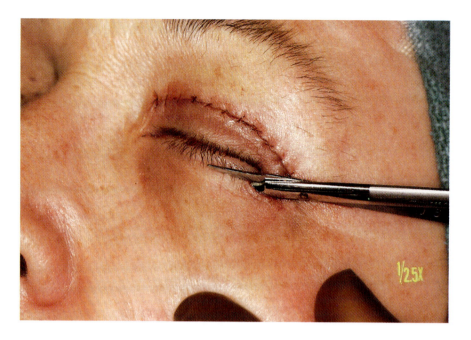

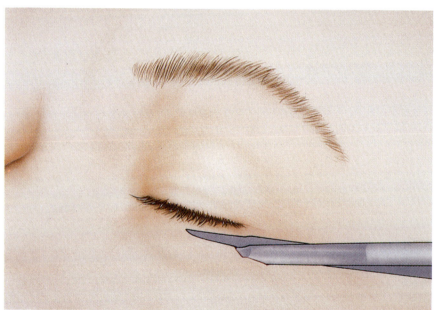

Figure 10-45
We ultimately complete the cutaneous incision at the margin by positioning one scissors blade into the dissected submuscular plane and cutting medially to a point just short of the inferior punctum, with the curve of the scissors blade paralleling the lid curve. The scissors are angled during the cut to preserve a small segment of muscle on the tarsal plate to ensure blood supply preservation.

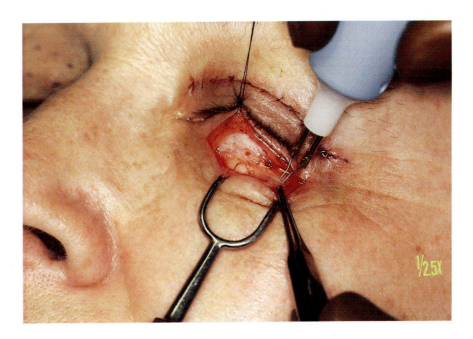

Figure 10-46
A useful alternative approach consists of limiting the initial incision to the skin only and completing the incision through the orbicularis with the Concept cautery 2 to 3 mm inferior to the skin incision; this results in a steplike configuration of the two incisions, is helpful in preventing any inferior retraction of the lower lid during postoperative healing, and provides superb hemostasis.

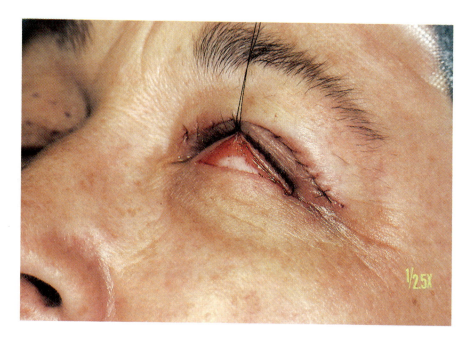

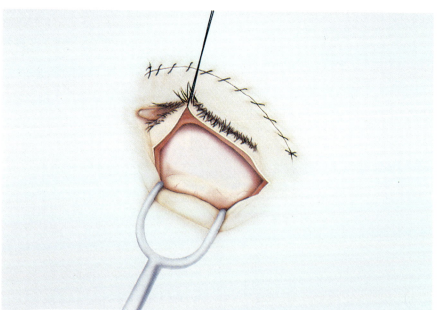

Figure 10–47
Meticulous hemostasis with the disposable or bipolar cautery renders the field absolutely dry. Wide exposure of the field is facilitated with a weighted traction suture of 6–0 silk passed through the wound margin superiorly as well as by a wide double-pronged skin hook on the flap below. At this point the attenuated orbital septum is clearly visible, often exposing through its semitransparent thickness the prominent fat pads of the *temporal, central,* and *nasal compartments.* Although the central and nasal fat prominences are generally confluent, the temporal fat pad exists in a more lateral, superior and isolated position.

CHAPTER 10 Aesthetic Blepharoplasty

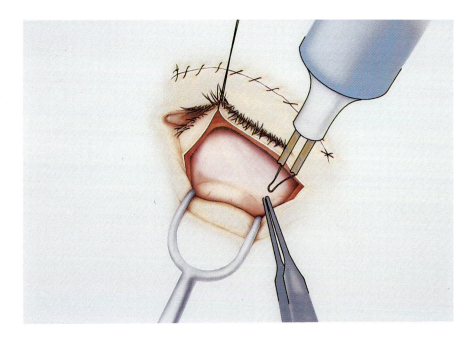

Figure 10–48
From this juncture on, essentially all lower lid dissection is completed with the use of the disposable Concept cautery, which ensures complete hemostasis and *accurate, direct-vision dissection*. After grasping the thin veil of connective tissue overlying the temporal fat pad, the fat is unveiled and freed with circumferential light cautery.

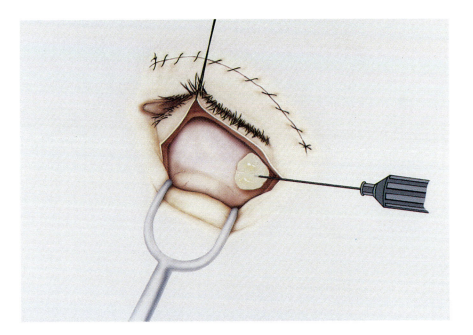

Figure 10–49
Plain lidocaine (0.1 to 0.2 mL) injected with a no. 30 needle renders the fat pedicle anesthetic for hemostat clamping of the base. Generally fat is removed to just below the superficial margin of the orbital rim. All fat above the clamp is scissors-excised with a generous cuff left for cauterization.

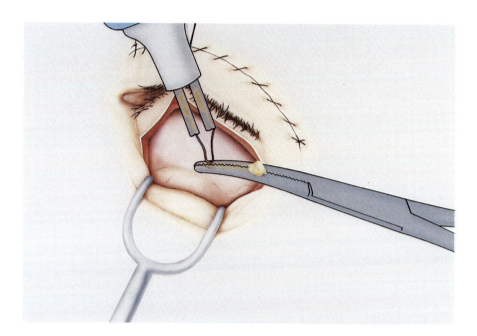

Figure 10–50
Absolute safety is once again promoted by securing the fat pedicle with delicate toothed forceps while releasing the hemostat, followed by final pedicle cuff cautery. *Only when hemostasis is absolute and complete is the pedicle released and allowed to withdraw into the orbit.*

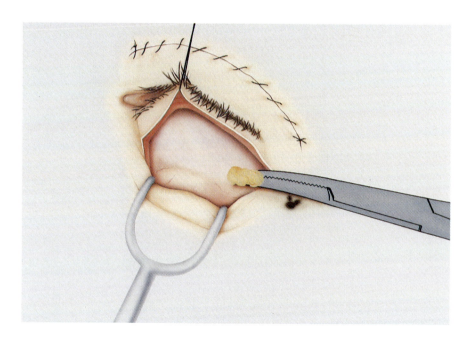

Figure 10–51
The cauterized fat pad is secured and meticulously inspected for any bleeding before release.

CHAPTER 10 Aesthetic Blepharoplasty

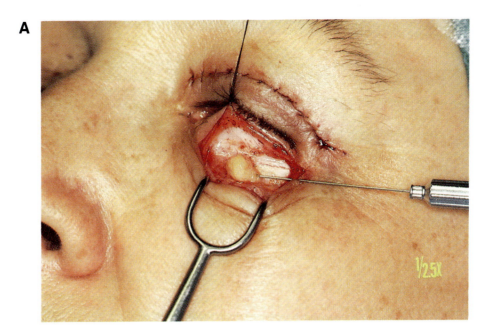

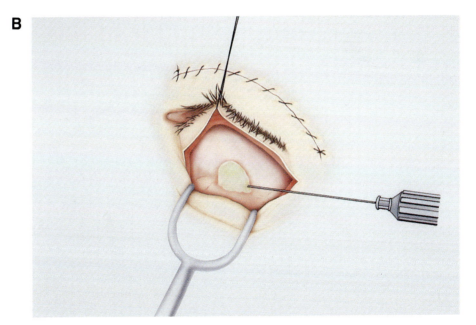

Figure 10–52
Gentle finger pressure on the globe further exposes the bulge of the *central* and *nasal fat compartments* lying medial to and at a slightly inferior level to the temporal pad. The central fat pad is managed in a manner similar to that just described: injecting its base, cross-clamping and excising excess fat, and securing the residual pedicle for hemostatic cauterization.

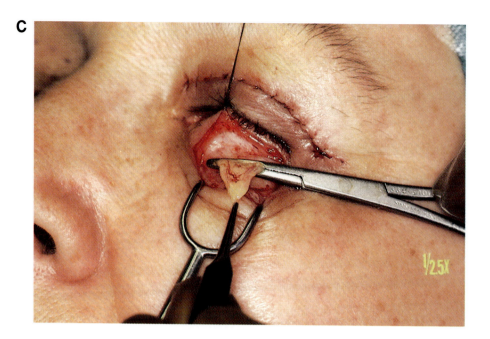

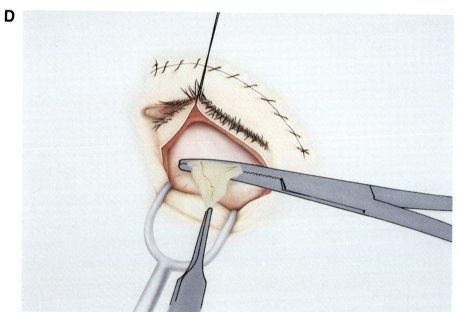

CHAPTER 10   Aesthetic Blepharoplasty

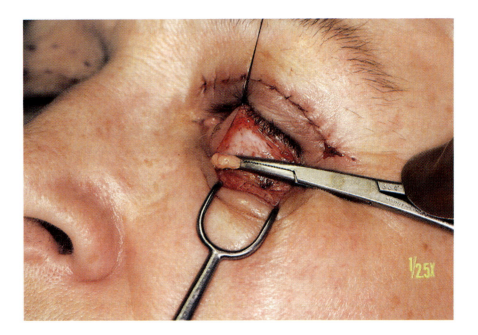

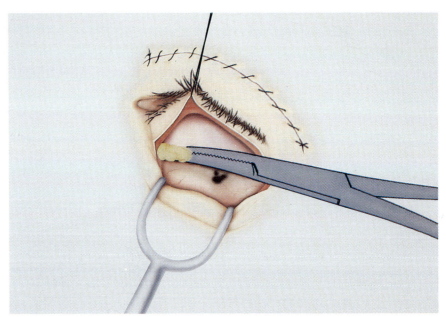

Figure 10–53
Rather than extend the lower lid incision medially to or near the inferior punctum, the medial extent of the more-limited lower lid incision provides excellent nasal fat pad exposure by retracting the medial extent of the incision toward the nose. Nasal compartment fat, often appearing lighter yellow in color, is teased out, clamped, excised, and cauterized.

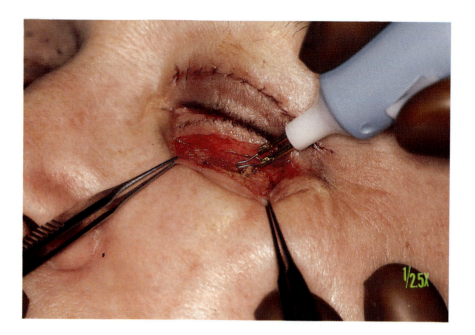

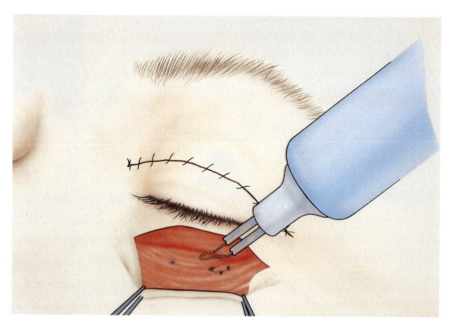

Figure 10-54
Seldom is the attenuated septum orbitale widely and completely opened—only small openings created by the Concept cautery are necessary for redundant fat pad access. Light cautery pinpoint scoring of the residual intact septum appears to firm and tighten this structure.

CHAPTER 10 Aesthetic Blepharoplasty

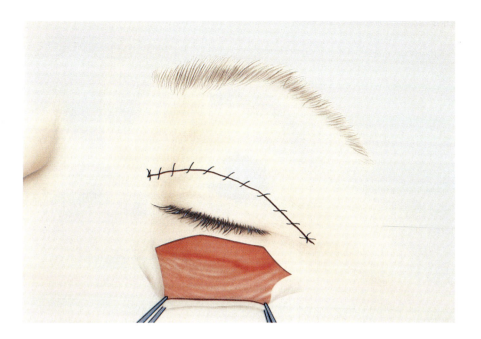

Figure 10–55
Prior to placement and tailoring of the skin-muscle flap, the surgeon and assistant evert the flap edge with fine forceps to expose the cut muscle and skin edge. Light cautery of the muscle edge and subcutaneous vessels aids in controlling even minor bleeding during trimming of the flap.

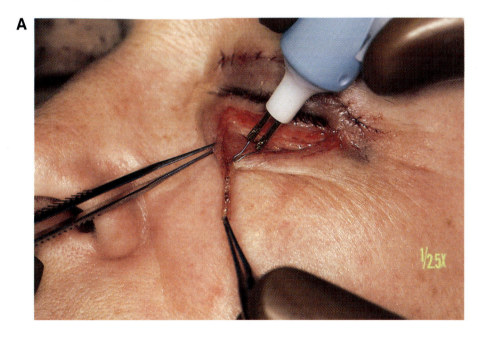

Figure 10-56
For legend see p. 270.

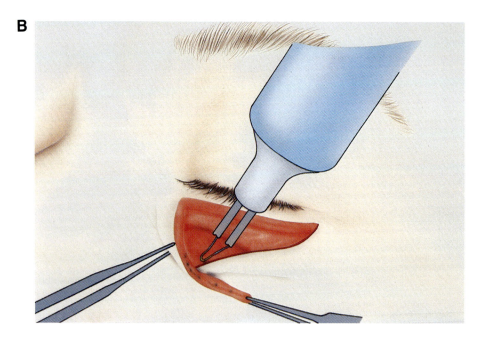

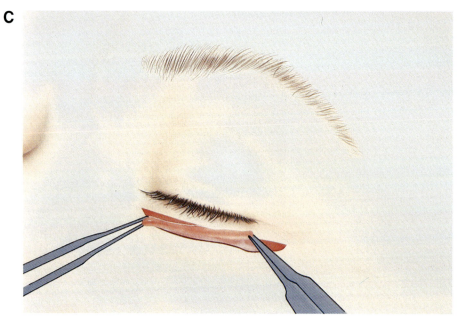

Figure 10–56 (cont.).
Excessive and redundant muscle may be excised by cautery if indicated to achieve a flatter, more natural lower lid appearance. Patients who exhibit a prominent horizontal bulge of orbicularis ridging (see Fig 10–23) benefit from excision of this excessive muscle.

CHAPTER 10 Aesthetic Blepharoplasty

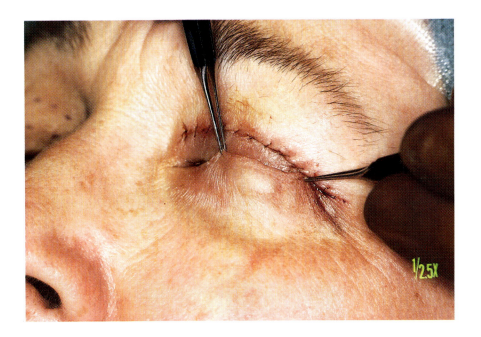

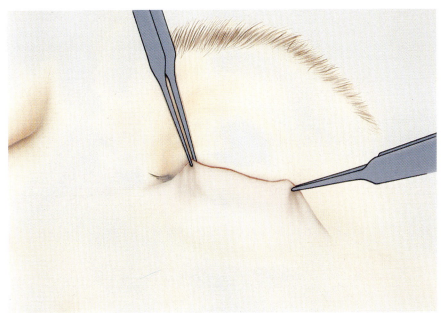

Figure 10–57
The flap is now allowed to fall back into its normal anatomic position and its surface smoothed in an upward direction with a moist cotton-tipped applicator. The goal of the excision of overlapping excessive skin and muscle is to develop a lower lid appearance of smoothness without resecting an excess of skin or muscle that could lead to a vertical shortening of the skin flap during healing contracture and create undesirable lid margin rounding, scleral show, and eversion or even ectropion.

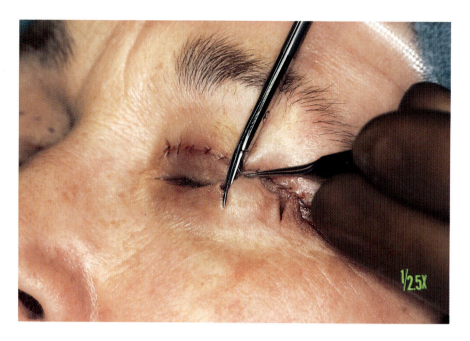

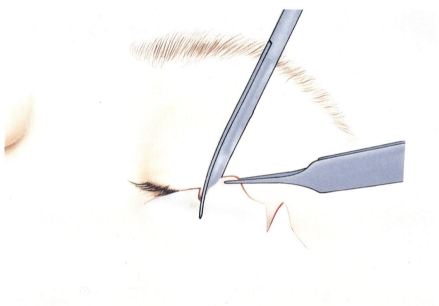

Figure 10–58
Removal of excess lower lid skin and muscle follows, often after creating several vertical cuts through the skin to guide the siting of the horizontal excision. It is frequently recommended in standard texts that the surgeon ask the patient to gaze upward and open the mouth during the estimation of lower lid excess to aid in avoiding excessive low lid resection; an experienced surgeon, however, finds little difficulty in judging the appropriate amount of skin-muscle flap excision if it is remembered that *sufficient skin must be retained to fall slightly into the new concavity created by excision of bulging lower lid fat* without resulting in any vertical pull on the lid margin.

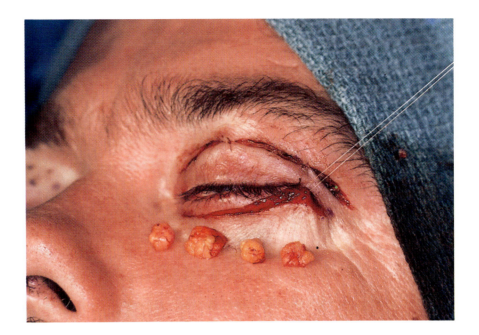

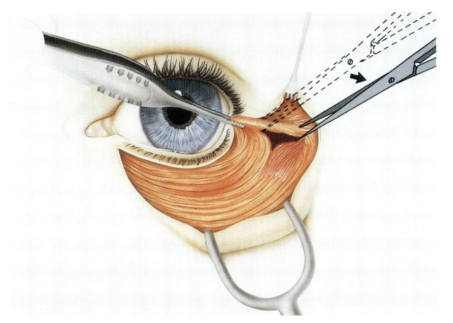

Figure 10-59
When the lower lid tissues are judged to be unusually heavy (common in males, less common in females), when secondary lower lid surgery is to be performed, and when a minor but important amount of horizontal lid shortening is indicated, the skin-muscle flap is suspended by suture from the lateral orbital periosteum with a single 5–0 clear nylon or PDS suture. After encircling a substantial amount of the lateral lower lid muscle, suspension and stabilization of the lower lid during the early healing process are effected by the buried suture as a result of its firm engagement to the lateral orbital wall periosteum. If muscle is judged extremely redundant, a segment is excised laterally and the cut edges reconstituted and again suspended by suture to orbital periosteum.

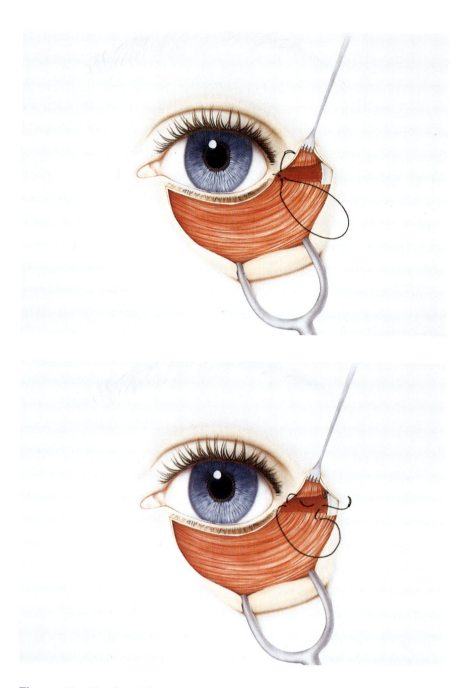

Figure 10-59 (cont.).

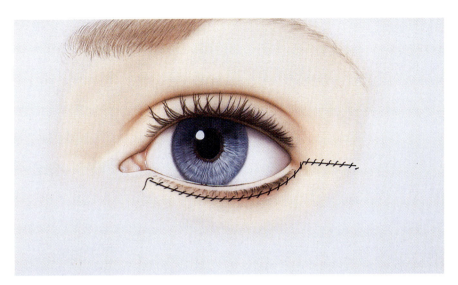

Figure 10–60
Lower lid incision closure ensues with a running 7–0 black nylon suture progressing laterally to medially; the suture remains untied as it exits the wound margins and simply lies free for simplified removal in 6 to 7 days. This is effective in creating a firm and complete closure of the lower lid incision. Steri-strip taping to further reduce tension on the healing lower lid may be employed over the lateral extent of the incisions.

Alternative Procedures

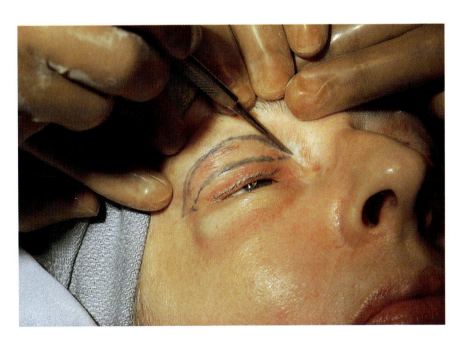

Figure 10–61
Direct excision of upper eyelid skin may be carried out with sharp knife incision and dissection if the upper lid skin excess is minimal; in secondary blepharoplasty excisions, generally little skin excess exists. Exacting four-point finger stabilization of the lax lid tissues facilitates accurate upper lid skin excision.

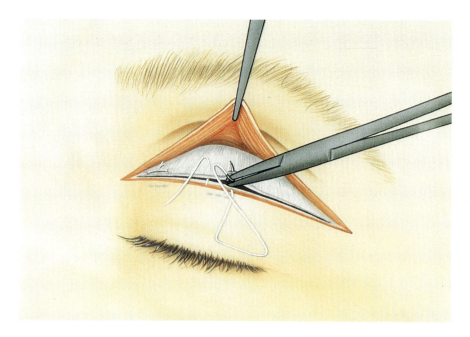

Figure 10–62
Suture fixation of the levator aponeurosis to the dermis of the upper lid inferior cut skin margin with four to five fine permanent sutures will increase upper lid skin crease definition and create a more defined skin fold. Certain types of Oriental eyelids may be favorably treated with this approach.

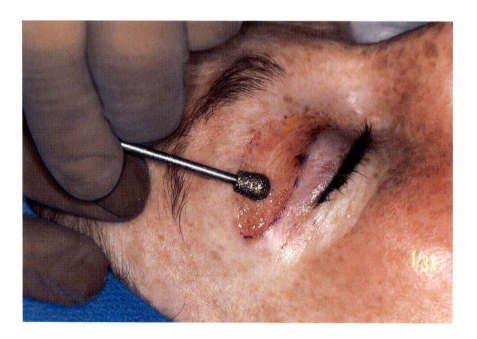

Figure 10–63
Orbits with heavy, overhanging supraorbital rims are improved by exposing the lateral orbital rim and reducing the heavy bone laterally with a sharp otologic rotating burr or thin chisel.

CHAPTER 10   Aesthetic Blepharoplasty

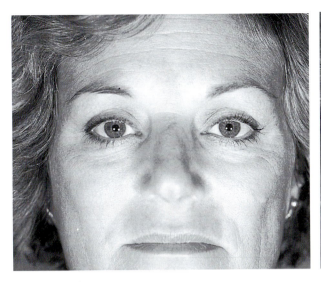
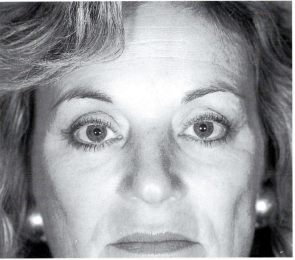

Figure 10–64
If the lower lid skin is highly wrinkled and excessive, initial sharp dissection of the skin flap only will aid in redraping the surgically reduced lid and provide an improved postoperative appearance. Invariably redundant muscle will require excision as well.

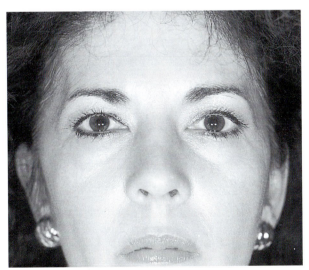
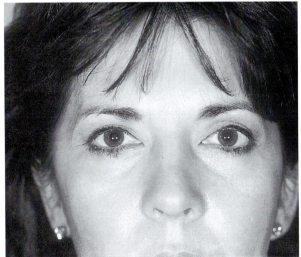

Figure 10–65
In young patients demonstrating abnormally excessive congenital fat herniation, no excess lower lid skin may be present, and simply redraping and suturing *without skin or muscle excision* after fat removal are required.

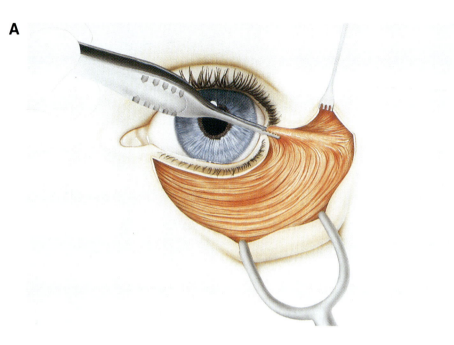

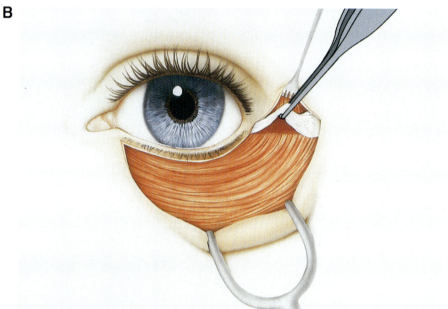

Figure 10–66
A, substantial loss of lower lid support may call for definitive horizontal shortening of the lower lid by a lateral canthal tendon shortening procedure. The tendonous thickening laterally is suspended horizontally for better definition. **B,** the tendon is isolated, stabilized by a single hook, and retracted laterally to plan the extent of removal required to tighten the lax lower lid.

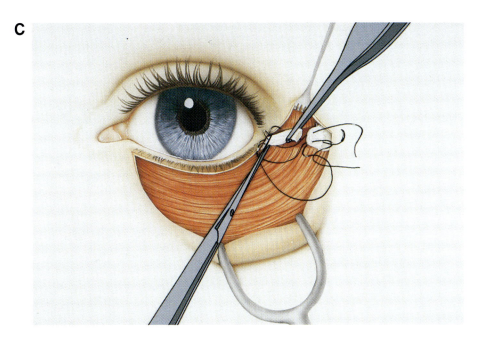

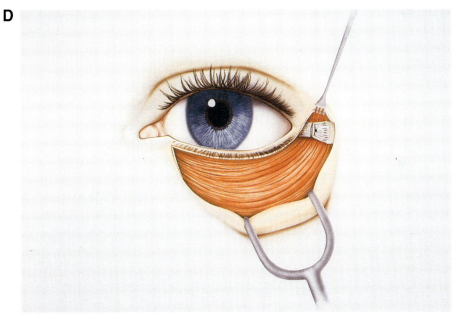

Figure 10-66 (cont.).
C, the tendon is divided, the excess excised, and suture reconstitution completed with 6–0 clear nylon sutures. **D,** suture repair of a shortened tendon.

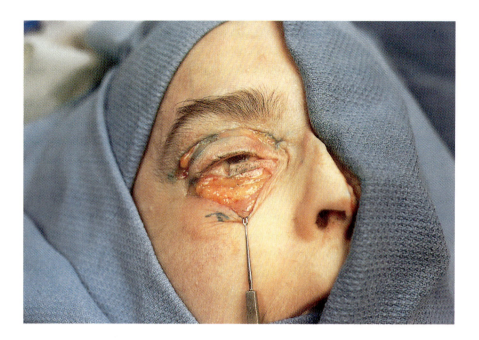

Figure 10–67
In senile lids, in particular, excessive lower lid fat is commonly poorly differentiated into the traditional three compartments. In such patients the attenuated septum orbitale is opened widely and all protuberant fat excised to the level of the orbital rim.

Postoperative Care

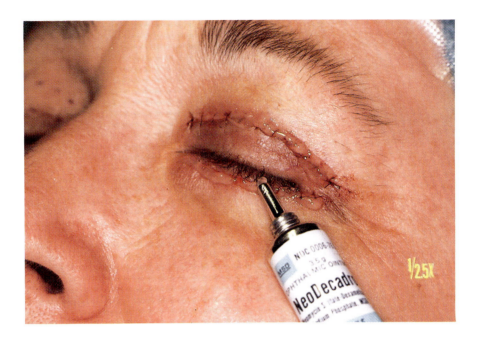

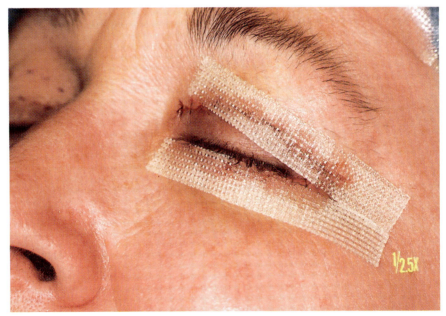

Figure 10–68
Blepharoplasty should result in an essentially *pain-free postoperative period*. Even minor pain should be reported and aggressively investigated to rule out corneal abrasion or intraorbital bleeding. The patient's head should be elevated and strenuous activities strictly curtailed. A double-layered strip of Adaptic gauze is applied to each suture line in the upper and lower lids and sealed in place with NeoDecadron ophthalmic ointment. The latter medication maintains a moist condition over the incision for 24 hours and, upon removal, facilitates easy cleaning of the wound with hydrogen peroxide. Light application of the ointment for 1 week following surgery facilitates healing and more rapidly diminishes wound redness.

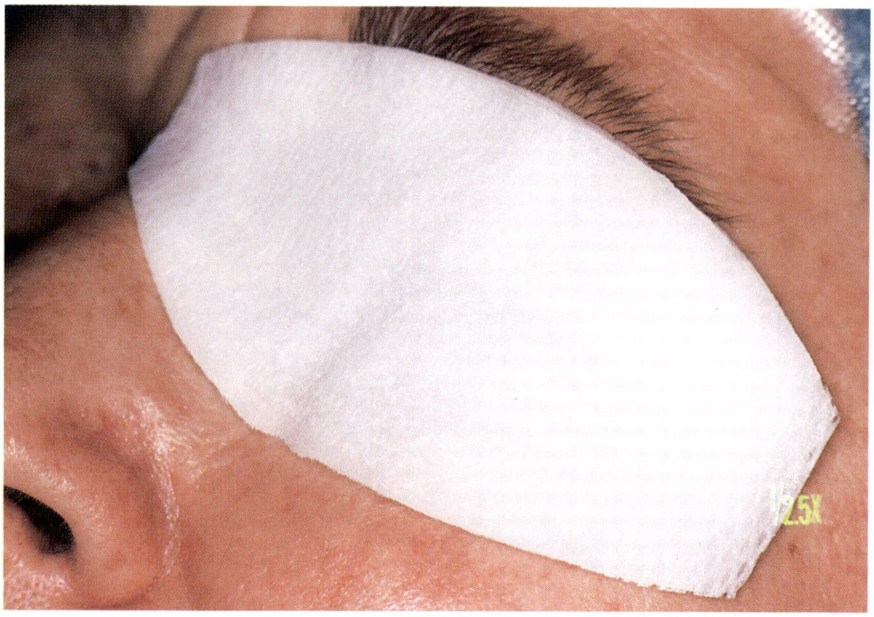

Figure 10–69
For 2 hours following surgery two cotton eye pads soaked in cold water are placed *without pressure* over the eyelids for comfort and protection from inadvertent injury by the patient.

Specific instructions are provided for home care, the most vital of which includes the avoidance of lifting, straining, and vigorous exercise (Fig 10–70). Contact lenses must be avoided until incision healing is sufficient to tolerate manipulation of the lower eyelid. Artificial tears are seldom needed but represent invaluable protection to the cornea if even slight irritation or dryness is detected.

Suture removal occurs at 7 to 9 days since the 7–0 monofilament nylon displays little propensity for creating suture tunnels, suture scars, or milia. This policy negates the potential wound separations infrequently seen when sutures are removed at 3 to 4 days. NeoDecadron ophthalmic ointment applied sparingly to the incision twice daily for 3 weeks diminishes wound redness and involves the patient in his own postoperative care.

CHAPTER 10   Aesthetic Blepharoplasty

PATIENT INSTRUCTIONS FOLLOWING BLEPHAROPLASTY
(EYELID SURGERY)

1. Sleep on your back or side with the head elevated.

2. Blepharoplasty usually causes little if any postoperative pain. If you notice significant sharp or dull pain that persists, notify my office immediately.

3. Cold compresses (ice–cold washclothes) may be used over your eyes for 20–30 minutes six times per day if you wish. Ordinarily, however, no cold compresses are necessary or of great value.

4. Take no aspirin or aspirin-containing pain medications. Tylenol, Darvocet N-100, or other mild pain relievers prescribed are safe if needed.

5. You may use your eyes for reading or TV viewing as frequently as you wish.

6. Apply the ointment provided to the incision twice a day. Use *sparingly*, and place only a *tiny amount* on the incision lines.

7. Do not use contact lenses for at least 2 weeks. Pulling on the eyelids while inserting or removing lenses may interfere with precise incision healing. Glasses may be used at any time.

8. Do not use mascara, eyeliner, or eye shadow until approved by us (usually 10–14 days). Minimal makeup applied to any bruising of the lower lid is acceptable at any time, but do not pull on the lids or incisions.

9. Any apparent redness of the whites of the eyeball is only a form of bruising and will subside during the early healing process.

10. Do not engage in vigorous exercise or sports for at least 3 weeks or until approved by us.

11. Stitches are removed at different times after surgery depending upon the extent of surgery carried out, the type of stitches, and the type and quality of your skin. We will advise you accordingly.

12. It is not abnormal to feel slight itching and tightness of the eyelids during the early healing period.

We greatly appreciate the confidence you have shown in us by allowing us to assist you in improving your appearance and health, and you may be assured of our best efforts to achieve the most satisfactory surgical result possible for your particular individual anatomy and condition.

Figure 10–70
Typical postoperative guidelines for patients following blepharoplasty.

PART II   FACIAL AESTHETIC AND LIFTING PROCEDURES

Results and Outcomes

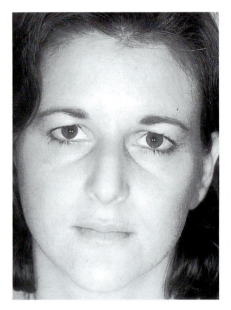 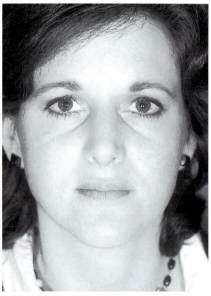

Figure 10-71
Young patient with congenital fullness and redundancy of the upper lids resulting in upper lid skin resting on the upper lid lashes, hooding, and a fatigued appearance. Low-positioned eyebrows compound the sad appearance. Moderate lower lid fat excess is removed with preservation of all lower lid skin. Upper and lower lid blepharoplasty restores an appropriate upper eyelid crease and brightens the entire facial expression. Subtle rhinoplasty further improves the overall facial appearance.

Figure 10-72
Patient demonstrating excess upper lid skin with abundant fat in both the upper and lower lids. Brow position is normal. Abundant skin, fat, and a 4-mm strip of orbicularis muscle have been removed from the upper lid. Fat excision without skin excision improves the lower lid appearance.

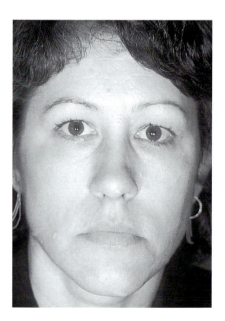 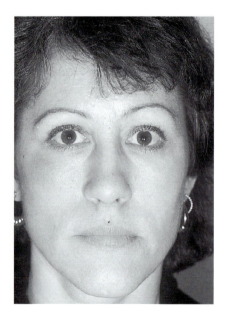

CHAPTER 10 Aesthetic Blepharoplasty

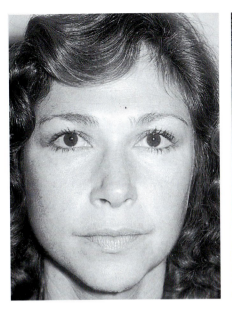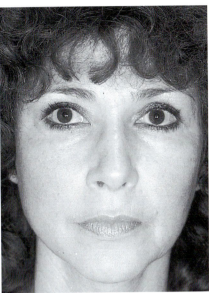

Figure 10–73
Early aging characteristics illustrated here include ptotic, redundant, hooded skin in the upper lids, with excess fat apparent in the mid and lateral lid regions. Early fat protruberance exists in the lower lids. Youthful lid appearance is restored with excision of excess fat in the upper lids and excision of a 3-mm horizontal strip of orbicularis muscle. Abundant lower lid fat required excision along with 2 mm of excess lower lid skin.

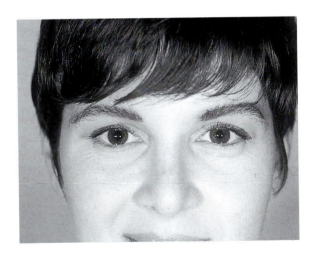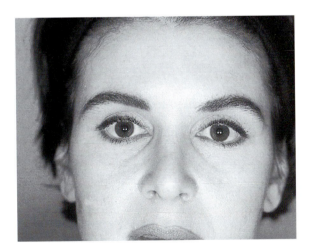

Figure 10–74
Early aging lid findings in a model characterized by the loss of a definitive upper lid cleft and prominent muscle ridging of the lower lids (more profound on patient's left) appearing upon even slight animation. Correction included excision of excess upper lid skin with resection of a 5-mm strip of lower lid orbicularis muscle to correct the muscle ridging.

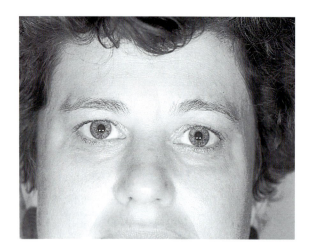 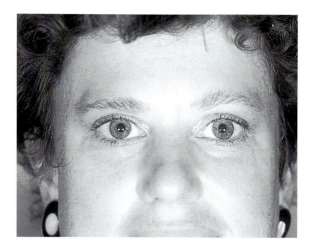

Figure 10–75
Midlife patient concerned about a "tired" appearance created by excess hooding of the upper lid skin and "bags" of the lower lids. Note the low-positioned brows with a horizontal character. Improvement required excision of excess skin and fat in the upper lids with removal of abundant fat and 2 mm of excess skin in the lower lids through a skin-muscle flap approach. A forehead-lift to correct the low-positioned brows was declined.

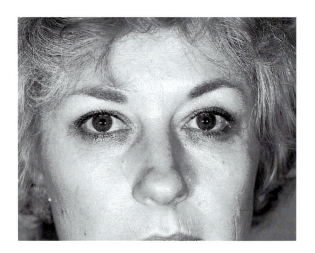 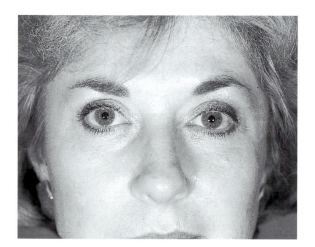

Figure 10–76
Middle-aged patient concerned about aging appearance around the eyes, specifically concerned that the eyes look "smaller" than earlier in life. Upper lid blepharoplasty combined with fat removal in the lower lids (greater on the patient's left) provides the appearance of larger eyes and a brighter expression. Through a skin-muscle flap, 2 mm of lower lid skin and muscle was excised.

CHAPTER 10 Aesthetic Blepharoplasty

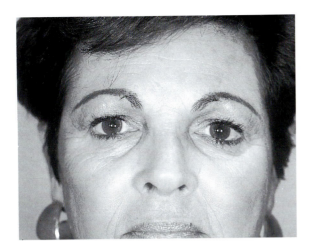 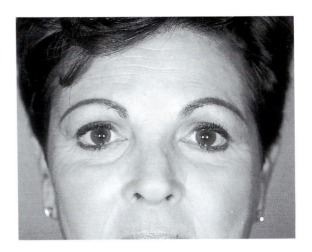

Figure 10-77
Older patient with significant solar skin damage, upper lid skin excess, deep lid creasing, and a lateral downward slant to the eyes. The eyes are deep-set with prominent orbital ridges. Upper lid skin excision along with a combined skin-muscle flap and skin flap approach to the lower lids has improved the patient's appearance by tightening the lower lids. Because of laxity of the lower lid the lateral orbicularis was suspended by suture to the periosteum of the orbital sidewall.

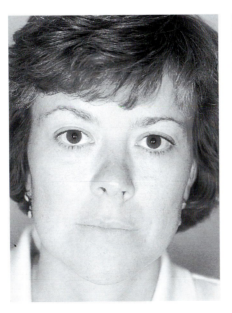 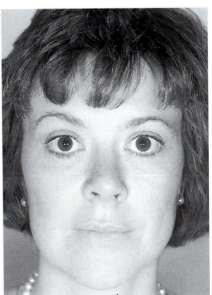

Figure 10-78
Beginning of aging orbital changes in a patient in midlife. The patient demonstrates slightly greater scleral show as a familial characteristic. Upper and lower lid blepharoplasty restores a larger, more youthful, and interesting eye appearance.

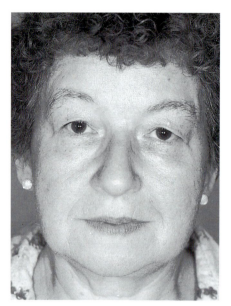
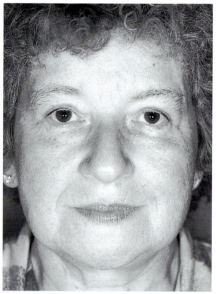

Figure 10–79
Older patient with asymmetrical hooding of the upper lid skin, a temporal visual field deficit, slight eversion of the lower lid margins with excess lower lid tone, and prominent fat protuberance. Upper lid creases are restored by removal of excess skin and orbicularis muscle, followed by a skin-muscle flap approach to the excess lower lid fat and laxity. Suture shortening and tightening of the lateral canthal tendon with suture suspension to the lateral orbital wall improve the appearance and function of the lower lids.

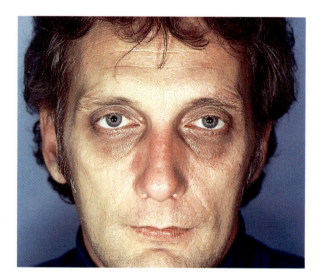

Figure 10–80
Excess familial hyperpigmentation in the orbital aesthetic unit. Blepharoplasty in such individuals may result in prolonged excess ecchymosis.

CHAPTER 10 Aesthetic Blepharoplasty

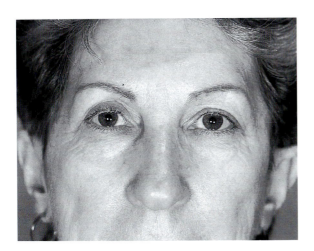
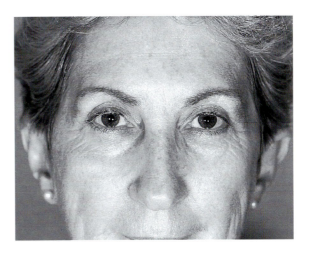

Figure 10–81
Marked asymmetry of the upper lids, probably the consequence of an increased orbital volume on the right combined with a slight difference in length of insertion of the levator aponeurosis. Differential upper and lower lid blepharoplasty restores near symmetry to the appearance, but the outcome of both eyes will never be completely the same. Asymmetries are the rule rather than the exception in patients requesting eyelid surgery, and candidates should be carefully informed *before* corrective surgery.

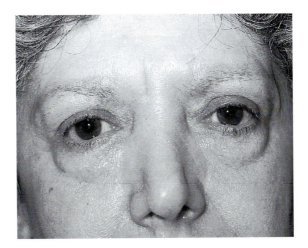

Figure 10–82
Residual lower lid fat protuberance 1 year following blepharoplasty elsewhere.

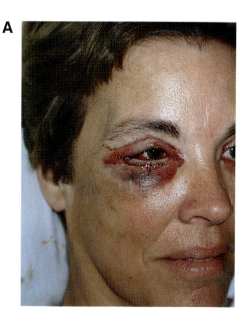
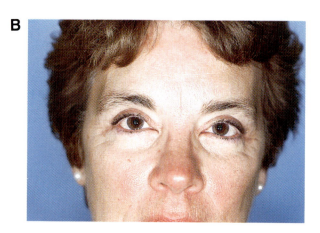

Figure 10–83
A, developing orbital hematoma forming abruptly 3 hours following uneventful blepharoplasty. *Immediate* return to surgery, exploration of the wound, and control of the bleeding vessel in the orbicularis muscle margin controlled the progressive bleeding. **B,** 1 year following surgery, the outcome is satisfactory and symmetrical.

CHAPTER 10   Aesthetic Blepharoplasty

Sequelae and Complications

Sequelae

- Blepharoplasty *scars* are permanent; careful siting by utilizing the principles outlined and meticulous incision closure are thus critical for ideal scar camouflage.
- *Fine rhytids* present preoperatively in the lateral canthal aspect of the orbital skin as well as in the lower lid will largely persist after blepharoplasty surgery.
- *Persistent ecchymosis* may develop in patients with hyperpigmented skin (see Fig 10–80); many months may pass before this condition returns to normal.
- *Malar bags* and *festoons* remain unaffected by blepharoplasty and require direct excision with irregularization scar camouflage techniques.
- *Slight visual blurring* resulting from minor conjunctival edema (in a small number of patients) or from overgenerous application of suture line ointment (the majority of patients) is a short-lived phenomenon.

Postoperative Complications

- *Prolonged ecchymosis* may develop if intraoperative bleeding has been excessive or occasionally in patients with hyperpigmentation of the eyelid skin.
- *Lagophthalmos and ectropion,* as discussed, are totally avoidable by the techniques recommended.
- Upper lid *ptosis* may be present temporarily (2 to several weeks) following upper lid techniques that involve suture fixation of the levator aponeurosis.
- Slight eyelid *asymmetry* is not infrequent following blepharoplasty (see Fig 10–81, A and B), despite careful surgical attempts to achieve perfect symmetry, particularly if significant asymmetry exists before surgery. Patients must be informed early about asymmetrical lids, unequal orbital shapes, and facial disharmonies.
- Loss of lashes is possible if the incisions are sited too close to the lash line or, more commonly, if there is thermal injury to the hair follicle. In our experience significant lash loss is rare; any lashes lost have been slowly but permanently replaced by regrowth.
- *Persistent fat pad herniation* results from a failure to accurately diagnose the extent of excess fat prior to local infiltration of anesthetic with subsequent incomplete removal (see Fig 10–82). Occasionally, patients who have massive fat herniation in the lower lid will continue to demonstrate some fat herniation even after extensive fat excision to a level posterior to the orbital rim. In such patients, a highly weakened and ineffective atrophic orbital septum simply fails to contain the protrusion of additional orbital fat.
- *Intraorbital hemorrhage* with *partial or total blindness* has been reported and is a disastrous complication never encountered by the authors. Meticulous hemostasis with blood vessel control *before* vessel division profoundly diminishes the risk of this optic nerve injury. Any postoperative bleeding demands immediate wound exploration and bleeding control (see Fig 10–83, A and B).

CHAPTER 10   Aesthetic Blepharoplasty

Suggested Reading

- McKinney P, Cunningham BL: *Aesthetic Facial Surgery.* New York, Churchill Livingstone, 1992.
- Putterman A: *Cosmetic Oculoplastic Surgery.* Philadelphia, W.B. Saunders, 1993.
- Putterman AM, Urist ML: Surgical anatomy of the orbital septum. *Ann Ophthalmol* 1974; 6:290–303.
- Smith B, Petrelli R: Surgical repair of prolapsed lacrimal glands. *Arch Ophthalmol* 1978; 96:113–114.
- Smith BC, et al: *Ophthalmic Plastic and Reconstructive Surgery.* St Louis, Mosby–Year Book, 1987.
- Tardy ME, Klingensmith M: *Facelift surgery: Principles and variations,* in Roenigk RR, Roenigk HK (eds): *Dermatologic Surgery.* New York, Marcel Dekker, 1989.
- Tardy ME, Thomas R, Fitzpatrick ME: *Facial Rejuvenation Surgery.* Memphis, Tenn, Richards Smith-Nephur Co.
- Webster RC: Blepharoplasty, in Smith BC (ed): *Ophthalmic Plastic and Reconstructive Surgery.* St Louis, Mosby–Year Book, 1987.
- Wolfley DE: Blepharoplasty: The ophthalmologist's view. *Otolaryngol Clin North Am* 1980; 13:237.

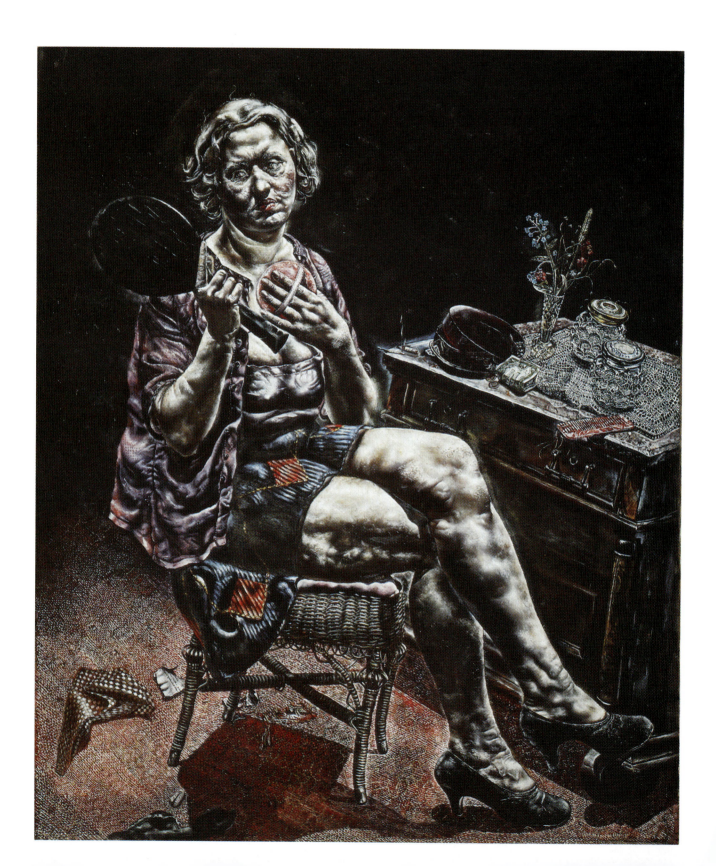

CHAPTER 11

 The Facelift Operation: Principles and Techniques

> *Oh! grief hath chang'd me since you saw me last; and careful hours, with time's deform'd hand, have written defeatures in my face.*
>
> **William Shakespeare**

Diagnosis and Candidate Selection

Facelift operations, like rhinoplasty, vary in extent and technique as required by the individual anatomy. While some patients may need lifting and repositioning of tissues in all of the aesthetic units of the face and neck, others (usually younger individuals) are better served by more limited segmental facelifts. "Minilifts," however, mistakenly popularized by the lay press, provide less-than-ideal outcomes and short-term improvement. They should be clearly differentiated from secondary facelifts (or "tuck-up" operations), which, although a more modest procedure necessitating reduced undermining and less skin resection, result in highly effective improvement of lasting value.

In one sense the facelift operation, when compared with the entire gamut of aesthetic operations, might be viewed as the least ideal rejuvenation procedure. It is inevitable that some of the favorable early postoperative result progressively deteriorates as the inexorable forces of gravity, aging, and constant facial animation counter the surgeon's lifting and repositioning efforts. Rhytidoplasty may best be characterized as a compromise with nature. Excessive sun exposure, wide swings in body weight, and poor skin care habits reduce facelift operation effectiveness and longevity. Thus patients chosen for a facelift must be willing participants in a total program designed to forestall the aging process and prolong the improvements of a well-performed facelift. The surgeon's responsibility, after recognizing the aesthetic shortfall, is to plan and fashion the best lifting and repositioning procedures possible consistent with the patient's wishes and anatomic limitations.

Since the operation is totally elective in nature, as few risks as possible should be taken to achieve the ultimate goal: a happy patient and proud surgeon. Heroic surgical attempts to achieve an extraordinary result must be balanced with the potential increased risks, since any complication, no matter how insignificant, represents a surgical failure (Fig 11–1).

The most successful facelifts are effected in patients in whom the aging process has not yet taken an overwhelming toll on the facial appearance (Fig 11–2). Chronologic age is an unreliable determinant factor since many diverse factors (genetic predisposition, sun damage, stress) have an influ-

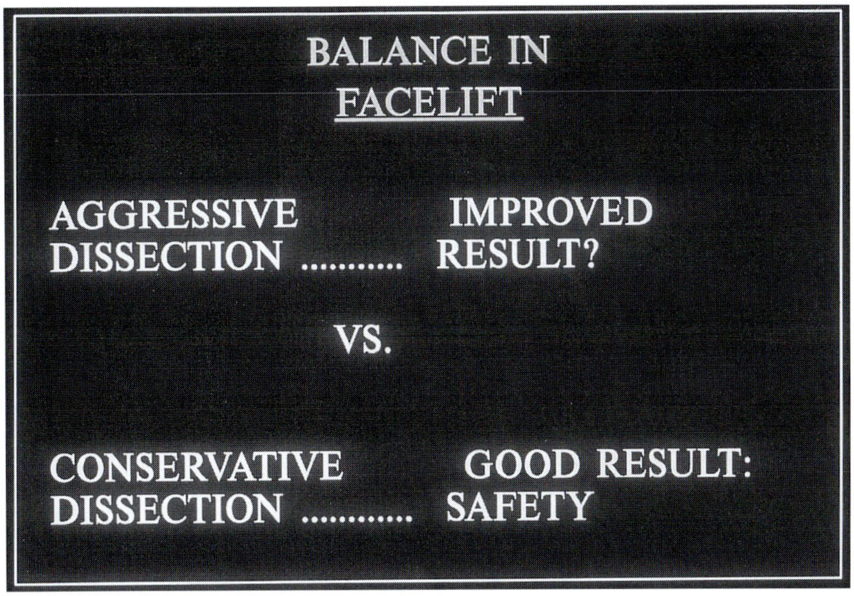

CHAPTER 11 The Facelift Operation: Principles and Techniques

Figure 11-1
A balanced approach must be considered in undertaking facial and cervical lifting procedures. In each patient fundamental decisions must be made: how aggressive must the surgical procedure be to ensure a satisfactory, lasting, and *safe* result? It remains unclear whether more extensive dissection procedures in a facelift are superior to more conservative approaches in terms of an improved outcome and rejuvenation of longer duration. Regardless of the approach, *safety without complication* remains the critical essential. In the majority of procedures the individual patient's anatomy and degree of aging will dictate the appropriate procedure(s). In addition, careful selection of *ideal patients* for facelift procedures outranks all other criteria for achieving superior results.

ence on the age at which patients begin to express concern about clearly deteriorating facial appearance.

An ideal patient from the standpoint of anatomy might be described as an attractive healthy female between the ages of 40 and 60 years. Retention of facial skin elasticity with a lack of severe solar and other environmental skin damage is a favorable finding (Fig 11-3,A). The patient should not be overweight, particularly from the standpoint of excess deposits of fat in the facial and cervical areas (Fig 11-3,B). The facial skeleton should be angular and attractively developed, especially in the malar, mandibular, and hyoid-thyroid complex areas. Upon manipulation, the facial skin and underlying soft tissue should slide over the more static underlying facial skeletal features with relative ease and mobility (Fig 11-4,A-C).

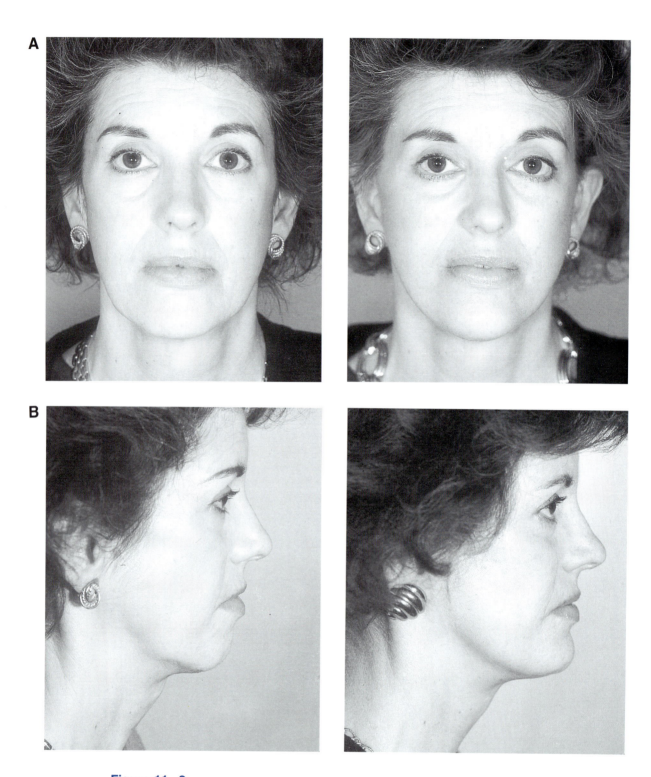

Figure 11–2
A and **B,** this patient who demonstrates early changes of facial aging is a near-ideal facelift candidate. At 2 years the outcome of facelift, blepharoplasty, and chin augmentation is favorable, with a natural appearance.

CHAPTER 11 The Facelift Operation: Principles and Techniques

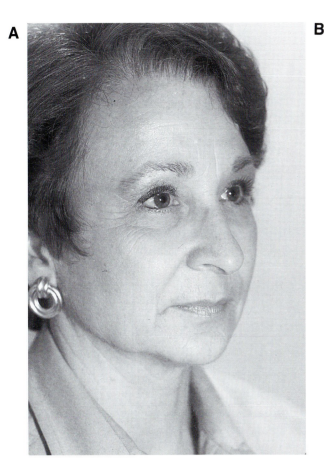
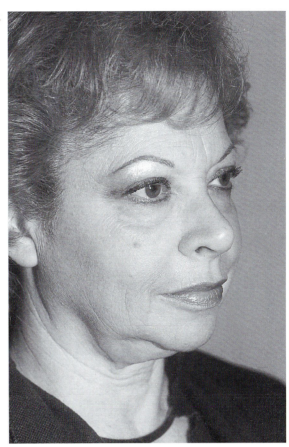

Figure 11-3
A, older patient with more advanced gravitational descent of the facial brow, lid, and cervical tissue. Good skin quality, the absence of excessive facial fat, and a favorable skeletal bone structure combine to make her a good candidate for successful rejuvenation procedures. **B,** a less ideal candidate for a facelift procedure. Excessive fat exists in the face, the bone structure is less than ideal, chin and submaxillary gland ptosis exists, and the neck is short with excessive medial and lateral submental fat. Improvement can be anticipated from rejuvenation surgery, but decided limitations exist.

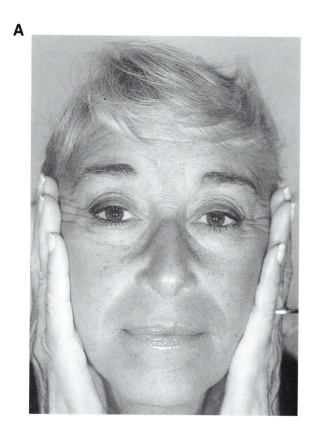 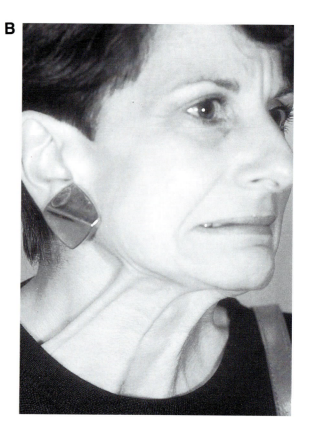

Figure 11-4
A, demonstration of favorable mobility of facial soft tissues—they glide loosely over underlying soft tissue and bony support structures. When mobility is poor or limited, the facelift result will be less favorable. **B,** forced facial grimace to further define the margins and conditions of the platysmal muscle bands during preoperative planning for a facelift.

Individuals who fall short of the above criteria in one or more categories are less ideal prospects for the fullest benefits possible from facelift surgery. However, adjunctive aesthetic procedures like chin augmentation, submental fat removal, suction lipectomy, and selective facial dermabrasion may partially compensate for initial anatomic shortcomings (Fig 11-5).

Patients commonly ask: How long will my facelift last? They are understandably unaware that no accurate response is possible since aging is a constant, inevitable, and progressive rather than an abrupt process. A satisfying and essentially accurate response may be helpful: "Aging is a continuing, progressive phenomenon strongly affected by gravity and your own personal genetically predisposed timetable for aging. For example, pretend you have an identical twin. The twin who undertakes rejuvenation surgery will likely always appear more youthful than the twin who does not, *but both will continue to age each year.*" Relatively conservative minor "tuck-up" or ancillary procedures carried out at 5- to 10-year intervals

CHAPTER 11 The Facelift Operation: Principles and Techniques

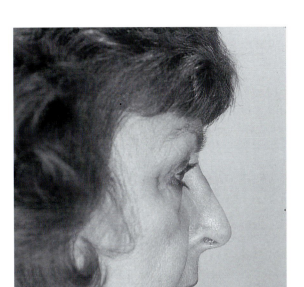
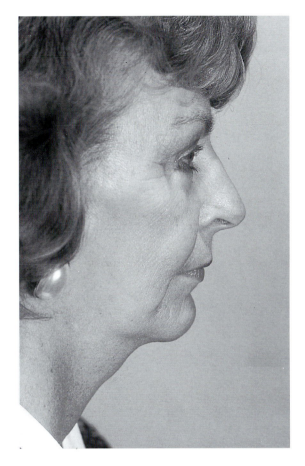

Figure 11–5
Less-than-ideal patient for a facelift because of retrognathia, excess submental fat, and a low-positioned hyoid. Significant lipectomy and chin augmentation were necessary in this facelift procedure.

are helpful in maintaining the best possible appearance. Most realistic patients understand and appreciate this simplistic but accurate analogy.

In our experience patients seeking a facelift are probably the most difficult group to satisfy completely with surgical rejuvenation, perhaps because of unvoiced, occult, and unrealistic expectations. Therefore a wise surgeon takes great care in the candidate selection process to ferret out with open-ended questions and attentive recognition of psychological clues and "body language" those individuals who are likely to be (and to *not* be) ideal candidates. Routinely more than one consultation is necessary to thoroughly discern true motivations and to inform and shape the patient's expectations about the seriousness of the operation, the need for complete cooperation during postoperative recovery, and the importance of thorough follow-up evaluation.

Indications for facelift surgery include the following:

- Healthy patient whose facial-cervical skin and muscle appear excessive, redundant, and ptotic and no longer conform firmly to the bony skeleton.
- Facial appearance characterized by a strong, angular bony skeleton with a normally positioned hyoid-thyroid complex.
- Patient at or near ideal weight for body type who possesses minimal facial fat and mobile facial skin with retained elasticity.
- Patient without deeply wrinkled, creased skin.
- Highly motivated patient who is aware that the goals of surgery are those of improvement and not perfection and who understands the anatomic and technical *limitations* of the planned surgery.

No amount of surgical cleverness can compensate for a poorly selected patient, a fact more true of the facelift operation than any other. Conversely, when facelift candidates are properly selected from both an anatomic and psychological standpoint, the surgical steps designed to ensure effective rejuvenation are straightforward and fundamental. These two preoperative considerations are all-important, since it is axiomatic that the most carefully selected patient from an anatomic aspect will be disappointed in even a superb surgical result if the operation is sought for the wrong psychological reasons.

Preparatory to facelift surgery the following evaluative procedures, laboratory studies, and planning aids are deemed essential:

- Thorough and complete verbal discussions with the surgeon as well as with the surgical nurse, who very effectively fills the role of "best friend" and ombudsman throughout the surgical experience.
- Consultation with and approval by patient's family physician when indicated.
- Consultation with interested and concerned family members (but only at the direct behest of the patient).
- Complete series of color transparency photographs in duplicate.
- Careful appraisal of all medications taken routinely or intermittently. *Aspirin and aspirin-containing medicines* must not be taken for 2 weeks prior to surgery.
- Assessment of any *drug allergies* or *sensitivities* known to the patient.
- Assessment of any nonnormotensive patient history that might have an adverse impact on intraoperative and postoperative blood pressure.
- Evaluation of the history of tobacco and its magnitude of use. Patients are advised to avoid tobacco for 2 weeks before and 2 weeks after facelift surgery. (Few do so. Although the surgical literature documents increased risk to healing, to date we have not experienced healing delay in smokers).
- Laboratory assessment of blood profile and coagulation studies. Other laboratory studies obtained are based on the suggestive history, including chest radiographs.
- Preoperative consultation and counseling by the anesthesiologist.
- Exact demonstration for the patient of the position of anticipated incisions (and ultimate scars) by marking the incision sites with a brow pencil.

CHAPTER 11 The Facelift Operation: Principles and Techniques

Goals of the Operation

- Cephalic and lateral positioning of ptotic facial and cervical soft tissues by the development of a large advancement-rotation flap anchored and supported internally by either plication or flap elevation and advancement/imbrication of the fascia of the superficial muscular aponeurotic system (SMAS).
- Creation of a rejuvenated facial appearance that is perceived as a natural nonoperated improvement characterized by well-camouflaged incision scars (Fig 11–6).
- Performance of an *atraumatic,* risk-free operation to promote rapid healing, significant improvement, and a satisfied, happy patient.
- Creation of a stable, lasting result by selecting the proper indicated techniques to correct the individual anatomic deficits present.
- Avoidance of a higher incidence of potential complications as the result of unnecessarily aggressive or nonindicated procedures.

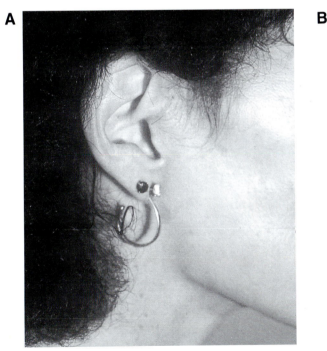
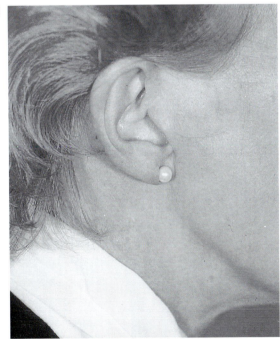

Figure 11–6
A and **B**, properly camouflaged preauricular scars 1 year following a facelift. We prefer the retrotragal placement of the incision whenever possible (most females). Note preservation of the preauricular temporal tuft of hair in the normal position.

Surgical Techniques

- Patients are advised to shampoo and wash the face and neck *gently* with pHisoHex soap the evening before and the morning of surgery, rinsing thoroughly. All makeup must be removed.
- Hair in the area of the incision is never trimmed or shaved; control is achieved through twist-tie bunching of hair segments or by moistening the temporal and postauricular hair with Bacitracin ointment.

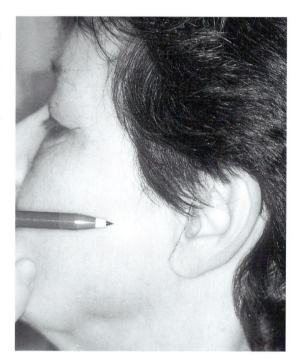

Figure 11–7
Prior to the administration of intravenous analgesia and local anesthesia, planned incisions are marked while the patient is in an *upright position*. Areas of fat to be removed are noted and marked.

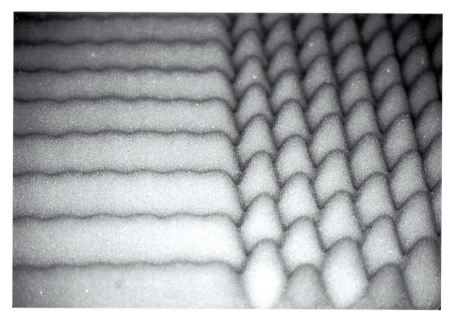

Figure 11–8
The patient is positioned on the operating table and cushioned by a foam mattress with the head elevated slightly. A narrow headrest facilitates easy access to the face and neck.

CHAPTER 11 The Facelift Operation: Principles and Techniques

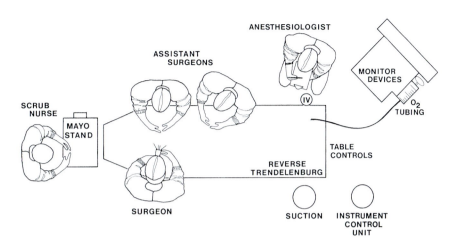

Figure 11–9
The operating room, operative assistants and essential equipment are positioned as indicated. Vital to the smooth, fluid execution of the facelift procedure is the management and coordination of the surgical team. Operating time is reduced, and technical safety is promoted when each member of the operating team participates in a well-orchestrated fashion by providing skin flap countertraction during undermining, securing exacting hemostasis, ensuring facile instrument coordination, and avoiding unnecessary or wasteful maneuvers.

Figure 11–10
Color slides of the patient in various views are projected to greater than life size on the operating room wall for constant reference.

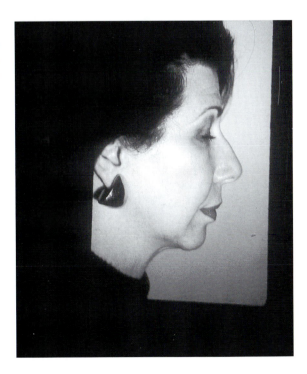

Figure 11–11
The essential instruments useful in facelift surgery.

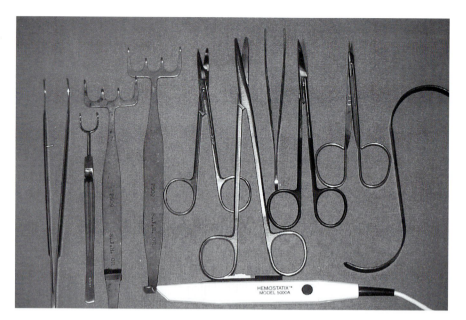

Figure 11–12
A, the Shaw thermal scalpel is considered invaluable because it creates a near-bloodless dissection, facilitating safer *direct-vision surgery* and minimizing surgical trauma and therefore postoperative edema and ecchymosis. **B,** control unit for the Shaw scalpel.

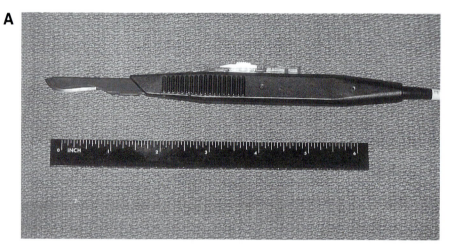

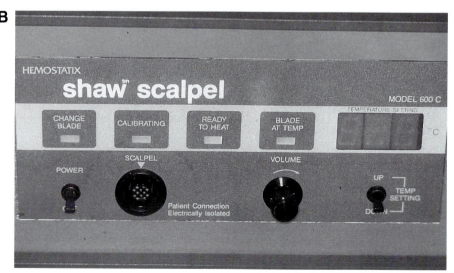

CHAPTER 11 The Facelift Operation: Principles and Techniques

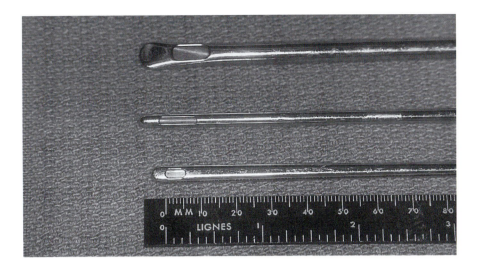

Figure 11–13
Small liposuction cannulas (3, 4, and 5 mm) connected to a strong vacuum are employed primarily to assist in cervical and submental suction lipectomy in selected patients. Removal of abundant submental fat by direct surgical dissection is preferred since we find it more accurate and considerably less traumatic than vigorous suction lipectomy. Facial fat removal, if indicated, is carried out with the Shaw scalpel.

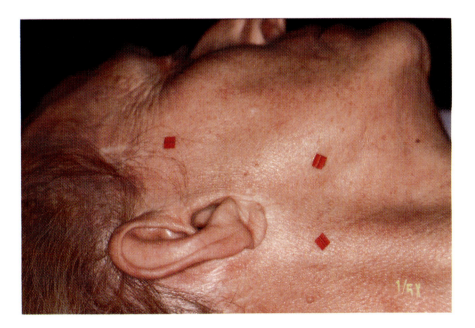

Figure 11–14
Key sites and areas important in facelift surgery are noted here and in Figures 11–15 to 11–25. Vital information and findings include the normal and variant course of the facial nerve branches (especially the frontal and mandibular branches), the anatomy of the tragus and auricular lobule, the variable distance of the postauricular hairline from the auricle, the prominence of the cheek-lip folds, the shape and projection of the mandible, the extent of submental fat, the condition of the submental platysma muscle, and the anatomic position of the hyoid-thyroid complex.

Specific Anatomic Considerations

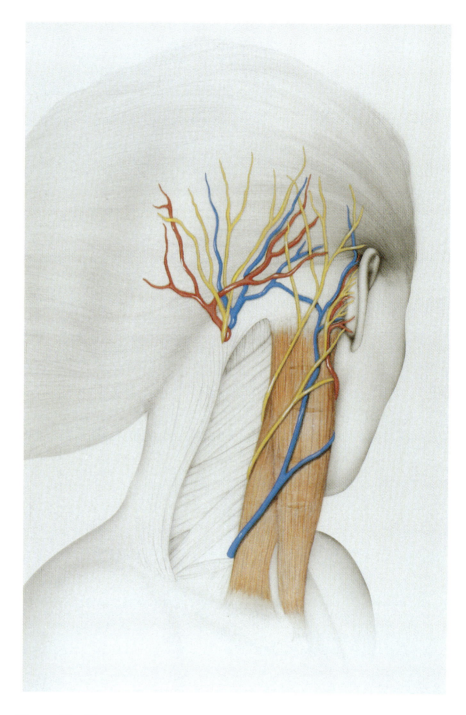

Figure 11–15
The great auricular nerve and the external jugular vein are important structures in the posterior triangle of the neck and postauricular region. To a lesser extent the posterior occipital nerves, artery, and vein may be found in the surgical field.

CHAPTER 11 The Facelift Operation: Principles and Techniques

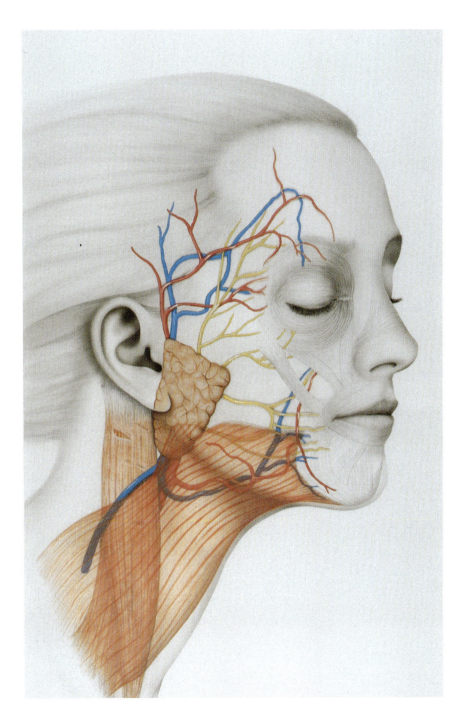

Figure 11–16
Pertinent anatomy of the face and neck in a facelift. The relationship of the facial nerve branches to the parotid gland, facial artery and vein, mandible, and platysma (cut away) are depicted. In aging patients, the marginal mandibular branch may course inferior to the mandible.

Figure 11–17
In the upper part of the face and temple, structures of importance include the superior temporal artery and vein and the frontal branch of the facial nerve.

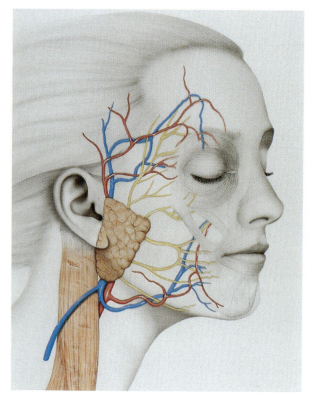

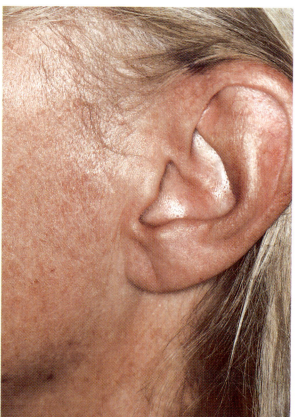

Figure 11–18
The shape, size, and characteristics of the external ear and earlobe, in association with the position and density of the preauricular and postauricular hairline, have an influence on accurate positioning of the various periauricular incisions for facelift surgery.

CHAPTER 11   The Facelift Operation: Principles and Techniques

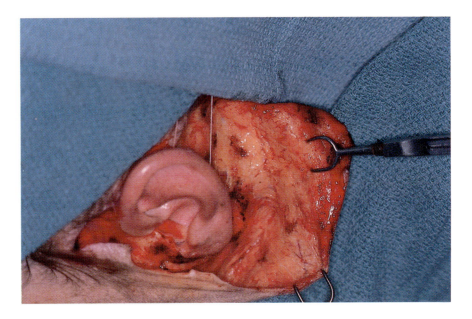

Figure 11-19
The dissection plane of a typical posterior facelift flap preserves this layer of subcutaneous fat on the skin flap to protect the subdermal plexus, while also avoiding the underlying dense fascia covering the sternocleidomastoid muscle. The great auricular nerve is visualized and preserved.

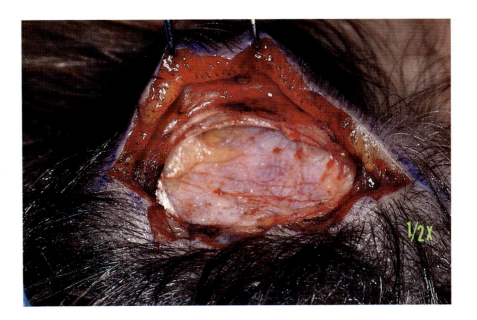

Figure 11-20
The temporal portion of the facelift flap is developed in a deeper tissue plane just superficial to the frontal nerve branch, and the dissection is carried much more superficial to the immediate subcutaneous tissue plane, or an undissected area of tissue is preserved over the frontal branch to protect it from injury.

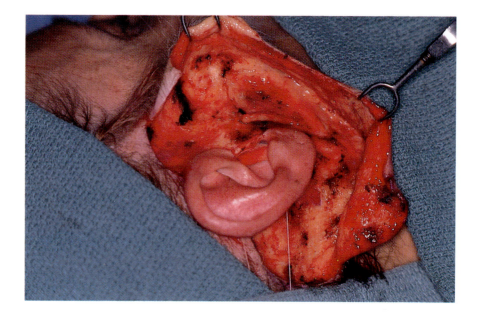

Figure 11-21
The facial flap tissue plane is developed by sharp dissection in the immediate subcutaneous plane, with a thin layer of fat preserved on the skin flap. Countertraction and flap transillumination during dissection facilitate this portion of the operation.

CHAPTER 11 The Facelift Operation: Principles and Techniques

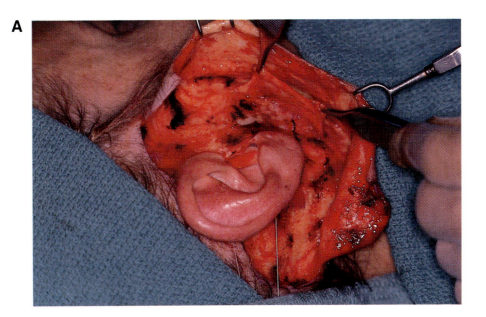

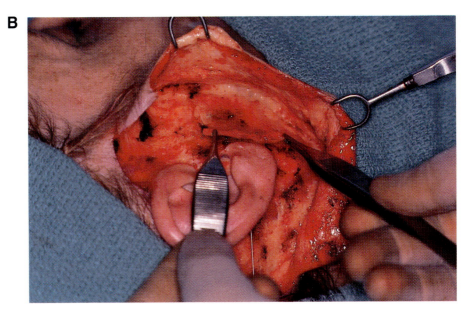

Figure 11-22
A and **B**, depending on individual patient needs, the deeper SMAS-platysma layer is sharply dissected as a distinct and separate fascia layer from the thin fascia protecting the parotid gland. Advancement, rotation, and suture plication or imbrication of this layer exert a strong, effective, and lasting lifting force to facial skin and subcutaneous tissues.

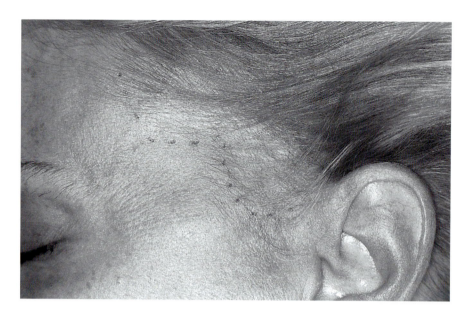

Figure 11–23
In most women a distinct "double tuft" of hair in the temporal and preauricular area is present. Incisions and flap vectors should be carefully planned to preserve this normal anatomy.

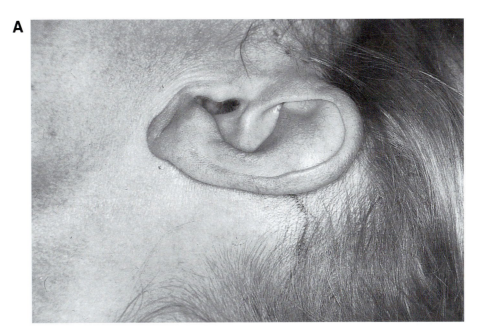

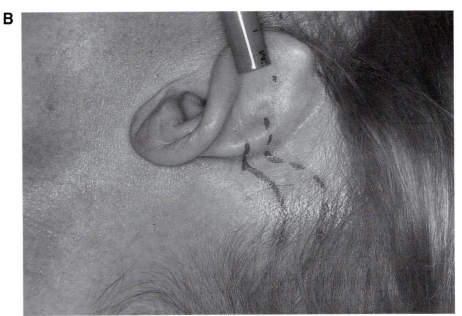

Figure 11-24
A and **B,** the cephalic extent of the postauricular incision will often depend upon the proximity of the postauricular hairline to the auricular helix. As a general principle, the point at which the curving posterior hairline intersects with the margin of the helical rim dictates the cephalic extent of the incision behind the ear (alternatives are shown here).

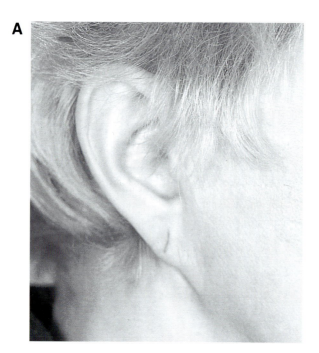
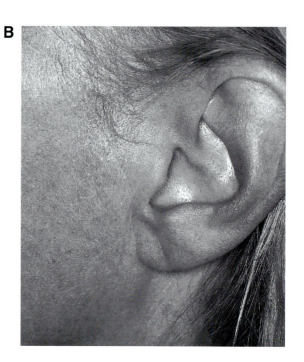

Figure 11–25
A, congenital satyr ear deformity with the absence of a typical, normal earlobe. **B,** more normal earlobe formation with recurving of the lobe into the face.

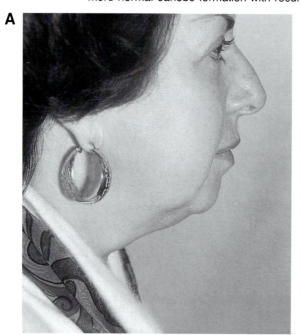
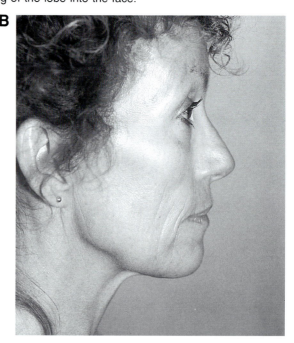

Figure 11–26
A, patient with gravitational aging of the facial-cervical tissues along with an unfavorably low position of the hyoid creating an obliquity of the cervicomental angle that is not totally correctable. **B,** aging face and neck associated with a normal position of the hyoid and minimal submental fat.

CHAPTER 11   The Facelift Operation: Principles and Techniques

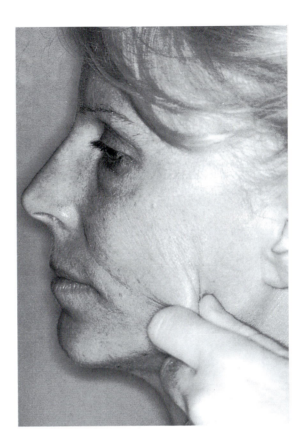

Figure 11-27
Mobility and manual advancement of the SMAS-platysma complex will often determine whether a full SMAS flap dissection is indicated. The quality, mobility, and retained elasticity of the skin along with the amount and location of subcutaneous fat are vital to an ideal surgical outcome.

Logical anatomic arguments have eloquently supported the *development of a separate SMAS-platysma flap in every case;* the tightened fascial flap (or split flaps) is sutured superiorly and posteriorward with the intent of improving both the degree of lifting improvement and the duration of such improvement.

Equally convincing arguments exist in the contemporary plastic surgical literature that extol the virtues of *plication (overlapping)* or *imbrication (edge-to-edge suture fixation) of the SMAS flap elevation;* the increased safety of the latter procedures and equivalent favorable outcomes are cited. Such differing philosophies clearly contain merit and should be thoroughly evaluated by every facelift surgeon.

Our own approach embraces a somewhat middle ground between these two extremes. Clearly it is immediately and ultimately helpful to reposition and tighten the underlying musculoaponeurotic tissues of the face and neck to achieve superior results that will resist gravitational deterioration. Whether SMAS overlapping and tight plication are chosen or whether SMAS flap undermining and elevation are selected *depends on the relative mobility and thickness of the SMAS-platysma complex* (see Fig 11-27).

Anesthesia

Figure 11–28
Beginning in the area of the great auricular nerve (2.5 cm below the earlobe) to establish a regional block, the facial and cervical skin is infiltrated with 1% lidocaine (Xylocaine) containing 1:200,000 epinephrine, freshly mixed to ensure proper proportions and pH. Only the first side is infiltrated, with infiltration of the contralateral portion of the face delayed until 12 to 15 minutes before dissection ensues. Time is thus allowed for the patient to metabolize the initial Xylocaine-epinephrine injection before adding more, thus reducing the risk. Twelve to 15 minutes should elapse before surgical dissection is begun to allow maximum vasoconstriction to develop.

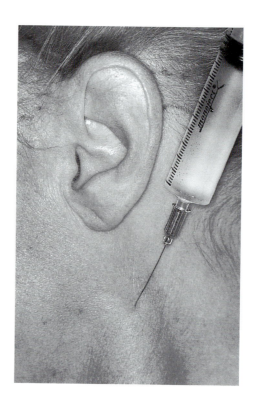

Preferred and Alternative Techniques

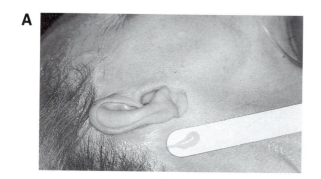
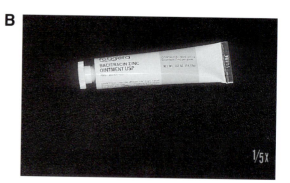

Figure 11–29
A and **B**, control of the hair is effectively accomplished with Bacitracin ointment. No hair is shaved.

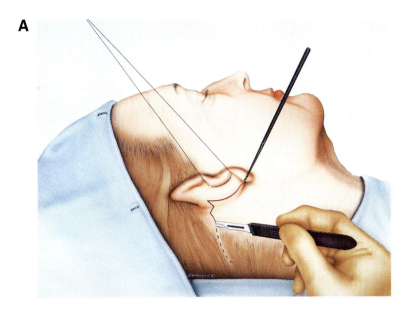

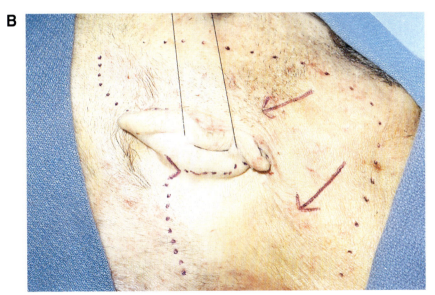

Figure 11-30

A, the right auricle is suspended under tension anteriorly with a temporary postauricular traction suture; countertraction is created inferiorly with a single skin hook positioned in an initial stab incision at the lobule-facial junction. Traction and countertraction applied to the skin flaps throughout the procedure by surgical assistants constitute vital dissection aids to the surgeon by facilitating safe, rapid, and uniform dissection in the preferred tissue planes. This team approach to facelift surgery greatly reduces operative time. **B,** *the postauricular incision* is carried through the skin with a no. 15 blade cephalically from the lobule in the auriculomastoid sulcus to the level of the junction of the postauricular hairline with the helical margin. For patients who will need minimal to up to 2 cm of skin removed in this region as a consequence of the facelift procedure, this incision is ideal. In very lax faces where more than 2 cm of skin will require excision, the hairline will be better preserved if the incision follows the postauricular hairline margin for most of its extent and is then carried into the finer hair above the junction of the hair with the neck skin. The incision next passes posteriorly into the hairline and inferiorly for a distance of 5 to 7 cm. As the incision sweeps posteriorly off the auricle, it is *irregularized* to improve ultimate camouflage and to avoid any possibility of a contracted bowstring scar developing in this anatomic concavity.

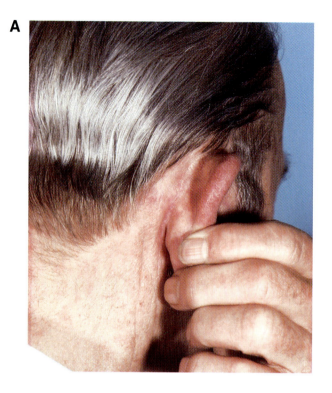

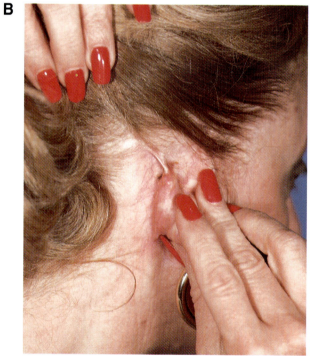

Figure 11-31
A, well-camouflaged scar 1 year following a facelift. The irregularized postauricular incision heals within the auriculomastoid sulcus without "bowstringing." **B,** contracted scar typical of healing of incisions traversing a concavity.

CHAPTER 11 The Facelift Operation: Principles and Techniques

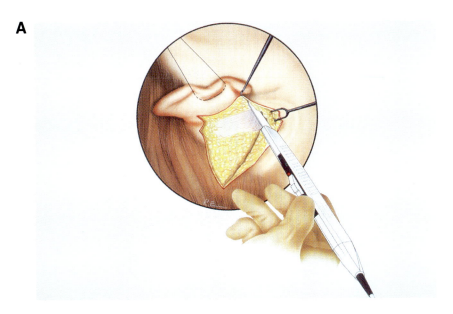

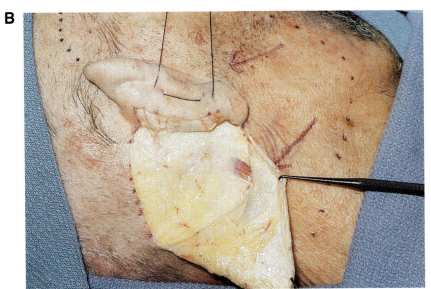

Figure 11–32

A and **B,** with traction provided by two wide double skin hooks suspending the flap skin edges, the postauricular flap is dissected inferiorly and anteriorly into the neck with the Shaw hemostatic scalpel until fibers of the platysma muscle are visualized. Broad, *slow,* sweeping strokes of the scalpel provide ideal dissection and maximal hemostasis. By employing the Millard double thimble-hook, the surgeon assists with traction in the flap margin while palpating the flap thickness with the adjacent ring finger. Near-absolute hemostasis is achieved throughout this dissection, substantially increasing surgical safety and ensuring perfect visualization. The great auricular nerve, often bifurcated or trifurcated, is routinely identified and protected from dissection or suture injury.

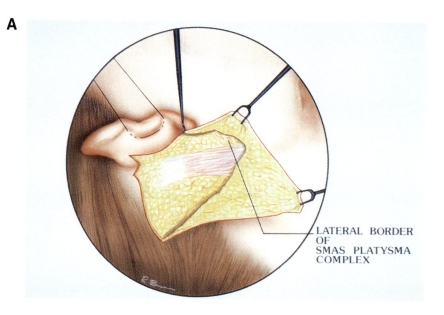
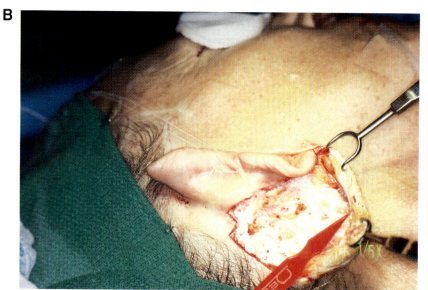

Figure 11-33
A and **B,** the depth of the dissection is quite superficial in this area, just deep to the hair follicles in the hair-bearing scalp and between the skin and the adherent dense fascia protecting the sternocleidomastoid muscle. A thin layer of fat is preserved on the flap undersurface to protect the subdermal plexus blood supply. Dissection continues into the anterolateral neck region to identify the posterolateral border of the platysma *(tip of pointer)* and beyond into the neck as necessary, superficial to the platysma fibers. Often this more anterior plane is amenable to gentle blunt dissection with a moist sponge. Hemostasis is secured and attention now turned to the temple area.

CHAPTER 11 The Facelift Operation: Principles and Techniques

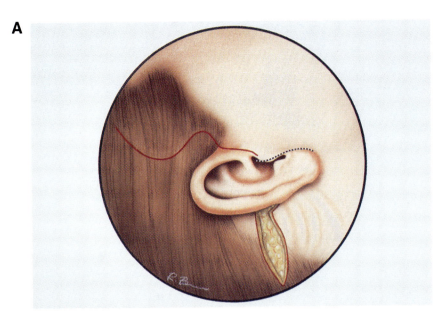

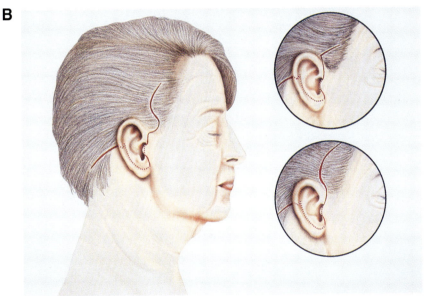

Figure 11–34

A, the *temple incision* varies according to the anatomic needs, hair distribution, and wishes of the patient. If the temporal aesthetic unit is ptotic and in need of lifting, the incision is begun at the junction of the superior helix with the temple and carried slightly posteriorly and upward within the hairline in a gently curved C configuration. Irregularization of the incision is a useful alternative if the hair is sparse. Undermining and elevation of the temporal unit are then ultimately effective in tightening the temporal unit and lateral canthal and brow area but necessarily elevate the temporal hairline to a variable degree. **B,** if the temporal unit needs little or no elevation, the temporal incision courses within the hairline from the superior helical junction obliquely anteriorly within the temporal hair approximately 30 degrees above the horizontal *(top right circled insert)*. This incision allows a triangle of hair-bearing skin to be excised after upward lifting of the face without significantly displacing the preauricular sideburn hair. We prefer to avoid pretrichal incisions in the temporal area.

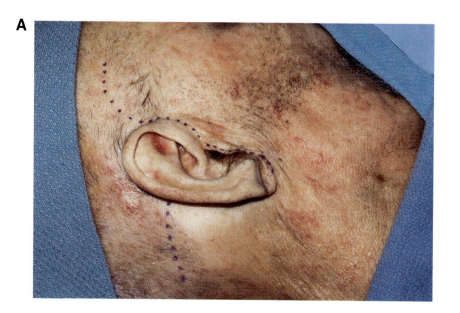

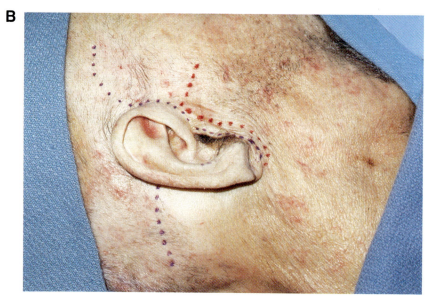

Figure 11-35
A and **B**, alternative facelift incisions utilized after evaluation of the individual hairline encountered and the degree of need for temporal unit elevation. The posttragal incision is preferred in women; in men the presence of the beard precludes the posttragal approach.

CHAPTER 11 The Facelift Operation: Principles and Techniques

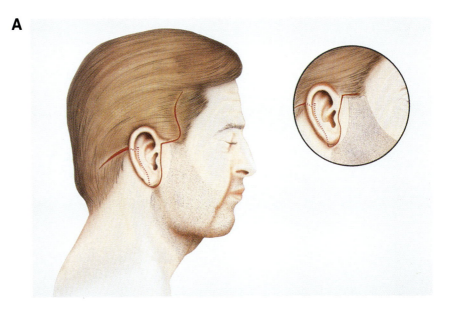

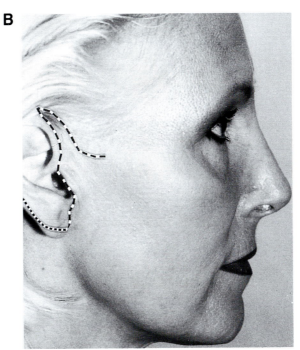

Figure 11-36
A, in men, the presence of the beardline requires modification of the typical facelift incision. At the lobule the incision is sited 2 to 3 mm *below* the lobule-facial junction, while in the preauricular area the incision follows a sinuous skin crease 3 to 5 mm anterior to the tragus. Frequently the cephalic extent of the preauricular incision in the male stops in a horizontal line along the inferior edge of the normal sideburn. **B,** alternative incision of Brennan that is used to preserve the sideburn in the normal position.

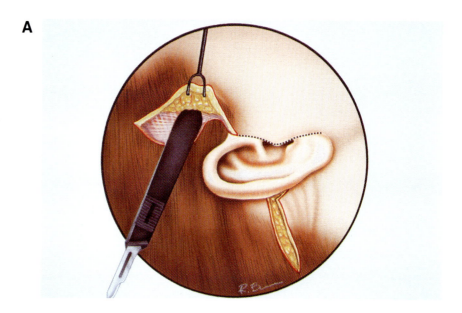
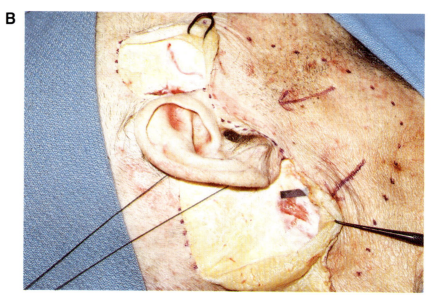

Figure 11-37
A and **B,** if the temporal aesthetic unit is to be elevated and tightened, elevation proceeds with relative ease and with little or no bleeding under direct vision with blunt finger or instrument elevation. The proper plane of elevation is deeper under this flap (just superficial to the dense temporalis fascia), preserves the base of the hair follicles, and traverses a natural loose areolar tissue plane over the fascia encasing the temporalis muscle. The inferior extent of this flap elevation should not violate the adherent tissues overlying the zygomatic arch in order to avoid placing the frontal branch of the facial nerve in jeopardy. It should thus be appreciated that the cheek flap and temporal flap, created in facial planes of different depths, will frequently not be joined in continuity (see Fig 11-40,B), a safety measure that does not limit the aesthetic result obtained unless profound temporal unit laxity exists. In **B** the temporal vessels are prominently displayed in the upper preauricular area.

CHAPTER 11   The Facelift Operation: Principles and Techniques

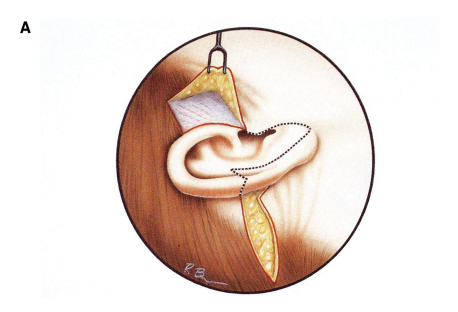

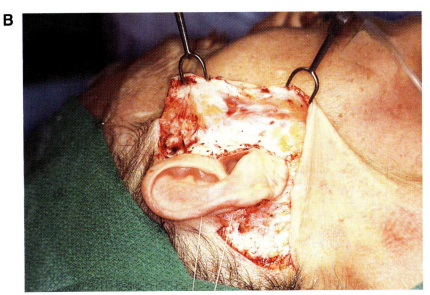

Figure 11–38
A and **B**, if the temporal unit does not require elevation and tightening, an alternative incision inside the temporal hairline is created in an obliquely slanting manner parallel to the direction of the hair follicles and the flap elevated under direct vision, ultimately to be brought into continuity with the elevated cheek flap. Again, this flap should be raised in the loose areolar tissue deep to the hair follicles.

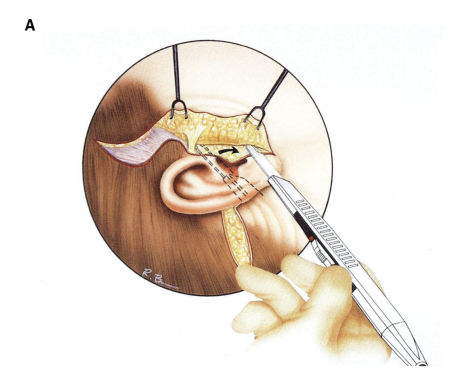
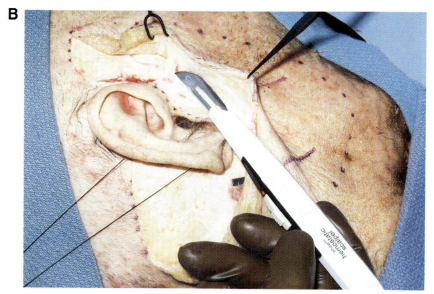

Figure 11-39
A and **B,** the *preauricular incision* curves inferiorly from the superior helix junction into the supratragal notch, courses along or behind the crest of the tragus (except in men), and curves in front of the lobule to join the initial stab incision created at the lobular-facial junction. Sharp, near-bloodless dissection with the Shaw scalpel under direct vision provides extreme safety.

CHAPTER 11 The Facelift Operation: Principles and Techniques

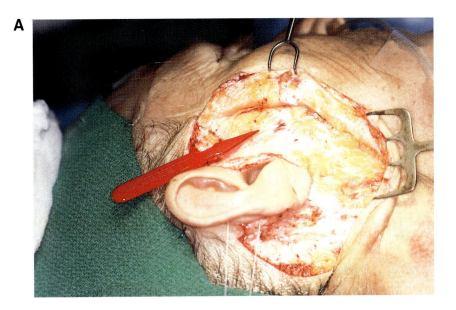

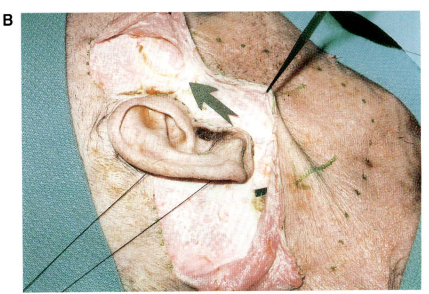

Figure 11–40
A and **B,** elevation of the large facial cheek flap in the midface *under direct vision* now ensues with the Shaw scalpel, with a thin layer of fat preserved on the flap to protect the subdermal plexus and ensure uniform redraping of the elevated skin. Gentle flap retraction by the assistant combined with delicate sharp knife dissection substantially reduces the trauma associated with traditional scissors flap elevation. Vessels perforating the subcutaneous fat layer are often easily visualized in the dry surgical field and may be cauterized with the Shaw scalpel before they are divided. Dissection must be kept superficial in the transition between the temple and cheek flap to protect the frontal branch of the facial nerve, (shown here at the *black arrow*).

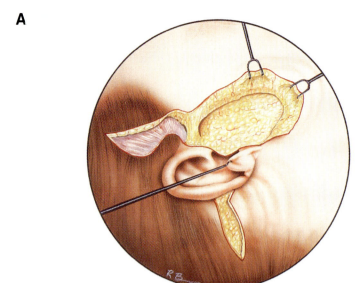
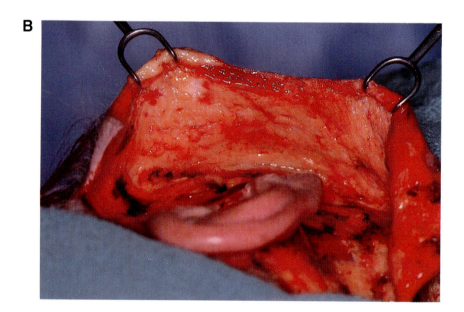

Figure 11–41
A and **B,** finger countertraction of the cheek skin medialward by the assistant facilitates elevation. The characteristic cobblestone appearance of the immediate subcutaneous fat adherent to the flap aids in creating a safe flap thickness. Transillumination with light shone through the flap from the facial side **(B)** is helpful in ensuring dissection of flap of uniform thickness.

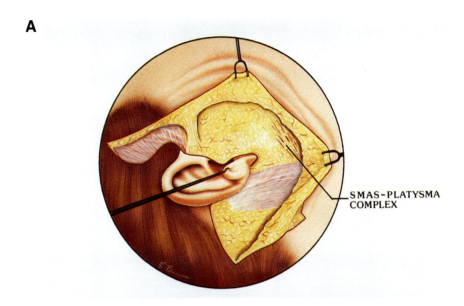

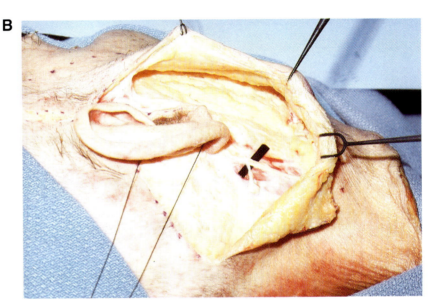

Figure 11–42
A and B, the flap length in the mid and lower parts of the face depends upon individual patient requirements. The anterior extent of the elevation of the cheek flap regularly extends well beyond the anterior border of the parotid gland but seldom beyond the nasolabial fold. With double skin hook traction upon both the cheek and postauricular flaps, the medial extent of undermining is further advanced as planned preoperatively, and the flaps are brought into complete continuity by dividing the bridge of subcutaneous tissue still remaining along the angle of the mandible between the facial and cervical flaps. It should be appreciated that all undermining to this juncture has ensued at a level *superficial to the platysma muscle,* thus protecting the mandibular facial nerve branch. Any excess fat remaining in the surgical bed is next removed with the Shaw scalpel or with open suction lipectomy. Since one phase of the aging process involves the progressive loss of subcutaneous facial fat and unpleasant hollowed skeletonization of the facial features, *we prefer to preserve sufficient facial fat to maintain smooth contouring.* Extensive removal of facial fat is always to be avoided. A trifurcated great auricular nerve is demonstrated in **B.**

Once skin flap undermining and elevation are sufficiently complete, decisions are now necessary regarding management of the *SMAS fascia and platysma muscle,* easily visualized and identified at varying distances in front of the ear. Surgeons of great experience differ markedly in their philosophy of management of the underlying musculocutaneous tissues of the facial skeleton.

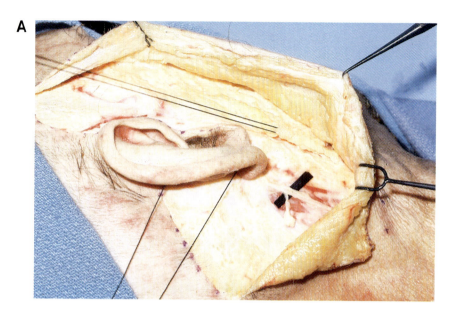
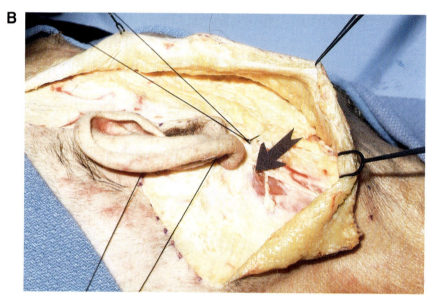

Figure 11–43
A and **B**, in *carefully selected* patients demonstrating easy mobility of the skin and SMAS, the skin flaps are elevated as described above, followed by identification of the SMAS fascia and posterior platysma for tight posterior *suture plication* (overlapping) to the dense fascia overlying the mastoid, sternocleidomastoid, and parotid.

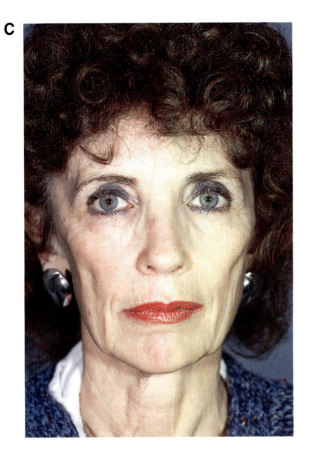
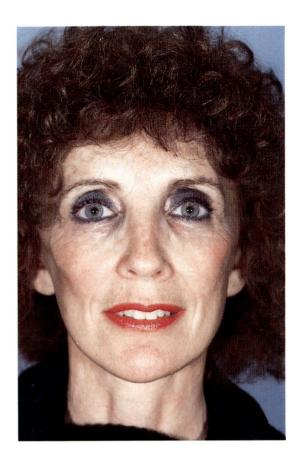

Figure 11–43 (cont.).
C, plication overlapping of lax facial fat and SMAS layer assists in filling hollow mid-cheek areas, effacing unsightly depressions.

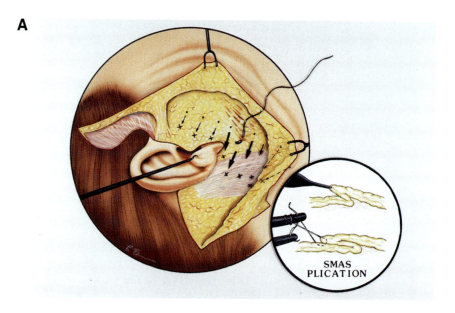

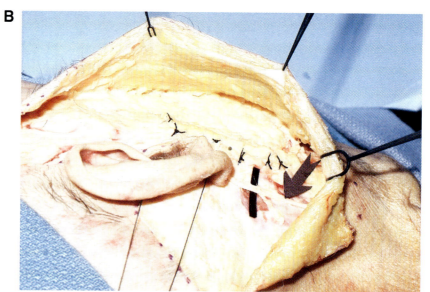

Figure 11-44

A and **B,** Eight to twelve 3-0 white Tevdek sutures are positioned to tightly suspend the fascia and muscle posteriorward and slightly cephalically. Suturing through or around the great auricular filaments must be avoided. We find that this "suspension rhytidectomy" creates improved immediate as well as long-lasting results as long as the SMAS-platysmal layer demonstrates good mobility and "slides" well over the underlying tissues. An effective tightening effect is visible on both the facial and cervical tissues with no concomitant skin tension whatsoever. Therein lies one of the virtues of this procedure: the underlying tissues may be repositioned under considerable tension while the skin flaps, after appropriate tailoring, may be sutured *under no tension at all*. In addition, the undermined subcutaneous tissue space is now diminished to a significant degree, a fact that facilitates rapid healing and diminishes the potential for postoperative bleeding.

Plication produces a further advantage in patients demonstrating early facial fat atrophy and unsightly cheek hollowness. Layering the fat and SMAS-platysmal layer in this fashion can substantially restore a smooth, more youthful cheek appearance. (Fig 11-43,C).

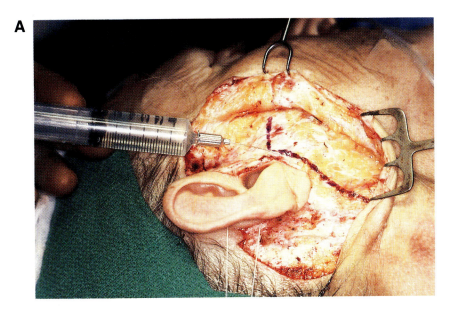

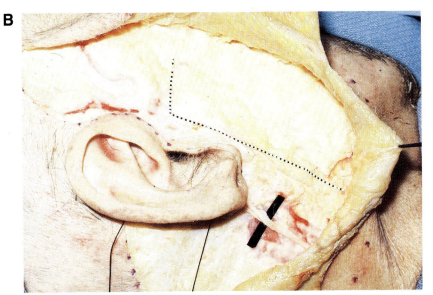

Figure 11–45

A and **B,** in patients possessing more limited skin and SMAS mobility and in the majority of secondary facelifts, *definitive SMAS flaps* are individually elevated, advanced and rotated posteriorly, and trimmed and permanent suture fixation established. Patients selected for this slightly more extensive procedure are those with less than ideal tissue mobility in whom SMAS plication alone is less effective in creating the desired cervicofacial definition. Intraoperative manipulation of the exposed facial fascia will confirm this judgment.

Elevation of a definitive SMAS flap begins by creating a horizontal incision in the SMAS tissues at the lower border of the zygomatic arch for a distance of approximately 3 cm. Additional local anesthetic infiltrated into the SMAS flap will be required to achieve full patient comfort.

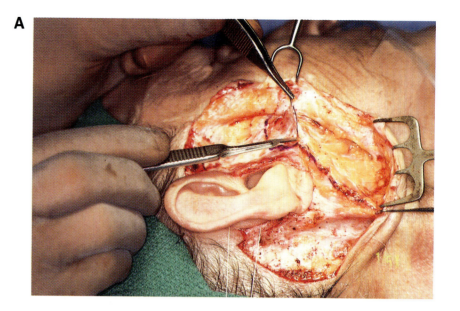

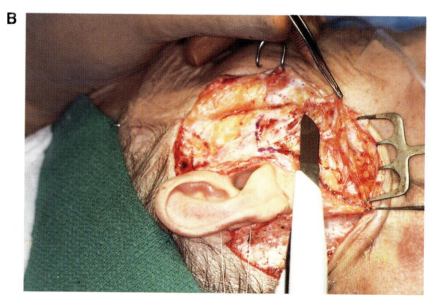

Figure 11-46

A and **B,** a superficial vertical incision 1 cm anterior to the preauricular incision extends from the zygomatic arch inferiorly to 4 to 5 cm below the mandibular border. Vertical inferior traction on the SMAS will then facilitate entry into the sub-SMAS plane with either sharp scissors or Shaw scalpel dissection. If bare parotid gland tissue is exposed, the dissection plane is too deep and must be reinitiated at a more superficial level.

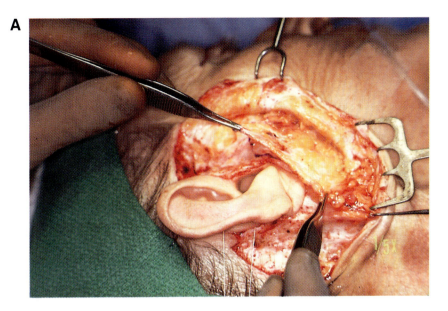

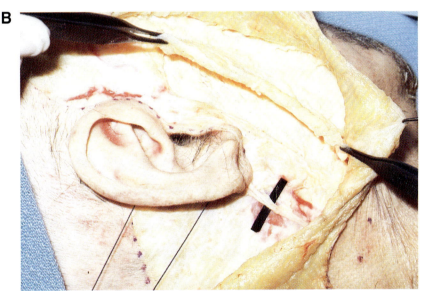

Figure 11–47
A and **B**, once elevated anteriorly for a distance of 1 to 2 cm, further flap development may be achieved with bloodless finger-sponge dissection. Vector forces are then exerted on the SMAS flap in a superior as well as posterior direction. If deemed more effective, the flap may be split near the auricular lobule and the inferior limb sutured onto the mastoid fascia for increased definition of the upper cervical area. The exact vector forces utilized will depend upon the individual anatomy encountered and the perceived effect of flap suspension upon the facial skin flap appearance.

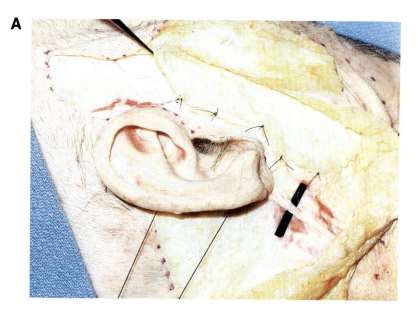

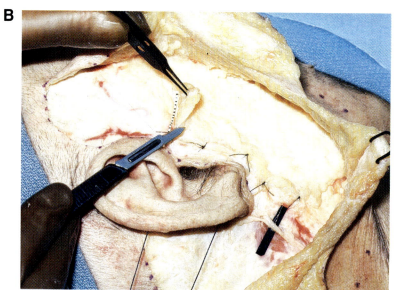

Figure 11-48
A and **B,** the SMAS flap is secured with multiple 3-0 white Tevdek sutures, the excess overlap trimmed, and edge-to-edge suture repair completed. The SMAS flap may be split horizontally at the mandibular border, with the inferior segment of the flap sutured to the mastoid fascia.

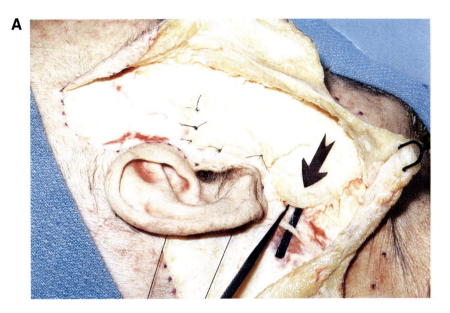
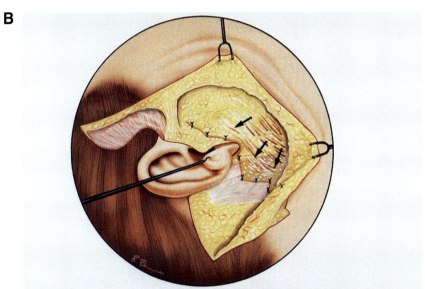

Figure 11-49
A and **B,** suture imbrication of the SMAS flap with multiple sutures exerts a profound lifting and tightening force on the facial and cervical skin and reduces the subcutaneous dead space significantly.

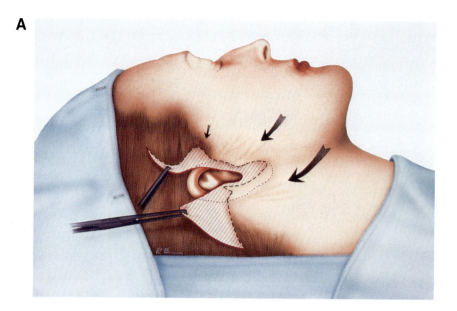

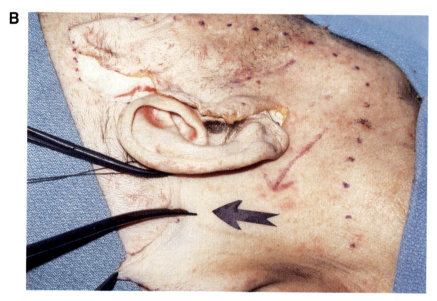

Figure 11–50

A and **B,** once undermining of the flaps is complete and suture repositioning of the deeper tissues has created satisfactory support and lifting effect, the skin flaps are placed on traction and the vector forces of skin flap repositioning assessed. It is obvious that if the flaps are rotated too cephalically, the sideburn and temporal hairline will be abnormally elevated. If the flap vector forces are simply advanced predominantly posteriorly with little or no upward rotation, then minimal lifting effect will be realized, particularly in the cheek and face. This dilemma is one of the *surgical compromises* peculiar to facelift surgery: an appropriate degree of both lateral advancement and cephalic rotation must be sought to provide the most improvement without distortion of the patient's hairline and facial features.

CHAPTER 11   The Facelift Operation: Principles and Techniques

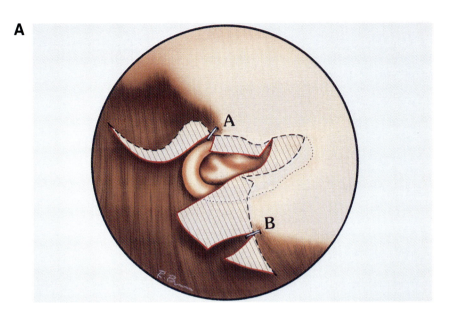

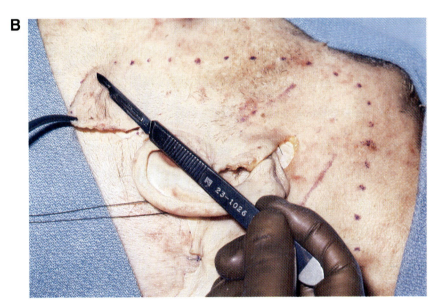

Figure 11–51
A and **B,** once this judgment is made, the skin is positioned *under no tension,* and the flap is incised to the limits of the scalp incision in two key positions: the first posteriorly at the junction of the scalp hairline with the non–hair-bearing expanse of postauricular skin and the second just above the helix of the ear in the temple incision.

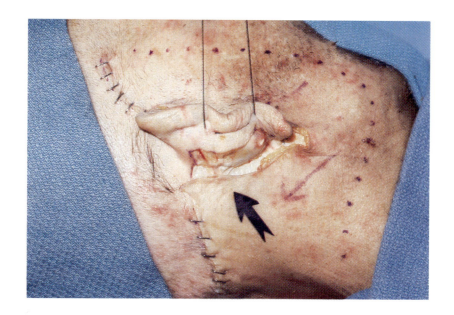

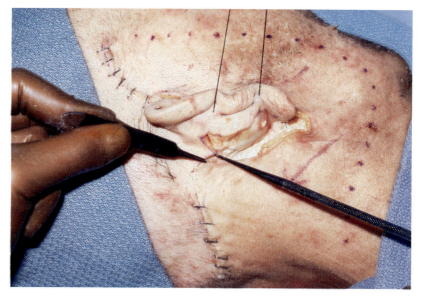

Figure 11–52
The flap is secured at each of these two initial fixation points in the hairline with a stainless steel surgical staple. The face is observed for smoothness without tension and the midportion of the flap incised obliquely down to the anterior aspect of the earlobe. Since the lobe has not been displaced by total division from the underlying facial tissues, recreation of the precise preoperative anatomic site of the lobular-facial junction is facilitated. A single key suture then secures this newly created junction, which should rest comfortably in the "sling" or "hammock" of the newly positioned facial flaps to avoid any later downward displacement. Lobular distortion following a facelift is an extremely significant and understandable source of patient distress. Where indicated or requested, however, the earlobe may be diminished or repositioned to achieve a more normal appearance.

The redundant and excessive skin in the hair-bearing portions of the flaps is now excised, hemostasis ensured, and closure effected in the hair-bearing areas with surgical staples. By advancing the posterior hair-bearing edge of the incision forward and upward the posterior hairline is matched up edge to edge for normal alignment. Because of the tension-reducing effect of the underlying deeper structure plication, the skin flaps may simply be gently approximated under *no* tension to facilitate rapid healing with well-camouflaged fine scars.

The majority of the skin in the immediate postauricular region is advanced *anteriorly (black arrow)* and preserved in order to recreate the auriculomastoid sulcus; repair in the postauricular area is effected with interrupted 5-0 collagen catgut sutures, which require no removal. The curving transverse incision in the hairless skin from the auricle to the postauricular hairline (including the inferior dart created in the sulcus) may be closed with fine suture or tissue glue or simply "steri-stripped" for the ultimate in camouflage. Staples should not be placed in this hairless skin.

CHAPTER 11 The Facelift Operation: Principles and Techniques

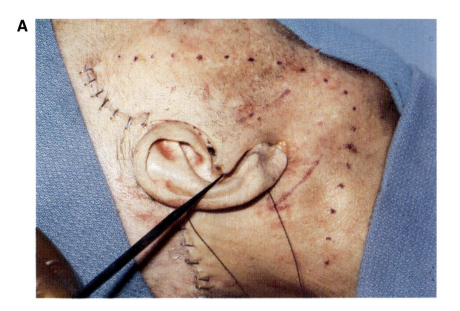

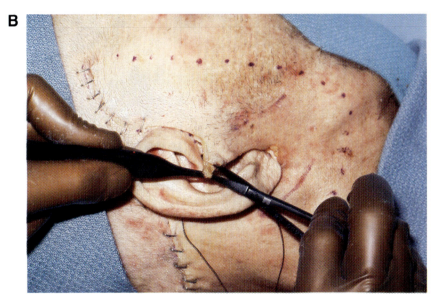

Figure 11–53
A and **B,** finally, careful attention is paid to the trimming and fine suture of the preauricular and retrotragal incision. Before proceeding with anterior flap tailoring and final suturing, time is taken to infiltrate local anesthetic into the contralateral side of the face to allow a sufficient period for vasoconstriction. A small but adequate flap of anterior flap skin is now fashioned to fit comfortably into the retrotragal incision, and the remainder of the anterior flap is assiduously tailored and defatted. The immediate pretragal region is defatted and tailored to restore the normal concavity found in the pretragal region of an unoperated patient.

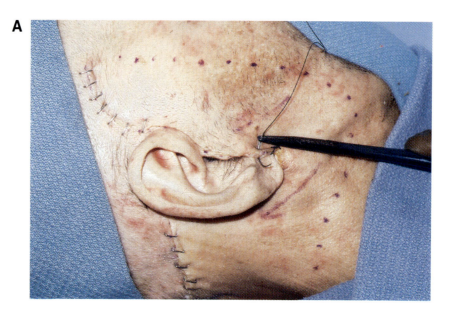
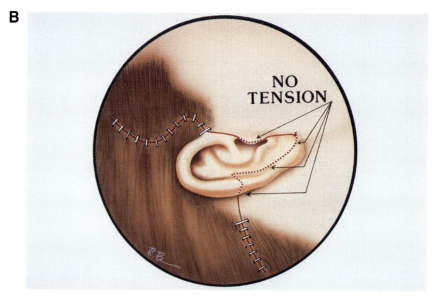

Figure 11–54
A and **B,** ideally the opposing edges of the skin should fall together easily and actually "push" each other slightly to effect the best possible scar camouflage. Preauricular incision closure ensues with a 6-0 blue Prolene continuous suture. Absolutely no tension should be present at the skin closure site.

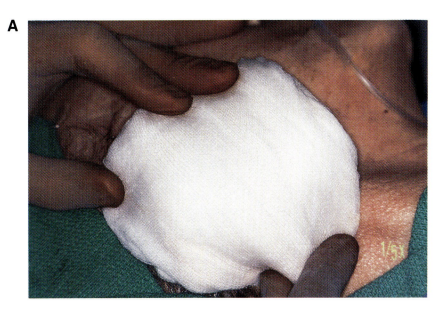
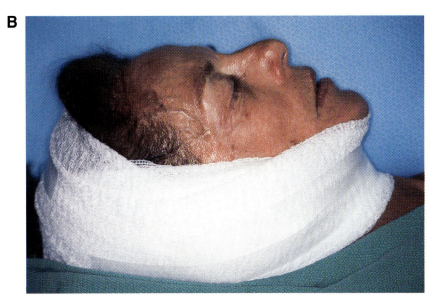

Figure 11–55
A and **B,** after insertion of a small Penrose drain into the postauricular incision (removed the next day), the wound margins are meticulously cleaned, anointed with NeoDecadron ophthalmic ointment, dressed with Adaptic gauze and moist 4 × 4-in. gauze fluffs, and supported with circumferential Kerlex gauze bandage. Tension and tightness of the bandage are unnecessary and undesirable.

If submental suction lipoplasty, direct fat excision, and/or platysmal band correction are required, it is best accomplished *before* the SMAS and skin flaps are suture-suspended since the latter maneuvers tighten the submental area markedly, reduce skin mobility, and allow little room to operate effectively.

Facial fat excision by direct removal or suction lipectomy techniques must be *conservative*, with strong emphasis placed on the *preservation* of a generous cushioning fat layer rather than aggressive (or excessive) fat removal.

Postoperative care is critical in facelift patients, with attention to relative immobility of the head and neck and bed rest for 24 hours and ensuring that normotensive blood pressure levels exist. Nausea must be prevented or promptly treated to avoid vomiting or retching. Anything other than mild discomfort is unusual in the early postoperative period. True pain is an infrequent complaint that varies with the motivation and pain threshold of the individual patient. Mild non–aspirin-containing analgesics are ordinarily sufficient to ensure comfort in the first 48 hours. Significant pain should alert the surgeon to the possibility of expanding hematoma development.

In the early postoperative period the following must be observed:

- The circumferential head dressing is replaced the morning following surgery with a smaller dressing maintained for 2 additional days to immobilize and "splint" the facial structures.
- Incisions are kept moist with NeoDecadron ophthalmic ointment twice daily for 1 week to eliminate crusting and hasten scar maturation.
- Oral antibiotics (cefaclor, 250 mg three times daily) are provided for 5 days.
- Gentle shampooing to cleanse the hair is allowed 48 to 72 hours following surgery.
- Physical activities (lifting, straining, sudden head motion) must be avoided for 1 week and then reinstituted only gradually.
- Suture removal commences at 6 to 8 days; staple removal occurs at 10 to 12 days.

CHAPTER 11   The Facelift Operation: Principles and Techniques

Results and Outcome

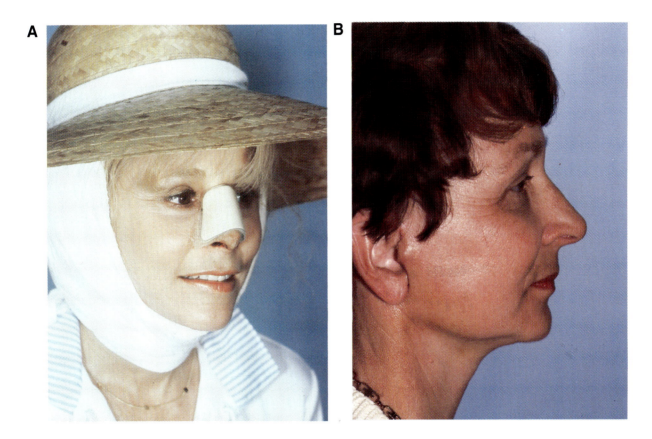

Figure 11–56
A, a patient 3 days after facelift and rhinoplasty demonstrates minimal edema and the ecchymosis typical when sharp dissection is performed with the Shaw hemostatic scalpel, which helps to limit intraoperative bleeding and thus postoperative bruising. **B,** patient 1 week following a facelift with minimal edema.

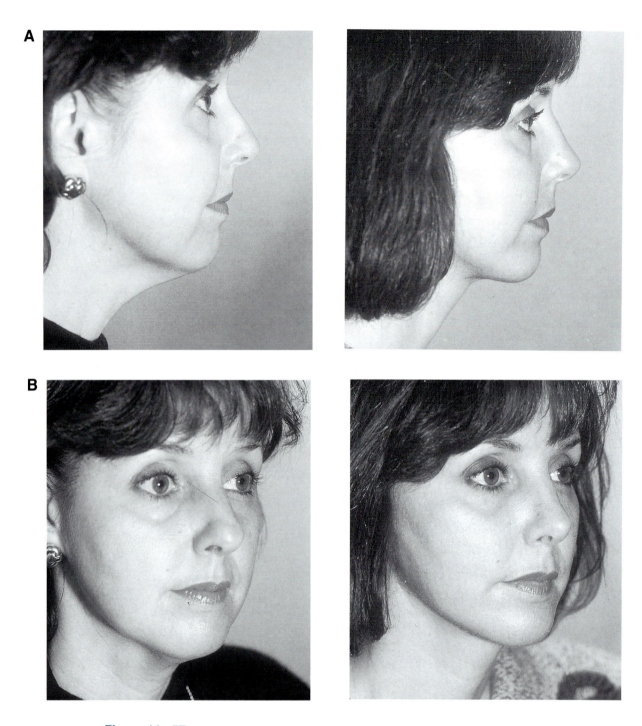

Figure 11–57
A and **B**, excess submental skin with an aging cervicomental obliquity primarily concerned this patient. Correction is dramatic in the lower part of the face and neck 6 months after a cheeklift plus necklift.

CHAPTER 11 The Facelift Operation: Principles and Techniques

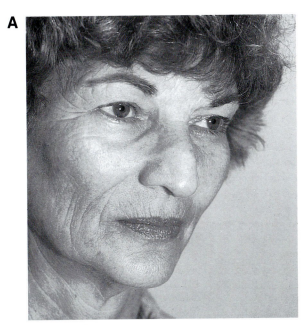
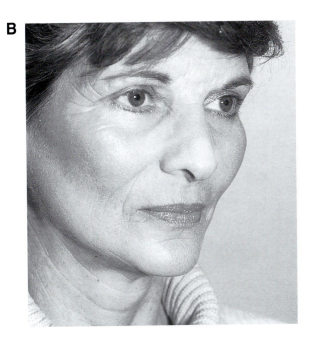

Figure 11–58
Significant sun damage to facial orbital and cervical skin poses limitations to rejuvenation in this older patient. An extended-flap facelift improves the facial appearance considerably, but deeply etched rhytids will always persist. The favorable outcome at 1 year is enhanced by blepharoplasty, a temporal-lift, and rhinoplasty. The patient's inherently good skeletal structure is revealed to great advantage following the rejuvenation procedures.

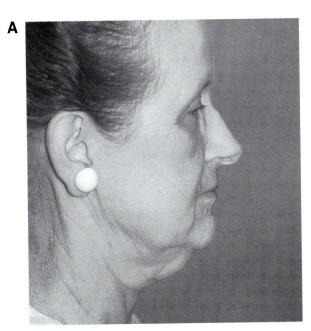
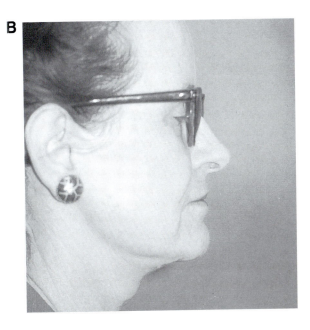

Figure 11–59
Individual who has long since passed the ideal time for facelift improvements. Significant weight loss through a strict diet has reduced facial-cervical fat predominance and left a marked excess of inelastic submental and cervical skin. An extended flap facelift creates significant improvement when combined with direct submental lipectomy, shown here 1½ years later. When significant cervical skin excess requires removal of more than 3 cm of skin postauricularly, the inferior descent of the postauricular incision is best placed at the hairline margin preperiorally and faded in the finer hair inferiorly, thus avoiding the creation of a large hairless region within the hairline.

In patients with markedly excess submental skin, a small excision of submental skin may additionally be necessary.

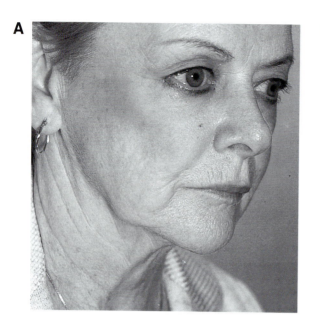
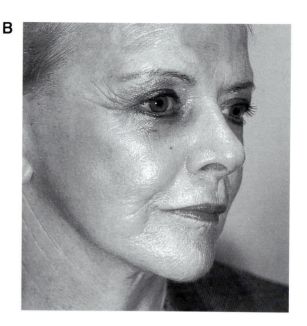

Figure 11–60
Improved appearance 1 year following a facelift and blepharoplasty. Deeply etched rhytids will persist, but the overall appearance and facial expression are favorable.

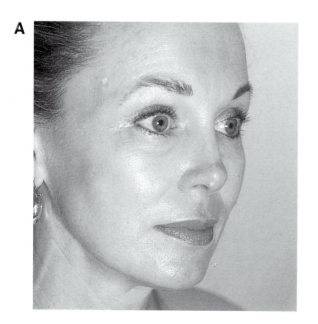
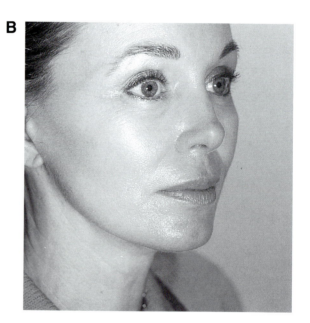

Figure 11–61
Many individuals prefer to correct aging characteristics before more profound changes occur. This logical form of "guardian maintenance" is highly useful; a long-term plan for maintaining a favorable, more youthful appearance can be established and rejuvenation procedures carried out at intervals as required and requested. Careful planning and conservation should dominate this theme in order that the surgeon not "burn any bridges" during the earlier lifting procedures.

CHAPTER 11   The Facelift Operation: Principles and Techniques

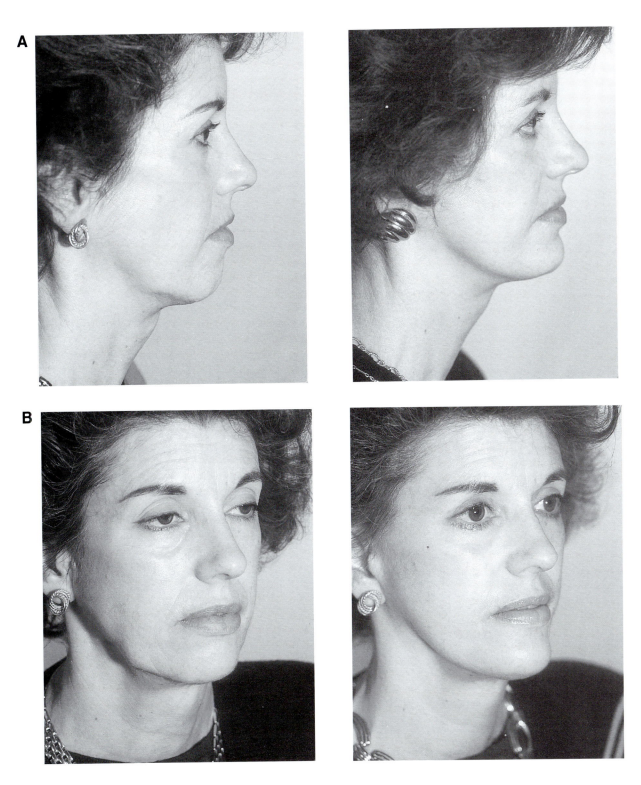

Figure 11–62
A and **B**, lifting procedures carried out earlier in the aging process tend to result in a longer lasting result because tissues are still strong and the skin still elastic. At 3 years, the patient shown here has maintained the favorable appearance created by a facelift with chin augmentation.

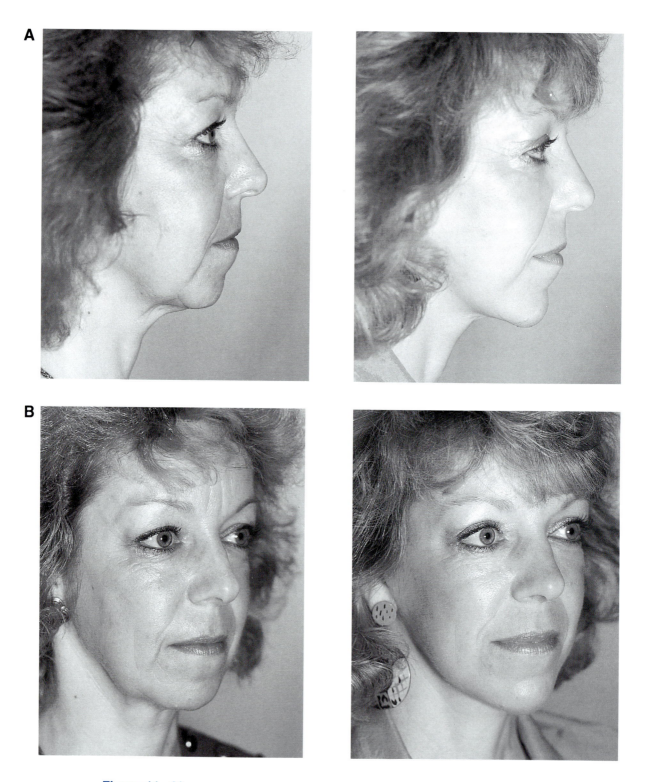

Figure 11-63
A and B, ideal facelift candidate with a natural, improved appearance result after a facelift, blepharoplasty, and augmentation mentoplasty.

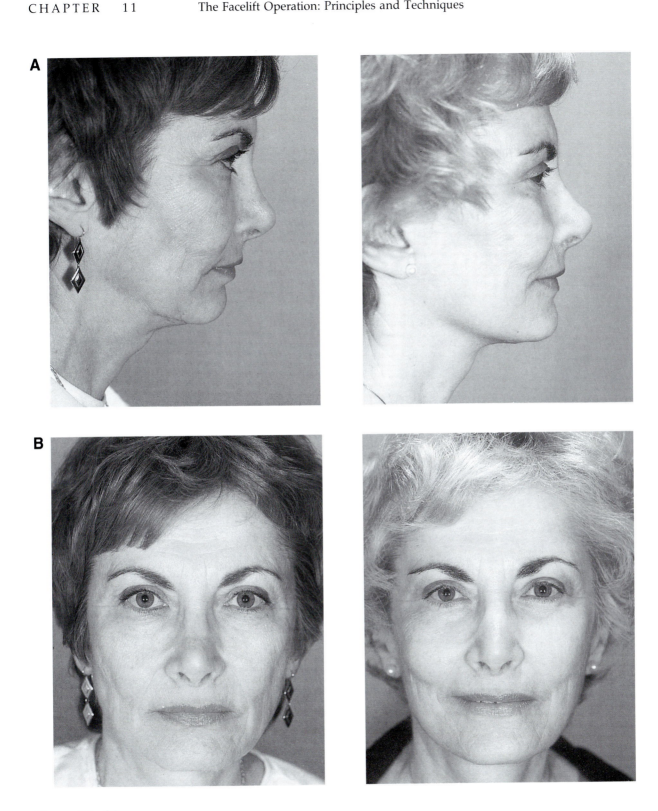

Figure 11-64
A and **B,** the presence of a favorable bone structure qualifies this patient as an excellent candidate for lifting procedures in the lower portion of the face and neck. One year following surgery utilizing SMAS plication, the result is natural with restoration of a cleaner neck and jawline. Scar camouflage is favorable.

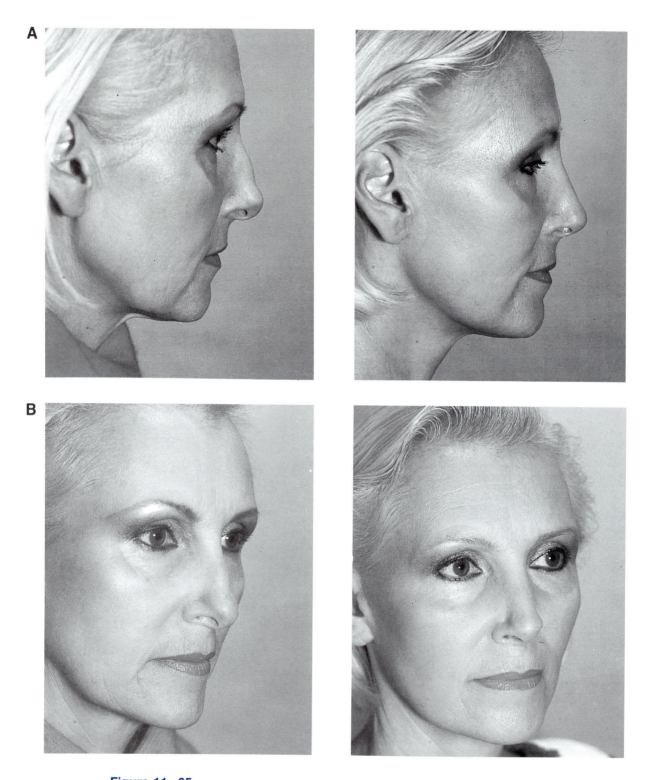

Figure 11–65
A and B, elegant skin quality and excellent bone structure exist in this ideal candidate. The favorable result, shown at 1 year, has been enhanced by rhinoplasty characterized by profile reduction and correction of an overly convex columella.

CHAPTER 11 The Facelift Operation: Principles and Techniques

Sequelae and Complications

Sequelae of facelift surgery include the following:

- *Fine scars* camouflaged in the hairline, preauricular creases, retrotragal area, and infralobular region.
- *Hypoesthesia* (temporary) in the regions undermined or deprived of sensory innervation as a consequence of skin incisions.
- *Bruising* in varying degrees for the early postoperative period.
- *Facial swelling,* which resolves in 1 to 2 weeks after surgery (the latter two consequences of surgery are substantially diminished or eliminated when the Shaw hemostatic scalpel is employed).
- *Pain* following a facelift should be minimal or nonexistent. Patients may complain of moderate soreness in the postauricular or nuchal area for 24 to 36 hours, but thereafter anodynes are seldom required or requested. A significant pain complaint should prompt immediate investigation for possible hematoma formation.

Significant *complications* of facelift surgery are fortunately infrequent. The following are the most important:

Hematoma

An expanding hematoma in the first several hours following a facelift is a true surgical emergency (Fig 11-66,A-C). Very properly referred to as a "malignant" hematoma, prompt recognition and treatment significantly diminish any possibility of poor healing with loss of tissue. Even the most skillful surgeons undertaking rhytidectomy will experience some incidence of postoperative hematoma; how well these problems are managed is a true reflection of the surgeon's expertise.

Attentive care in the first 6 to 8 hours following a facelift is vital since most hematomas of consequence occur within this time frame. All personnel caring for facelift patients must be aware of the hallmark signs heralding hematoma formation: *pain, nausea, agitation, swelling, and blood pressure elevation.* Bleeding is not always a reliable indicator. Although some annoying postoperative discomfort (usually postauricularly) is common, true pain following a facelift indicates hematoma with progressive tissue swelling until proved otherwise. Immediate evaluation of the facial flap condition by a knowledgeable observer is mandatory (the nurse or resident inexperienced with facelift patients should be instructed to inspect the lips and lateral buccal region of the oral cavity—*bluish discoloration, hardness, and lip eversion* are sure physical signs that rapid emergent intervention is indicated (Fig 11-66,B). Bandages should be removed and immediate return to the operating room for hematoma evacuation and control of bleeding points carried out without delay lest flap blistering, edema, and necrosis ensue (Fig 11-66). Delaying or temporizing the decision to intervene places the facelift flap in extreme jeopardy. Promptly and adequately treated, patients experiencing a hematoma should have no serious long-term compromise of a satisfactory facelift outcome.

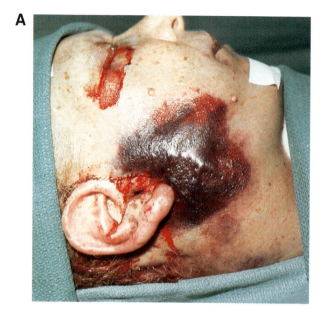
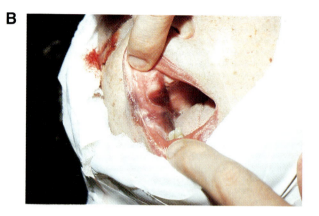
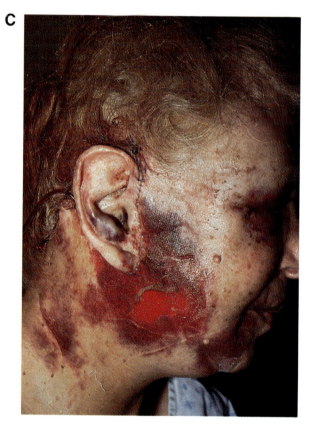

Figure 11–66

A, expanding hematoma developing abruptly 6 hours following a secondary facelift procedure by the senior author during which very little bleeding occurred (the usual circumstance in revision or secondary lifts). Hematoma onset was heralded by abrupt pain, facial swelling, bleeding onto the bandage, and lip edema. Note the skin blistering and epithelial injury occurring within minutes of the onset of "malignant" hematoma. **B,** in expanding hematomas the hallmark sign of buccal bruising from a hematoma is pathognomonic. All personnel caring for facelift patients should be familiar with this finding in order that prompt action can be taken. **C,** skin appearance 1 day after hematoma evacuation and control of the bleeding (single pumping arterial vessel from the identified or bleeding source). Superficial epithelium has sloughed, but healing was uneventful with no loss of full-thickness skin, and the outcome was favorable.

CHAPTER 11 The Facelift Operation: Principles and Techniques

In the majority of patients incisional anesthesia of the facelift flap permits hematoma evacuation under only mild intravenous sedation and minimal local anesthetic infiltration. Control of pain and blood pressure elevation improves the overall status of the patient while a search for the bleeding vessels is instituted. Evacuation of the hematoma followed by irrigation with sterile saline and hydrogen peroxide permits identification and control of the offending vessels. A complete view of the operative field under strong lighting is essential.

Once the hematoma is evacuated and bleeding controlled, suture closure of the skin margins ensues exactly as before. Drainage is instituted, but any pressure dressing is contraindicated. Modest postoperative sedation is usually comforting to the patient. Although edema and ecchymosis will be of a longer duration on the hematoma side, the ultimate result is usually uncompromised.

Hematomas occurring late in the postoperative course (after several days) are usually small in volume and localized (Figs 11–67 and 11–68) and present no emergent problem for treatment or danger to the flap integrity. Suction-aspiration in the office with a large-gauge needle or small 2-mm liposuction cannula may hasten resolution of the process and avoid delayed healing. In such patients hyperpigmentation of the overlying skin may persist for several months. Since employment of the Shaw hemostatic scalpel for facelift flap elevation in the past 12 years, the senior author has experienced less than a 1% incidence of early postoperative hematoma. Meticulous intraoperative hemostasis combined with patient stability and comfort provided by outstanding anesthesia colleagues facilitates this innocuous postoperative experience.

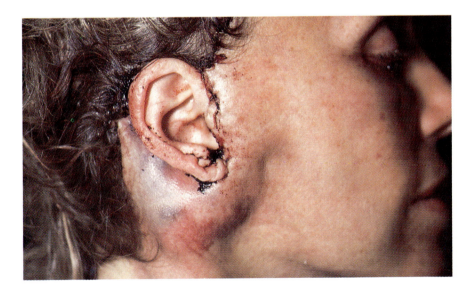

Figure 11–67
Small hematoma developing after excess patient exertion 6 days following facelift surgery. At this stage suction-aspiration resulted in early healing without complication.

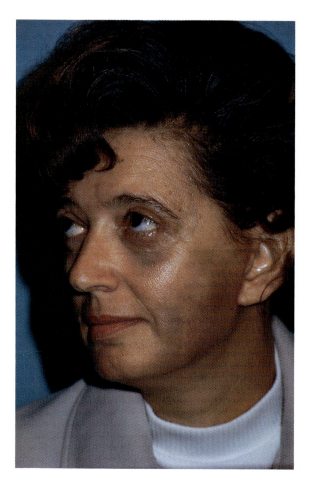

Figure 11-68
Midface hematoma that developed abruptly 11 days after facelift surgery during excessive exertion. No treatment was necessary; the condition resolved quickly with favorable surgical results.

Infection

Localized infection following a facelift is rare; only two such patients have been encountered in two decades. Both responded rapidly to wound drainage without intervention and oral antibiotic therapy with cephalosporin. Infection is usually heralded by localized pain, swelling, redness, fluctuation, and wound drainage. Palpation and inspection confirm the diagnosis. Since ordinarily no wound drainage occurs after 48 hours following a facelift, drainage reported by the patient thereafter should raise the suspicion of an actual or impending infectious process. Facelift surgery should be deferred in any patient demonstrating active external otitis until the infection is completely controlled. We have not experienced infection (or impaired flap circulation) in diabetic patients following facelift surgery, although caution should clearly be exercised in these patients to ensure adequate blood supply to the facelift flap by maintaining a thicker flap during dissection.

Nerve Damage

All patients experience hypoesthesia for 4 to 12 weeks following facelift surgery; sensation loss for longer periods may indicate division or ligation of a portion of the great auricular nerve. Large and occasionally bifid or even trifid, the great auricular nerve is easily identified and preserved during posterior flap elevation. It is probably more commonly injured by monopolar electrocautery or suture ligation during advancement of SMAS tissues. In time hypoesthesia and dysesthesia generally diminish or disappear completely. A difference in sensation in the two sides of the face is always a source of great concern to patients and correctly so.

Motor nerve damage to the facial nerve branches is reported to occur most frequently to the marginal mandibular and frontotemporal branches (Fig 11–69), although injuries to the buccal branch have been reported. To date, we have experienced no facial nerve injuries following facelift surgery. Flap elevation in proper tissue planes, meticulous hemostatic surgery under direct vision, and blunt dissection in areas of known danger to the facial nerve should provide complete protection for this vital structure. Before a facelift, particularly before revision surgery, surgeons should inspect the face carefully for pre-existent weakness or asymmetry of the muscles of facial expression and document them clearly with photographs in repose as well as in animation.

Figure 11–69
Unilateral forehead paralysis resulting from surgery performed elsewhere—4 months postoperatively.

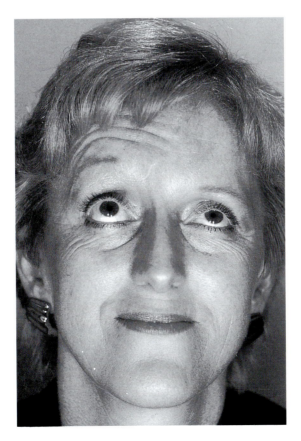

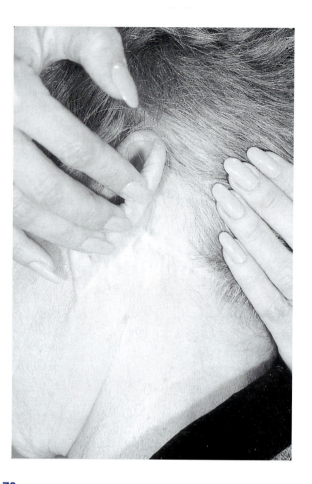

Figure 11–70
Poorly positioned postauricular scars in a patient requesting revision surgery. The incision has been placed far too caudally; permanent suture marks further compromise adequate scar camouflage.

Depression

Although the vast majority of patients fare exceptionally well during the early postoperative period, particularly those who have been well prepared for the minor annoyances of healing, it is not uncommon for an occasional patient to have a transition period of mild depression (similar to the classic "postpartum blues" phenomenon). Strong psychological support by the health care team and family is vital during this period while a favorable self-image returns as the benefits of surgery emerge. As facial ecchymosis and edema fade, mild depression routinely gives way to pleasant satisfaction in the vast majority of *carefully selected* patients.

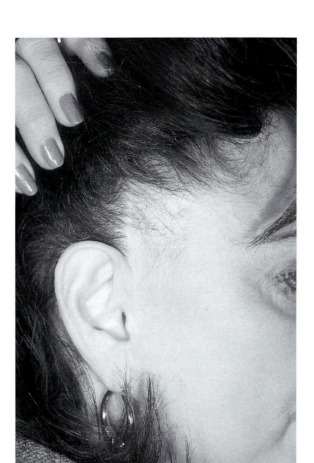

Figure 11–71
Distortion of the temporal and preauricular hairline in a patient requesting corrective surgery. Apparent alopecia further compromises scar camouflage.

Poor Scars

Widened, depressed or even hypertrophic scars are possible after facelift procedures (Fig 11–70 and Fig 11–71), but are rare if the aforementioned principles are respected.

Suggested Reading

- Adamson JE, Toksu AE: Progress in rhytidectomy by platysma-SMAS rotation and elevation. *Plast Reconstr Surg* 1981;68:23.
- Anderson JR: The tuck-up operation: A new technique of secondary rhytidectomy. *Arch Otolaryngol* 1975; 101–739.
- Aston SJ: Platysma muscle in rhytidectomy. *Ann Plast Surg* 1979;3:529.
- Baker DC: Complications of cervicofacial rhytidectomy. *Clin Plast Surg* 1983;10:543.
- Baker DC, Conley J: Avoiding facial nerve injuries in rhytidectomy. *Plast Reconstr Surg* 1979;64:781.
- Baker TJ, Gordon HL: Rhytidectomy in males. *Plast Reconstr Surg* 1969;44:218.
- Baker TJ, Gordon HL: *Surgical Rejuvenation of the Face.* St Louis, Mosby–Year Book, 1985.
- Connell BF: Cervical lift: Surgical correction of fat contour problems combined with full width platysma muscle flap. *Aesthetic Plast Surg* 1978;1:355.
- Courtiss EH: *Male Aesthetic Surgery.* St Louis, Mosby–Year Book, 1982.
- Davis RA, et al: Surgical anatomy of the facial nerve and parotid gland based upon a study of 350 cervicofacial halves. *Surgery* 1956;102:385.
- Dedo DD: A preoperative classification of the neck for cervicofacial rhytidectomy. *Laryngoscope* 1980; 90:1894.
- Dingmen RO, Grabb WC: Surgical anatomy of the mandibular ramus of the facial nerve based on the dissection of 100 facial halves. *Plast Reconstr Surg* 1962;29:266.
- Ellenbogen R: Pseudoparalysis of the mandibular branch of the facial nerve after platysmal face-lift operation. *Plast Reconstr Surg* 1979;63:364.
- Fodor PB: Platysma-SMAS rhytidectomy. *Aesthetic Plast Surg* 1982;6:173.
- Goin MK, Burgoyne RW, Goin JM, et al: A prospective psychological study of 50 female facelift patients. *Plast Reconstr Surg* 1980;65:436.
- Gonzalez-Ulloa M: Facial wrinkles: Integral elimination. *Plast Reconstr Surg* 1982;29:658.
- Gordon HL: Rhytidectomy. *Clin Plast Surg* 1978;5:97.
- Guerrero-Santos J, Espaillat L, Morales F: Muscular lift in cervical rhytidectomy. *Plast Reconstr Surg* 1974;54:127.
- Gurdin MM: Should the subcutaneous tissue be plicated in face lift (letter)? *Plast Reconstr Surg* 1975;55:84.
- Hoffman S, Simon BE: Complications of submental lipectomy. *Plast Reconstr Surg* 1977;60:889.
- Kamer FM: The two-stage concept of rhytidectomy. *Otolaryngol Head Neck Surg* 1979;87:915.
- Lemmon M, Hamra ST: Skoog rhytidectomy: A five-year experience with 577 patients. *Plast Reconstr Surg* 1980;67:283.
- McKinney P, Maywood BT: Camouflage of the postauricular scar in rhytidectomy. *Plast Reconstr Surg* 1982;69:352.
- Mitz V, Peyronie M: The superficial musculoaponeurotic system (SMAS) in the parotid and cheek area. *Plast Reconstr Surg* 1976;58:80.

- Rees TD: *Aesthetic Plastic Surgery*. Philadelphia, WB Saunders, 1980.
- Rees TD, Aston SJ: A clinical evaluation of the results of submusculo-aponeurotic dissection and fixation in face-lifts. *Plast Reconstr Surg* 1977;66:851.
- Regnault P, Daniel RK: *Aesthetic Plastic Surgery*. Boston, Little, Brown, 1984.
- Skoog T: *Plastic Surgery*. Philadelphia, WB Saunders, 1975.
- Tardy ME, et al: *Surgery of the Aging Face*. Memphis, Tenn, Richards Medical, 1981.
- Tardy ME, et al: Surgical correction of facial deformities, in Ballenger JJ (ed): *Diseases of the Nose, Throat and Ear,* Philadelphia, Lea & Febiger, 1977.
- Tardy ME, Klingensmith M: Face-lift surgery: Principles and variations, in Roenigk RK, Roenigk HH (eds): *Dermatologic Surgery: Principles and Practice*. New York, Marcel Dekker, 1989, pp 1239–1288.
- Tenta LT, Tardy ME, Pastorek NJ: Buccal lipectomy, in Conley J, Dickinson JT (eds): *Plastic and Reconstructive Surgery of the Face and Neck*. Stuttgart, Thieme, 1972.
- Tipton JB: Should the subcutaneous tissue be plicated in a facelift? *Plast Reconstr Surg* 1974;54:1.
- Webster RC, Davidson TM, White MF, et al: Conservative face-lift surgery. *Arch Otolaryngol* 1976;102:657.
- Webster RC, et al: Cosmetic platysmal surgery. *Facial Plast Surg* 1987;4:97.
- Webster RL, Smith RC: *The Aging Face and Neck*. New York, Field, Rich, 1985.

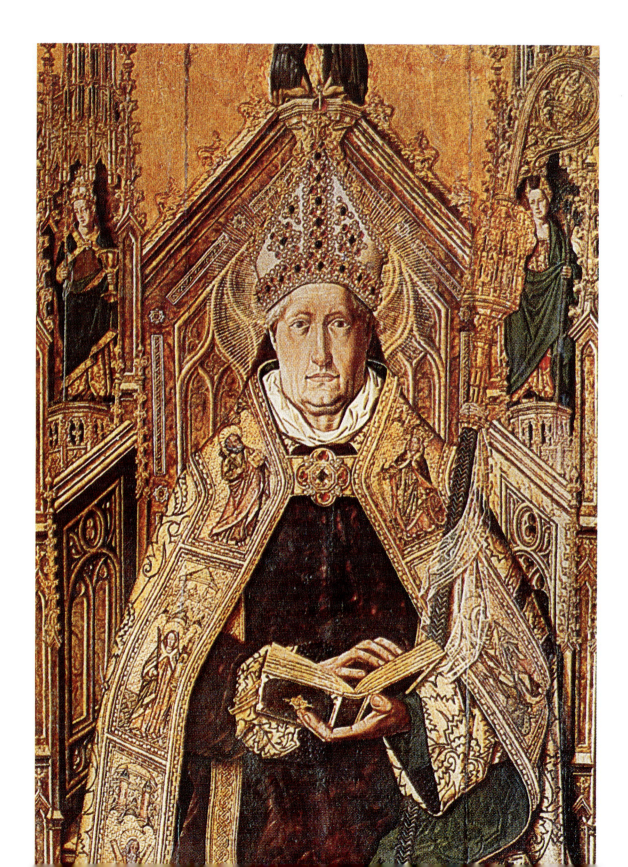

CHAPTER

12

  Secondary and Revisional Facelift

*Our years
Glide silently away.
No tears, no loving orisons repair
The wrinkled cheek, the whitening hair.
That drop forgotten to the tomb.*

Horace

Diagnosis and Candidate Selection

It is inevitable that the beneficial effects of the facelift operation deteriorate inasmuch as gravity and aging result in tissue relaxation characterized by redundant skin and muscle. No precise prediction of facelift longevity is possible since patients age at different rates because of individual genetic predispositions combined with detrimental environmental factors. Repeated weight gain and loss are clearly detrimental, as is excessive sun exposure; each may accelerate the need for a secondary facelift. All surgeons encounter a small but significant percentage of patients whose excessive skin laxity and redundancy herald the inevitable requirement for an early additional tightening procedure 12 to 18 months following the primary facelift—the "tuck-up" or two-stage rhytidoplasty. Recognizing this possibility and carefully informing such patients *prior* to undertaking the initial facelift is vital for ultimate patient satisfaction.

Our experience indicates that well-performed facelifts in patients who are ideal candidates generally provide lasting patient value for 5 to 10 years before any additional surgery need be contemplated. It is simply not possible to predict exactly "how long a facelift will last" since much depends upon the patient's evolving perception of his personal image and appearance. A useful, easily understood explanation of facelift longevity invokes the following analogy: "if you possessed an identical twin sister and you elected to undergo rejuvenation surgery, you will probably always look better than your nonoperated sister, *but both of you will continue to age and grow older.*" Without question, patients who undergo facelift surgery earlier in the aging process, before profound skin elasticity is lost, maintain facial appearance longer than those who delay their surgery until skin elasticity is severely compromised.

The benefits of facial lifting surgery may be enhanced by improved skin care and sun avoidance—we counsel each patient undergoing facelift surgery to adopt a much more stringent regimen regarding care of the skin and urge avoidance of sun exposure, weight control, and proper selection of moisturizers and cosmetics.

CHAPTER 12   Secondary and Revisional Facelift

Surgical Goals

In secondary facelift surgery a cardinal principle prevails and should be respected: the facial-cervical skin is ideally *redraped, reoriented,* and *redistributed* over a surgically tightened, subcutaneous soft tissue bed and attempts avoided to simulate the primary facelift procedure in which significant amounts of redundant skin may of necessity have been sacrificed. Certainly if a decade or more has separated the primary and secondary lifting procedures, significant additional skin may require removal, but in the majority of revisional procedures it is vital to avoid producing a potential overtightened, mask-like appearance from attempts to pull facial skin too vigorously. Instead, significant and long-lasting appearance improvement is best achieved by firm tightening of the underlying facial superficial musculoaponeurotic system (SMAS) in conjunction with the layer of "favorable fibrosis" scar tissue plane resulting from the primary facelift. If the primary lift has been well performed, the elevated facial skin now in essence represents a delayed pedicle flap possessing all the virtues of delay. As such, one generally encounters much reduced bleeding while elevating this delayed flap and tightening the underlying scar and SMAS layer, a surgical advantage of no little consequence. Generally little or no swelling and ecchymosis result, the result is quickly apparent, and patients resume normal activities much more quickly. Secondary rhytidoplasty thus carries significantly less risk than a primary facelift.

As long as the surgeon adheres to the vital principle of *reorientation* and *redistribution of skin* rather than unjudicious resection, revisional facelifts may be safely repeated at intervals in patients who possess good skin and strong skeletal structures and wish to forestall the ravages of aging as much as possible. As a practical matter, it is unusual for us to carry out more than two secondary procedures on any individual patient.

Surgical Techniques

As in a primary facelift, revisional surgery requires a varying degree of exposure and extent of dissection depending upon the degree and sites of sagging. In each patient the procedure must be individualized. In more limited situations, simply tightening the preauricular SMAS and scar tissue plane will substantially lift the midfacial area, jowl, and cervical regions favorably. If mandibular and cervical laxity appear to be more profound, complete excision of the entire extent and length of the primary facelift scar may be required with substantial exposure of the entire cervicofacial soft tissues and SMAS. The degree of undermining to establish favorable skin redistribution evenly may be similar to that required in a primary facelift.

A revision facelift provides an opportunity for improvement in the siting and camouflage of primary rhytidoplasty scars. We prefer, in women, to site the facial scar in the retrotragal region and to place the postauricular incision, insofar as possible, as cephalic as possible at the hairline–helical rim junction.

Generally, a secondary facelift requires only local infiltration anesthesia performed as an outpatient procedure. If extensive dissection is required, additional comfort and sedation may be achieved with the addition of intravenous anesthesia.

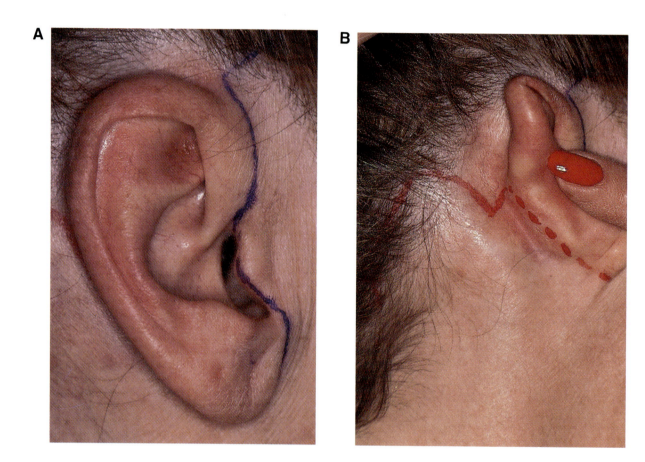

Figure 12–1
A, the extent of the periauricular incision will depend upon the extent and site of the laxity of cervicofacial tissue. No skin (or scar) is initially excised until the underlying soft tissues are lifted and tightened since only a paucity of skin may require actual removal after reorientation of the dissected skin flap. A nasal tampon is placed in each ear canal to prevent blood from entering the ear canal and creating annoying crusts. **B,** a more extensive secondary facelift incision necessary for the lower part of the face and cervical lifting.

CHAPTER 12 Secondary and Revisional Facelift

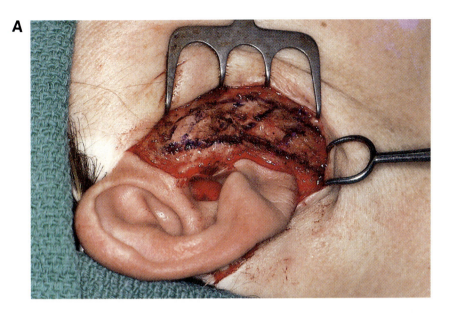

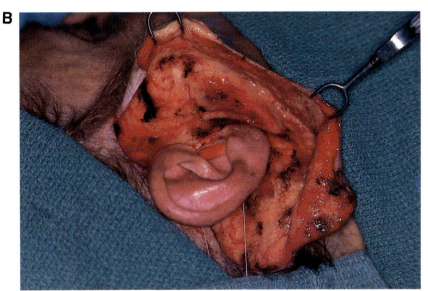

Figure 12-2
A, hemostatic scalpel elevation of the facial or cervicofacial flap proceeds toward the midface until the desired exposure of the SMAS and scar tissue plane is realized. Seldom does any significant bleeding occur when flap development is created in the desirable subcutaneous, favorable fibrosis plane. **B,** more extensive flap elevation in a secondary facelift in which wider undermining of the facial and cervical flaps is required to repair sagging facial and cervical skin and muscle.

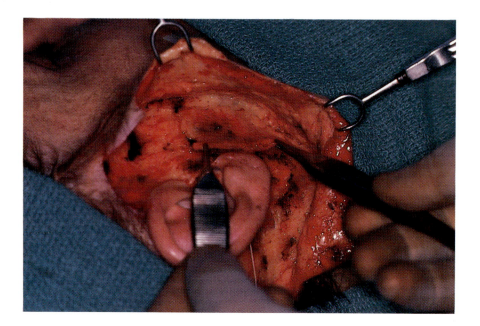

Figure 12–3
Mobility of the SMAS-scar tissue bed is assessed while noting the desired lifting effect transmitted to the overlying skin. Any wrinkling or creasing created by pull placed on the SMAS-scar is relieved by further skin undermining. In patients who for whatever reason have apparently not undergone SMAS tightening by their primary surgeon, plans must be made to create a definitive SMAS-scar flap for improving the lifted face.

CHAPTER 12 Secondary and Revisional Facelift

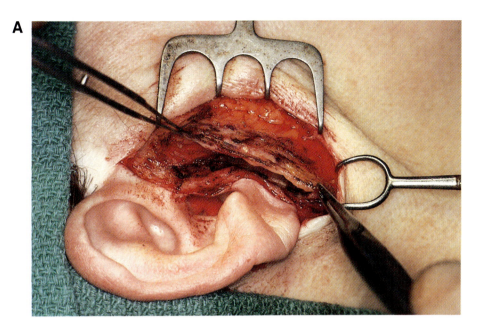

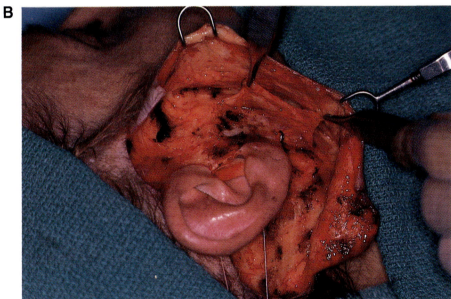

Figure 12–4
A, after creating a vertical incision 1 cm in front of the ear, the SMAS-scar flap is elevated by sharp dissection from the parotid fascia and retracted laterally and slightly cephalically. **B,** larger SMAS-scar flap elevated in a patient requiring more extensive undermining.

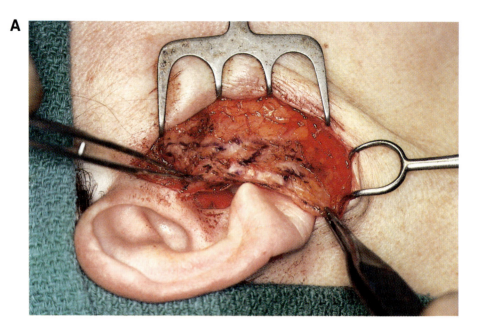

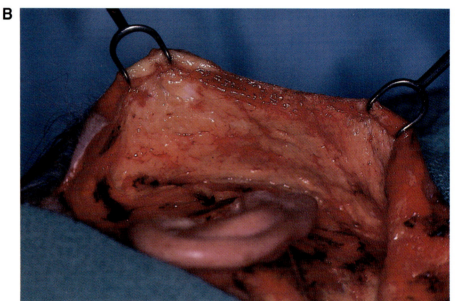

Figure 12-5

A, the overlapping excess is trimmed and discarded; multiple imbricating sutures of 3-0 white Tevdek secure the flap to the strong preauricular SMAS-scar complex. Any excess created cephalically is excised by extending the SMAS incision horizontally anterior, just below the zygoma. **B,** suture-imbrication of the SMAS-scar flap in a patient requiring more extensive undermining. Redundant excess facial skin to be excised is now evident. Note that the wound dead space has almost totally closed.

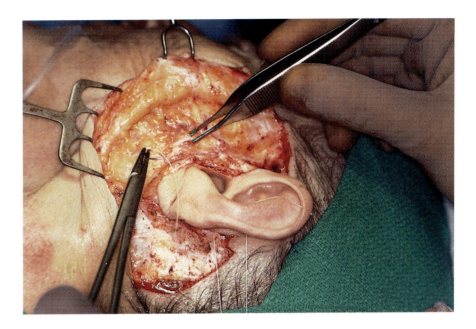

Figure 12-6
Occasionally patients are encountered who demonstrate a hollow ridging and soft-tissue atrophy in the preauricular and cheek area. Plicating (tissue overlapping) instead of excising and imbricating the excess SMAS-scar flap will allow improved contouring and filling of such depressions, thereby improving the overall appearance.

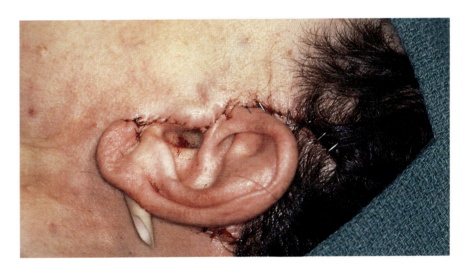

Figure 12-7
Excess skin (usually very limited in extent) trimming follows and the defect repaired with surgical staples in hair-bearing scalp areas, 5-0 chromic in postauricular skin, and 6-0 blue Prolene for preauricular closure.

We prefer a small circumferential lightly compressing dressing overnight to absorb any small amount of drainage encountered. Small postauricular Penrose drains, if used, are removed in 24 hours, after which no further dressing is generally required. Perioperative antibiotic (cefaclor) is given orally for 5 days.

Results and Outcome

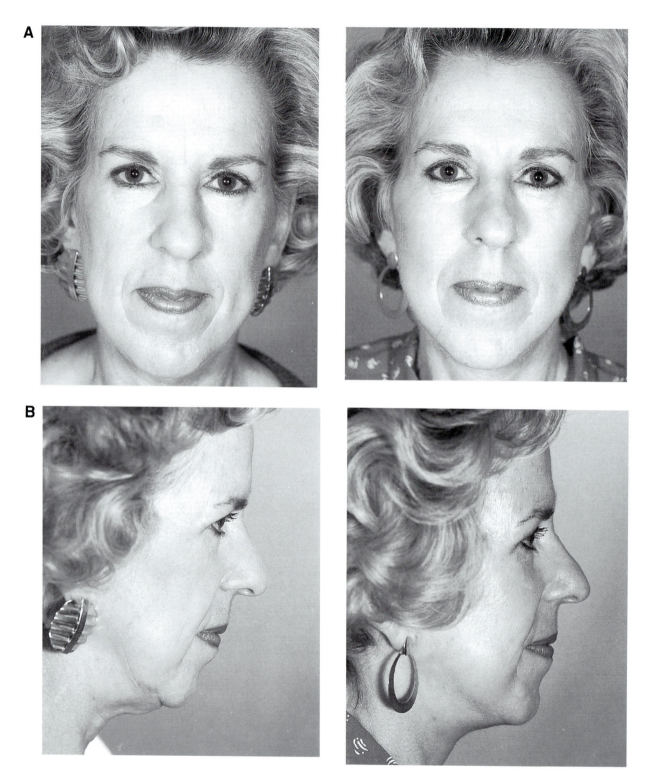

Figure 12–8
A and **B**, cervicofacial secondary facelift procedure 5 months after surgery.

CHAPTER 12 Secondary and Revisional Facelift

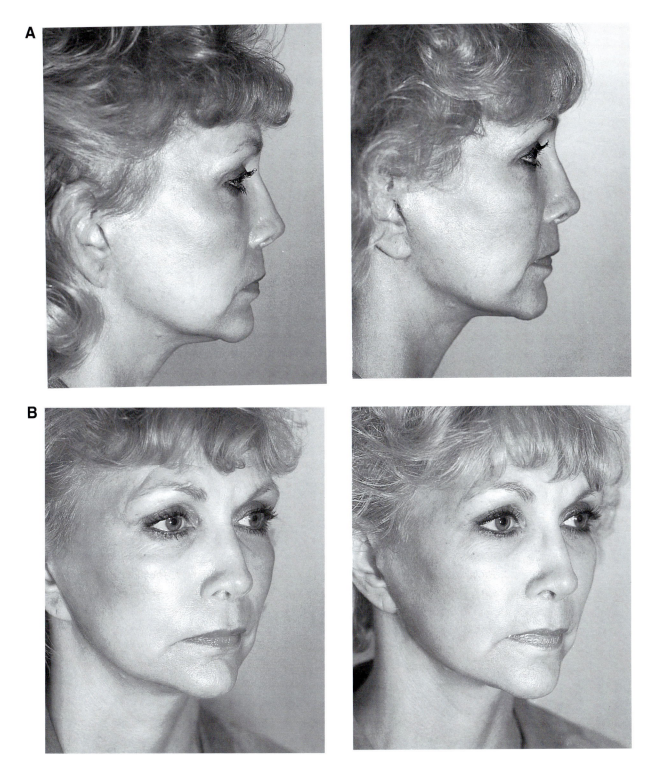

Figure 12–9
A and **B,** secondary correction of sagging cervical skin, poor scars, and satyr ear deformities.

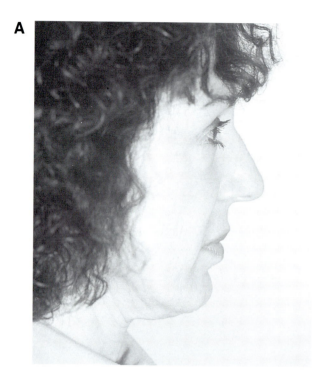
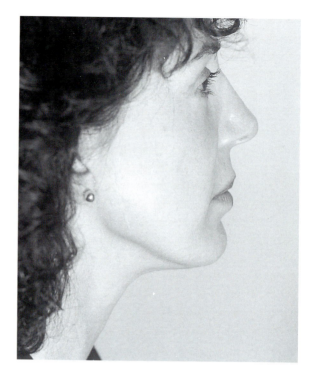
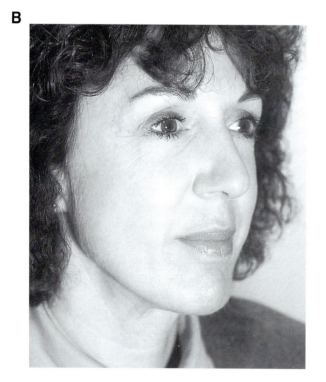
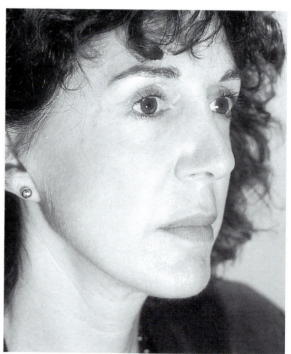

Figure 12–10
A and **B,** improved lower portion of the face and cervical regions following a more extensive cervicofacial lifting procedure.

CHAPTER 12   Secondary and Revisional Facelift

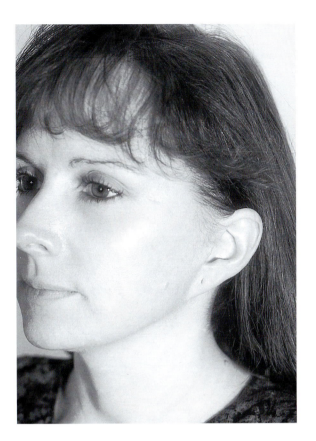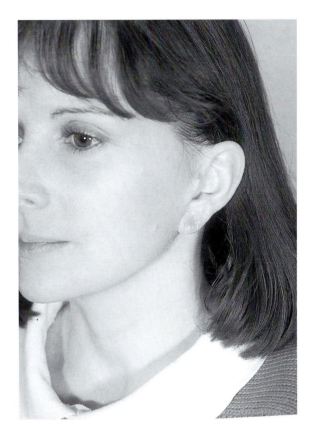

Figure 12–11
Correction of a severe satyr ear deformity complication in a young patient who underwent facelift surgery elsewhere at an unusually young age. Rejuvenation of the face with earlobe reconstruction is shown 3 months following repair.

Complications and Sequelae

Any of the potential sequelae and complications of a primary facelift may develop after secondary and revisional procedures. Because flap dissection is generally less extensive and bleeding usually minimal, significant complications are indeed rare.

Unique to secondary facelift surgery is the possibility of creating an overlifted, mask-like face appearance if the principles cited above are not followed carefully. Overlifting with excess tension invariably leads to poor scar camouflage or scar contracture producing the possibility of widened, displaced incisions and tragal eversion, a completely avoidable complication.

Secondary facelift surgery in which significant cervical skin requires removal may lead to elevation or irregularization of the postauricular hairline. Careful attention to flap redraping and hairline alignment is thus necessary.

Suggested Reading

- Kamer F: Sequential rhytidectomy and the two-stage concept. *Otolaryngol Clin North Am* 1980;305:320.
- Mitz V, Peyronie M: The superficial musculoaponeurotic system SMAS in the parotid and cheek area. *Plast Reconstr Surg* 1976;58:80.
- Skoog T: *Plastic Surgery.* Philadelphia, WB Saunders, 1975.
- Skoog T, Ellenberg J: Skoog technique of facelift. *Aesthetic Plast Surg* 1989;721:723.
- Webster RC, et al: Comparison of SMAS plication with SMAS imbrication in facelifting. *Laryngoscope* 1982;92:901.

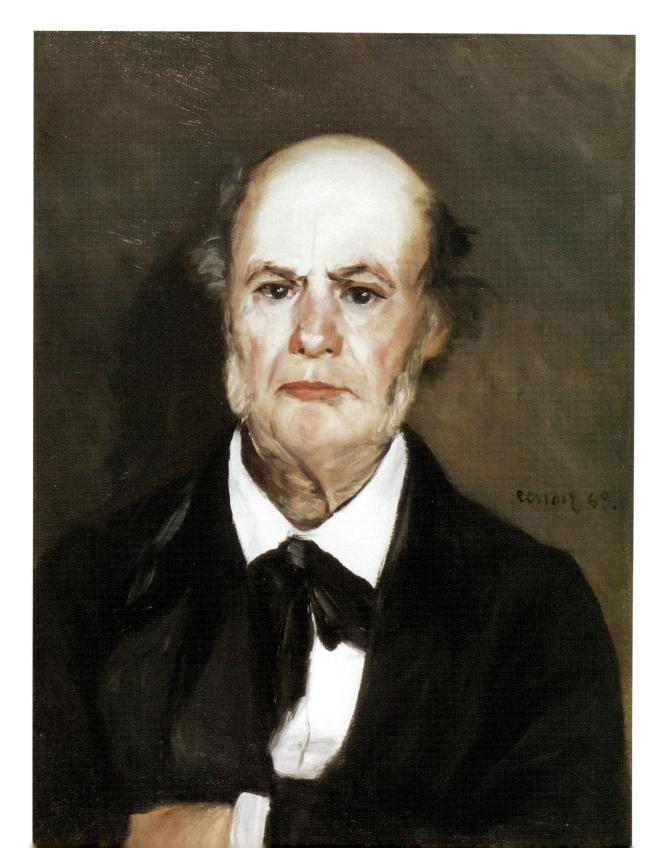

CHAPTER 13

 Aesthetic Surgery of the Aging Neck

> *Senescence begins*
> *And middle age ends*
> *The day your descendents*
> *outnumber your friends.*
>
> **Ogden Nash**

Wide anatomic variations exist in patients with evidence of aging in the submental and cervical areas. In the normal time frame of the aging process the submental cervical region suffers early deterioration in appearance. Patients requesting facelift operations are uniformly concerned with improving the appearance of the submental area and complain of a fatty fullness that is resistant to diet, loose skin, and hanging vertical folds. The aging condition in this area is indeed characterized by a variable degree of relaxation and redundancy of the medial platysmal borders, an accumulation of excessive fat both superficial and deep to the platysmal decussation (commonly present in even teenage and very young patients), and on occasion ptosis of the submandibular glands. Oblique and transverse creases appear and are worsened by sun exposure. The youthful cervicomental angle becomes more obtuse as the above factors partially obliterate the anatomy of the columnar neck. The most favorable surgical management of the medial cervical region will depend upon which combination of these factors must be surgically corrected and to what degree. Except in the most early stages of cervicofacial support loss, the platysma muscle often requires surgical tightening and repositioning from both its posterolateral and medial aspects. This anatomic judgment is ideally completed prior to surgery and included in the overall surgical "game plan" for facial appearance improvement.

Significant skeletal limitations to complete rejuvenation exist when a low-positioned hyoid/thyroid complex will not allow sharp surgical definition of the cervicomandibular angle; overdeveloped, thick musculature may likewise limit ideal surgical production of an ideal contour.

If the patient accepted for rejuvenation facial surgery demonstrates relatively early ptotic skin changes with little or no medial platysmal banding and minimal unsightly submental fat accumulation, then a facelift operation incorporating posterior platysmal plication or imbrication will effectively improve cervical definition and contour.

Unsightly, prominent vertical platysmal bands with excessive submental fat and skin, however, demand a direct approach to the area through a short curvilinear incision, preferably placed slightly posterior to the submental crease. Suction lipectomy with direct excision submentoplasty is ideally carried out prior to initiation of the facelift operation, before the

CHAPTER 13 Aesthetic Surgery of the Aging Neck

facial skin and musculofacial flaps have been repositioned and tightened. Thus, in order to dissect in the neck under no tension and to excise or reposition the medial platysmal fibers precisely with direct-vision surgery, we prefer to undertake the major correction of the submental anatomy *before* facelift dissection and skin flap advancement ensue, eventually refining the submental surgery following cervicofacial lifting by "feathering" the borders of the submental dissection. Firming this area first improves the repositioning of the facelift flaps over a tightened and defatted submental and submandibular region.

Extreme conservation should be exercised by surgeons in removing any more than a very slight amount of submental skin in all but the most aged of patients. The creation of a greatly improved cervicomental angle requires the retropositioning of "excess" submental skin into the angle. What may initially appear to be excess skin before surgery often becomes nonexistent when the facelift skin–superficial musculoaponeurotic system (SMAS) flaps are advanced and rotated, particularly if chin augmentation has accompanied the more major rejuvenation procedures.

If initially excessive submental skin is aggressively removed, surface contour deformities and even "bowstring" submental scars traversing the submental concavity may develop and frustrate future repair efforts. For this reason in most patients we defer final closure of the submental incision until all other facial procedures are completed. Judgments about final submental skin tailoring are thereby enhanced.

Neck Rejuvenation

Diagnosis and Candidate Selection

Patients concerned about the appearance of the neck and submental region commonly require more than cervicofacial lifting techniques to provide satisfactory and lasting cervical rejuvenation. In assessing the cervical aging characteristics, it is helpful to consider and evaluate the *individual cervical anatomic components* that deprive the neck of its youthful appearance. These variably deteriorating or congenital anatomic components, considered from external to internal levels, consist of the following:

Skin. Redundancy and excess skin develop, with a loss of skin tone and elasticity. Permanent horizontal and oblique creases appear.

SMAS. Loss of support and tone is manifested by sagging of the skin and platysma muscle, with ptosis of the contents of the upper part of the neck.

Fat. Excessive submental fat appears (or persists from accumulation in youth) and may consist of a large superficial subcutaneous fatty accumulation as well as excessive subplatysmal fat (denser and generally more vascular in nature).

Platysma Muscle. Progressive degrees of sagging and muscle banding occur, with diastasis normally developing between the anterior decussation of the muscle fibers. The cervical contents become ptotic, no longer well supported by the youthful firm and well-toned platysma.

Hyoid-Thyroid Complex Location. A low anatomic position of the hyoid-thyroid cartilage structures contributes to an aesthetically undesirable obliquity to the upper cervical region, effectively defeating surgical efforts to achieve an ideal well-defined cervicomental angle.

Mandibular Length. Retrognathia, whether minimal or profound, congenital or progressively acquired, contributes to the appearance of aging in the cervical region; chin augmentation in conjunction with submentoplasty procedures profoundly improves the overall cervicofacial appearance. Ptosis of the chin pad accentuates the cervical aging characteristics and requires cephalic repositioning to correct this support deficiency. Deepening of the submental crease accentuates this aging appearance. Incisions for submental access placed directly within the crease may accentuate its depth, an undesirable result.

Just as in rhinoplasty, the contribution of each of these cervical anatomic components and subcomponents must be individually and accurately assessed in order to orchestrate the appropriate cervical surgical measures. Correction of these various aging deformities may be carried out concomitantly (as an integral part of the facelift operation) or individually as required and will depend upon which of the aging components requires repair. Precise diagnosis and planning are facilitated by classifying patients into commonly encountered clinical categories and *adapting the appropriate and effective surgical manipulations to the individual anatomic variations encountered.* Variations are certainly encountered in any large series of patients, but the following grading system has been found helpful and effective in preoperative analysis. As the extent and complexity of the encountered deformity increases, progressively more involved surgical procedures are required for correction.

CHAPTER 13 Aesthetic Surgery of the Aging Neck

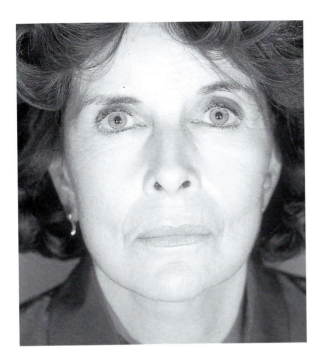
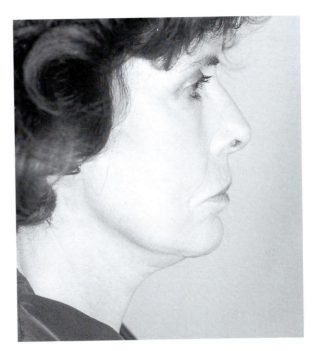

Figure 13–1
Grade 0.—Early facial skin excess and redundancy with little lax neck skin and minimal submental fat, good platysmal-SMAS support, and normal hyoid position.

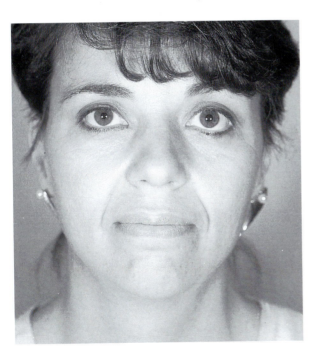
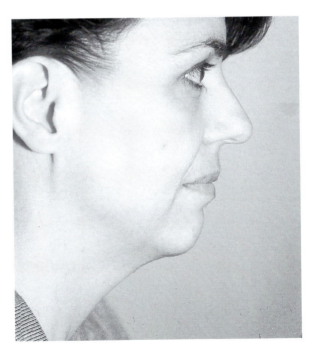

Figure 13–2
Grade 1.—Minimal but visible cervical skin excess, minimal submental fat, little or no midline platysmal separation and banding, and normal hyoid position.

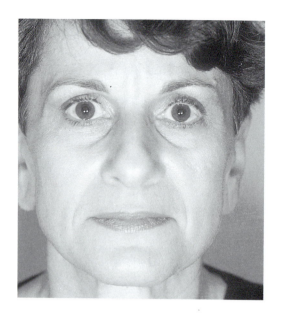
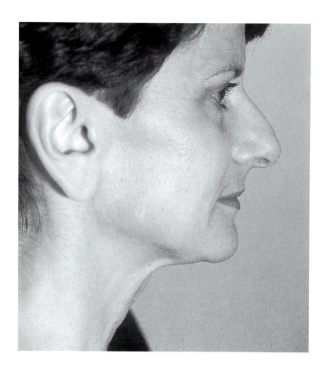

Figure 13–3
Grade 2.—Moderate to severely ptotic submental skin with obvious platysmal banding and midline diastasis, little submental fat, and normal hyoid position.

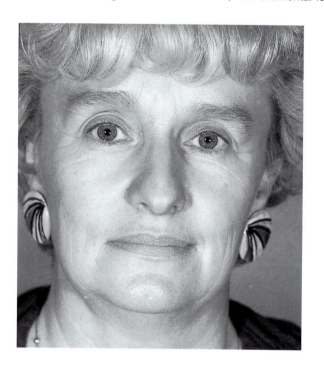
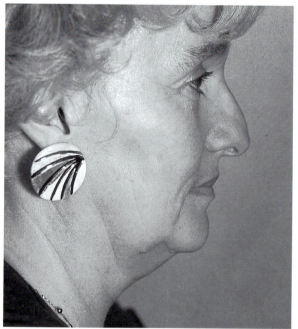

Figure 13–4
Grade 3.—Moderate to severely ptotic submental skin with platysmal banding, objectionable and obvious excess submental fat, and normal hyoid position.

CHAPTER 13   Aesthetic Surgery of the Aging Neck

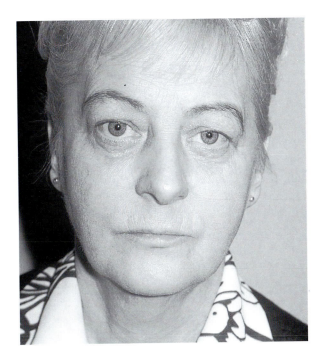
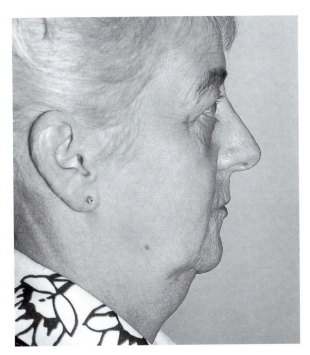

Figure 13–5
Grade 4.—Ptotic, toneless cervical skin, significant excess submental fat, redundant and stretched platysma-SMAS layer, low-lying hyoid, retrognathia with an obtuse cervicomental angle, and a deep submental crease.

In any of these general categories, the mandibular length as well as the chin position and attitude may vary individually and suggest chin augmentation when indicated and desirable. Visible ptosis of the submandibular gland may be manifested as the investing SMAS-platysmal layer loses the capacity to support the neck contents in sling-like fashion. Excess and unsightly subplatysmal submental fat may be suspected preoperatively but is ordinarily diagnosed in its real extent during submental exploration.

Satisfactory and effective rejuvenation of the cervical region presently consists of a predetermined combination of a cervicofacial lifting procedure incorporating SMAS-platysmal cervical repositioning by plication or SMAS flap imbrication, precise submental suction and dissection lipectomy by excision and/or suction carried into the lateral submental region with lateral fat beveling, excision of a segment of the anterior cervical platysmal bands with suture reapposition in the midline, direct excision of subplatysmal submental fat, and suction lipectomy of the lateral cervical region, with chin augmentation or repositioning as indicated for more favorable delineation of the cervicofacial profile.

Although these procedures, individually or collectively, effectively rejuvenate the cervical region, the patient should be advised that the taut submental neck produced surgically in the immediate postoperative period will undergo a slight but definite skin relaxation as surgical swelling and edema subside. Permanent horizontal cervical creases will largely persist even after extensive surgical dissection. All patients are informed that aging is a continuous, steady, and unrelenting process and that the result achieved at the operating table will inevitably become less ideal over time. The concept of *serial rejuvenation procedures* carried out to provide a facial "guardian maintenance" is an important one to emphasize to patients keen to forestall the effects of aging on appearance.

Since cervical rejuvenation is usually carried out in conjunction with facelift surgery, the preoperative laboratory, clinical, and photographic studies necessary are essentially identical to those described in the chapter on facelift surgery. One helpful photographic view obtained consists of the "forced grimace" view in which the patient is asked to forcibly contract the platysma muscle by intensively pulling down the corners of the mouth. The fibers of the platysma are thus thrown into broad relief for additional diagnostic information (see Fig 11–4,B).

Surgical Goals and Planned Outcome

The planned outcome of surgical rejuvenation includes firming of redundant, lax cervical and submental skin, excision/sculpture of submental fat, elevation and tightening of the SMAS-platysmal supportive layer, restoration of a more defined cervicomental angle, and improvement of the mandibular contour with chin augmentation and/or reversal of chin pad ptosis. Suture tightening of the visible hanging anterior borders of the platysma muscle after excisional and incisional maneuvers combined with posterosuperior suture repositioning of the cervicofacial SMAS-platysmal complex is fundamental to the outcome of neck surgery. Elimination of

CHAPTER 13   Aesthetic Surgery of the Aging Neck

excessive submental fat and lateral cervical fat, when indicated, is a common goal, even in patients where submental fat does not appear to be excessive (commonly, cervicofacial lifting of the skin and SMAS-platysmal complex, demonstrated manually before surgery, will reveal the bulge of excessive submental fat) (Fig 13–6). Correction of retrognathia frequently requires chin augmentation, which significantly normalizes the mandibular-neck appearance.

In no instance do we choose to transect the platysma muscle *completely* horizontally as advocated by some authors, since the incidence of contour deformities produced by the retracted cut borders of the platysma is objectionable.

Overaggressive skin removal in the submental area may result in an insufficient length of residual skin to comfortably and smoothly cover this now elongated submental area from anterior to posterior and create the complication of an obliquity of skin from the upper submental area to the midneck, a totally preventable but common sequela of overaggressive skin excision. Similarly, excision of a large triangle of submental skin with subsequent closure in a "T" configuration, advocated by others, can lead to unsightly depressions, tissue bunching, and unacceptable hypertrophic or contracted scarring. Always, care must be taken to not remove excessive fat in the submental triangle, which can lead to an unsightly depression ("cobra") deformity.

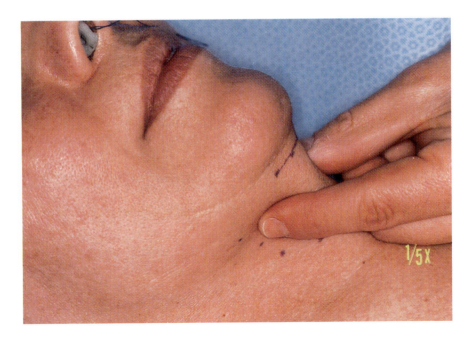

Figure 13–6
Evaluation of extent and distribution of excess submental fat may be assessed by palpation of the subcutaneous tissues with the educated thumb and forefinger. Subsequent serial palpation during suction lipectomy provides a guideline to the amount of fat removed and to that intentionally left behind.

Surgical Techniques

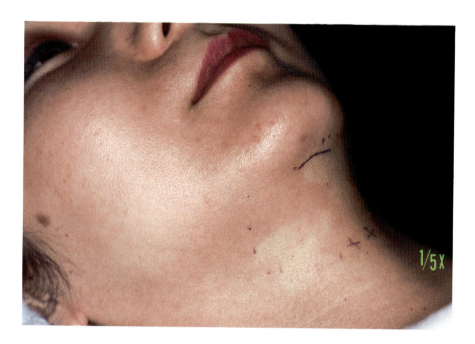

Figure 13–7
The preferred submental incision is best created within or several millimeters *posterior to* the submental crease in order to not deepen the crease further. The incision length will vary, depending upon the degree of exposure required for dissection (2.0 to 3.5 cm), but should never be extended to the lateral aspect of the mandible since advancement-rotation of the facelift flap might pull the lateral corners of the incision out of the submental area and render it visible. Despite the validation of liposuction techniques in the submental area in younger patients with elastic skin (see Chapter 17), in older individuals who require modification of the medial aspect of the platysma, direct-vision excision-sculpture of the submental fat often provides a superior and more reliable surgical result. Concomitant suction lipectomy may be helpful in beveling or "feathering" the lateral regions of the submental fat.

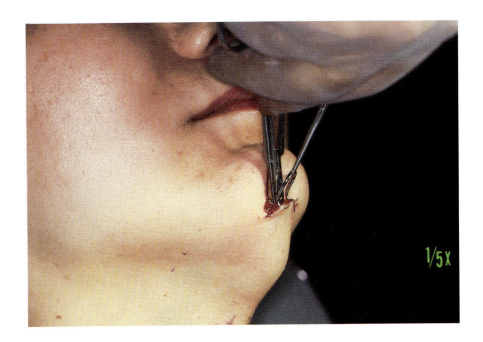

Figure 13-8
With countertraction applied to the inferior margin of the submental incision, dissection is facilitated with sharp scissors in a spreading and cutting manner to gain access to the superficial and deep layers of excess fat. Undermining of the cervical flap ordinarily proceeds to the level of the hyoid bone. Visualization is enhanced with fiberoptic headlight lighting. The fat found superficial to the platysma is relatively bloodless save for a few vessels penetrating into the submental musculature. Fat beneath the platysma near the floor of the mouth is highly vascular and requires a more delicate dissection with strict attention to perfect hemostasis.

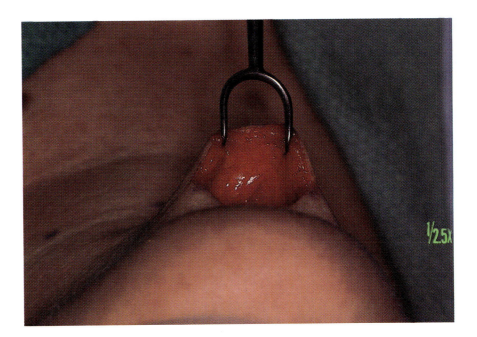

Figure 13-9
Sufficient fat (often as much as 1 cm) should be left on the undersurface of the submental skin flap to avoid creating an unaesthetic submental depression, which further accentuates early ptosis of the chin pad.

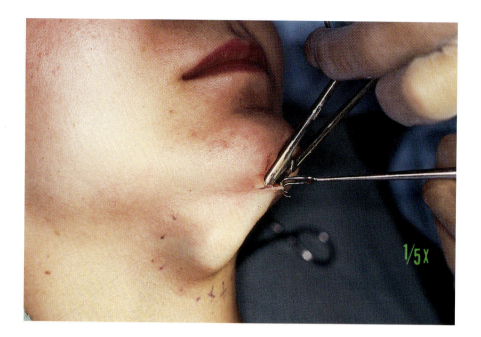

Figure 13-10
Sculpture of the fat laterally to blend into the contours of the lateral aspect of the mandible and cervical soft tissues requires some skill and experience but is vital to achieve the best results and avoid an abnormal submental appearance. The region of the hyoid-thyroid cartilage complex is ordinarily the inferior extent of fat excision; a feathering sculpture may also be required here. Absolute bipolar hemostasis is critical since hematoma development in the submental area will substantially prolong satisfactory healing.

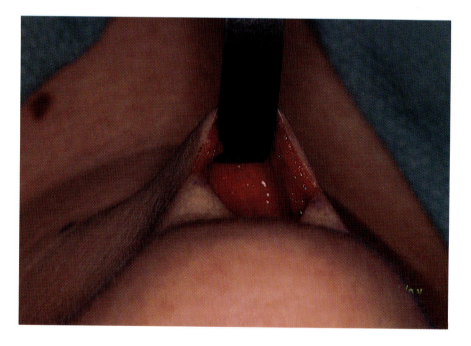

Figure 13-11
Exposure is facilitated by using the ebonized narrow S-shaped Cummings retractor (Smith-Nephew Co., Memphis, Tenn).

CHAPTER 13 Aesthetic Surgery of the Aging Neck

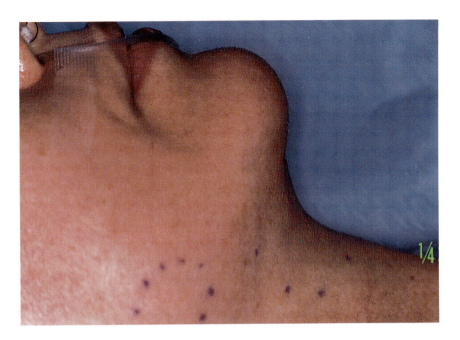

Figure 13–12
Fat is removed in gradual increments until manual repositioning of the submental cervical flap demonstrates restoration of a more normal cervicomandibular angle.

Once fat sculpture is complete and hemostasis ideal, the condition of the medial borders of the platysma may be evaluated and a treatment plan determined depending upon the exact anatomy encountered. The "sling effect" created by decussation and interdigitation of the medial platysmal fibers in the young patient gradually diminishes during the aging process and results in deterioration of support and a variety of medial platysmal configurations. The fibers may have departed the midline with diminished or minimal decussation, they may hang in asymmetrical ptotic early folds along with their attached overlying skin, or thick prominent vertical bands may result in a typical "turkey gobbler" neck deformity (see Figs 13–2 to 13–5).

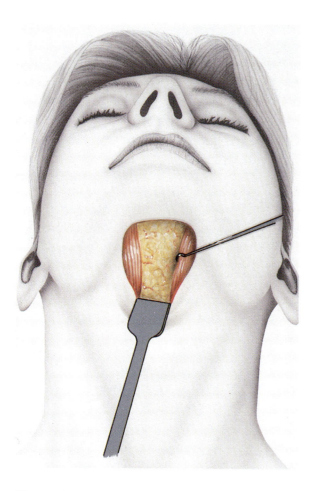

Figure 13–13
The medial borders of each platysma muscle (previously marked on the skin preoperatively in the sitting position) are grasped with a single hook near the level of the hyoid bone.

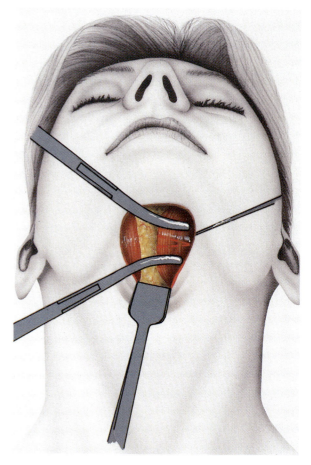

Figure 13–14
The free muscle margins are clamped at the hyoid level and above. A 1.5- to 2.5-cm wedge segment of the ptotic bands is excised between the clamps.

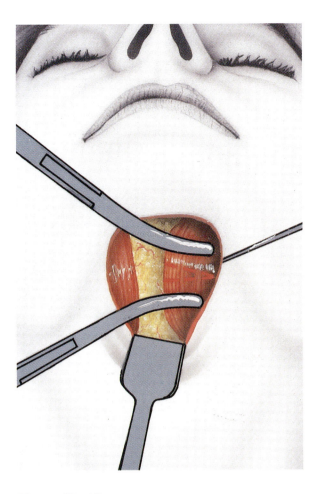

Figure 13–15
Bipolar cautery of the muscle stumps for absolute hemostasis.

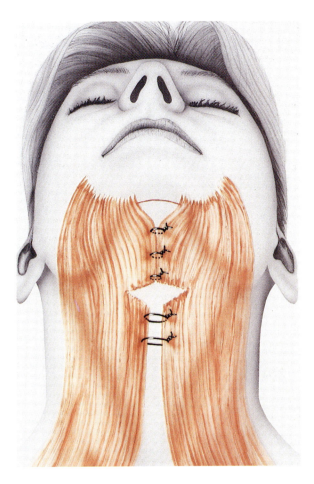

Figure 13–16
The proximal (cephalic) margins of the medial platysmal borders above the point of muscle excision are securely plicated together in the midline with 4-0 polydioxanine sutures, effectively initiating the tightening of the submental neck and restoring a more youthful cervicomental angle by creating a supportive sling effect. Redundant platysma muscle distal to the sites of muscle excision will be tightened by the skin-SMAS facelift procedure to follow. If severe upper platysmal redundancy is present, the vertical medial borders of the muscle may be trimmed to avoid irregularities after suture plication.

Before closure of the submental incision, the cervicofacial lifting procedure (facelift) is carried out to further define the extent of improvement possible in the submental region and any final fat sculpturing or additional hemostasis is attended to.

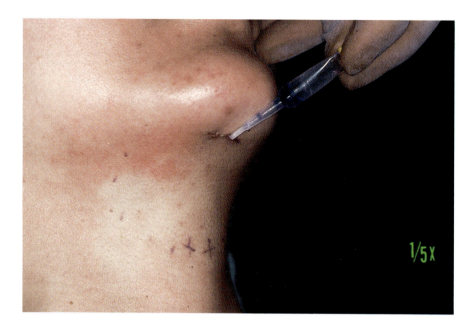

Figure 13–17
Incision closure ensues with subcutaneous 5-0 absorbable polydioxanine suture followed by a running intradermal 6-0 Prolene closure of the skin incision reinforced by Histoacryl glue.

Postoperative Care

Attentive and sympathetic postoperative care of the patient undergoing rejuvenation shares equal importance with the technical operation itself. In the first few days following the operation, strong support is necessary by the surgeon, his staff, and family members in order to reinforce a positive patient attitude.

Anything other than mild discomfort is unusual in the early postoperative period, with true pain being an infrequent complaint varying with the motivation and pain threshold of the individual patient. If chin augmentation has been performed, mild non–aspirin-containing analgesics are ordinarily useful in the first 48 hours to reduce any discomfort. No other special medications are given or appear to be useful.

A neck and facial dressing of Conform and Kerlex gauze provides support and light compression to the submental region and is changed at 24 to 48 hours. Patients are encouraged to wear a supportive elastic cervical dressing for 1 week thereafter. Prophylactic perioperative antibiotics are employed for patients undergoing chin augmentation. All incisions are cleaned gently with hydrogen peroxide and kept sparingly moist with Neo-Decadron ophthalmic ointment twice daily during the first week after surgery; this provides the dual advantage of preventing crusting over the incision sites and hastening the resolution of redness.

Results and Outcomes

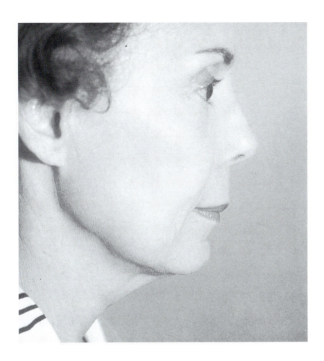
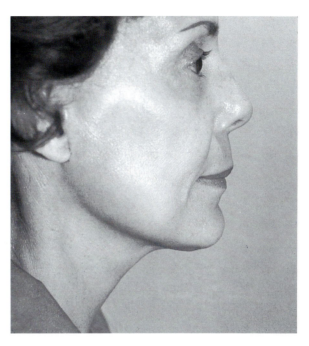

Figure 13-18
Patient with minimal preoperative submental fat and platysma deformity treated by direct removal of a small amount of submental fat combined with a facelift.

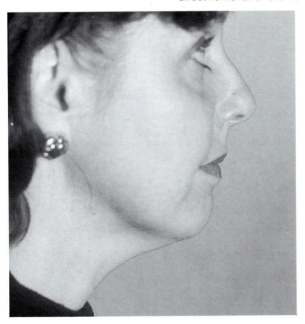
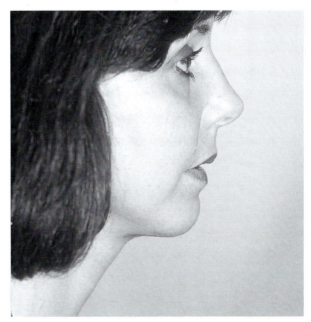

Figure 13-19
Surgical outcome in a patient in whom more generous submental fat removal was carried out; direct and suction lipectomy was combined with facelift surgery. Rhinoplasty enhances total outcome.

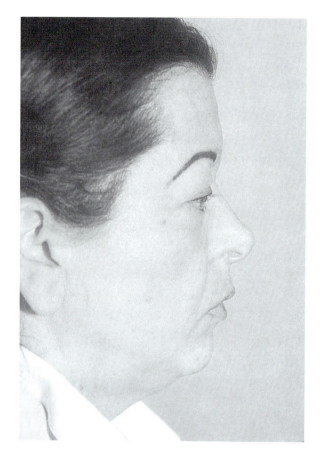 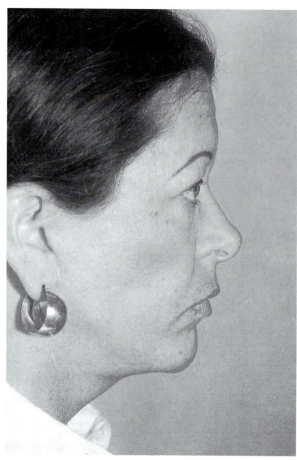

Figure 13–20
Substantial submental lipectomy performed by combining direct excision and suction lipectomy with facelift surgery.

The surgeon should be aware that substantial submental fat may mask ptotic, redundant platysmal borders; this will become apparent in the early postoperative period following lipectomy and spoil the cervical contour. Thus suture-plication of platysmal borders must be considered intraoperatively, even when platysma banding is not prominent preoperatively.

CHAPTER 13 Aesthetic Surgery of the Aging Neck

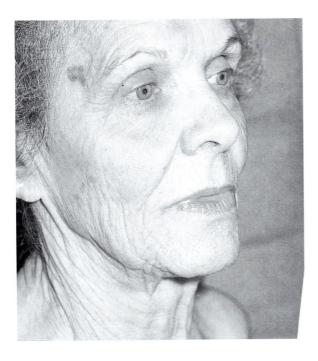
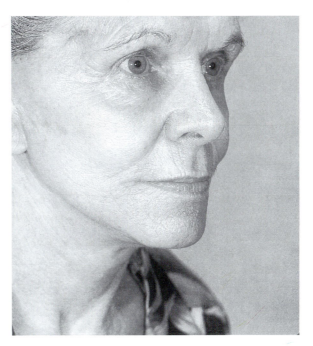

Figure 13–21
Patient demonstrating more prominent platysmal banding and less submental fat. Treatment was platysmal border segmental resection and suture-plication, minimal submental lipectomy, and facelift surgery.

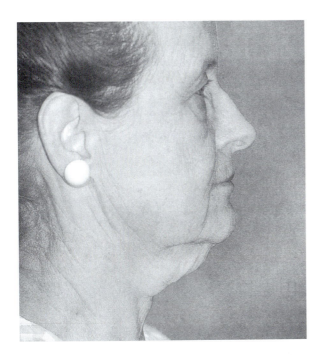
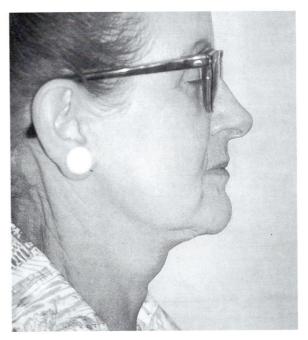

Figure 13–22
Surgical outcome following combined direct and suction submental lipectomy, along with platysmal suture-plication and facelift surgery.

Complications and Sequelae

The postsurgical cervical area remains initially hypoesthetic for 6 to 8 weeks; sensation returns totally thereafter.

Fat, damaged by scissors dissection or suction cannula trauma, continues to be absorbed for many weeks postoperatively. Thus it is vital to avoid *overexcision* of submental fat. A generous layer of cushioning fat must be left undisturbed on the flap undersurface.

Extensive suction lipectomy in the submandibular region may expose ptotic submandibular glands otherwise inapparent because of cervical fat excess. Patients must be warned of this possibility, particularly in the older age group with markedly diminished tissue support. Worse, overexcision of fat in the midline submental region can lead to an unsightly hollow or "cobra" deformity.

Submental hematomas, although rare, are serious problems and, when they occur in the immediate postoperative period, demand immediate wound exploration, hematoma evacuation, and hemostasis. Even small seromas or hematomas will slow the healing process and retard or diminish the favorable neck contours sought.

Assiduous intraoperative hemostasis combined with constant manual pressure during the associated facial procedures facilitates early and favorable healing that is free of excessive submental edema and swelling.

Damage to the marginal mandibular branch of the facial nerve is always possible but has not been encountered by the authors to date.

Combined Submental Fat and Skin Resection

Diagnosis and Candidate Selection

Submental contour deformities require surgical correction techniques that address the specific anatomic contributions. Excessive submental fat, a low-lying hyoid, dehiscent or redundant platysma, and finally, redundant, flaccid submental skin all produce anterior neck contours that represent less than the aesthetic ideal. While numerous procedures including liposuction have been described to correct the double chin or "pseudo–double chin" that results from excessive fat, few have addressed the particular abnormality of excessively redundant submental skin commonly called the "turkey gobbler" deformity (Fig 13–23,A).

Both men and women demonstrate accumulations of submental fat, a low-lying hyoid, or dehiscent and redundant platysma. However, the problem of excessive, flaccid submental skin independent of or out of proportion to the aging deformities occurs more frequently in men (Fig 13–23,B). When redundant submental skin is minimal or capable of eventual shrinkage, standard rhytidectomy combined with submental lipectomy and including, when indicated, resection, imbrication, or plication of the platysma muscle produces superior improvement in appearance.

CHAPTER 13 Aesthetic Surgery of the Aging Neck

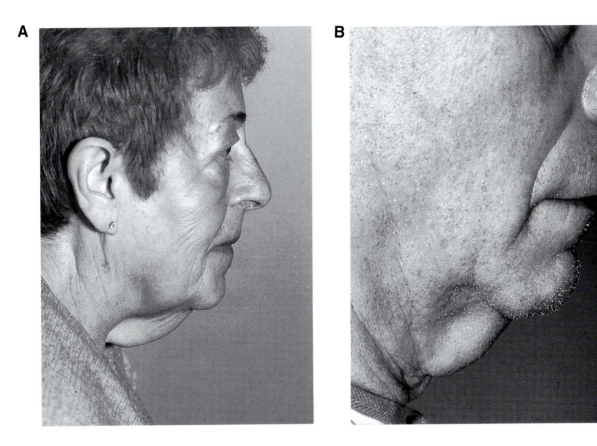

Figure 13-23
A, flaccid "turkey gobbler" deformation of neck in elderly woman. **B,** redundant skin, platysmal bands, and fat in submental region of male patient.

The "turkey gobbler" deformity, however, is not usually adequately corrected with a typical cervicofacial lifting procedure. In fact, in many patients who find this excess skin both cosmetically displeasing and a functional nuisance (tight collars and ties become impossible to tolerate), a full facelift is often neither desired nor aesthetically necessary. A submental skin W-plasty or T-Z-plasty possesses value when executed as an isolated procedure, or it may enhance the final favorable submental contour achieved during cervicofacial lifting procedures.

Surgical Goals and Planned Outcome

In our experience excessively redundant submental skin can be adequately removed and tightened by using a submental W-plasty (or multiple Z-plasty) closure that produces a more concealed scar confined to an area between the submental and suprahyoid creases.

The running submental W-plasty may be carried out in conjunction with a standard rhytidectomy but is most often applicable to male patients who exhibit exaggerated submental skin redundancy without the associated changes of aging that would warrant a full facelift. In fact, many men who are distressed by the appearance of a "turkey gobbler" neck and annoyed by the physical discomfort that this excess tissue can cause are not displeased with the "mature" look that other facial aging changes impart. It is for these selected patients that the running submental W-plasty (or Z-plasty) is a rewarding and helpful procedure for correction of an isolated submental contour deformity without the added morbidity of more extensive and often undesired cosmetic procedures. The resultant scar matures to an inconspicuous, aesthetically superior scar.

Surgical Technique

While sitting upright, the patient is examined, and the lateral borders of the skin redundancy are palpated and marked. Once supine, the anterior portion of the neck is infiltrated with 1% lidocaine (Xylocaine) with 1:100,000 epinephrine, and sterile preparation and draping are accomplished. The transverse submental crease is then marked, as is the suprahyoid crease (Fig 13–24). The transverse portion of the incision is often sited slightly proximal or distal to the natural crease to produce a smoother cervical contour. A W-plasty is outlined vertically, to one side of the midline along a perpendicular joining these two creases. Each limb of the W-plasty is kept less than 1.0 cm long. Skin undermining is next carried out laterally in both directions, with care taken to confine dissection to an

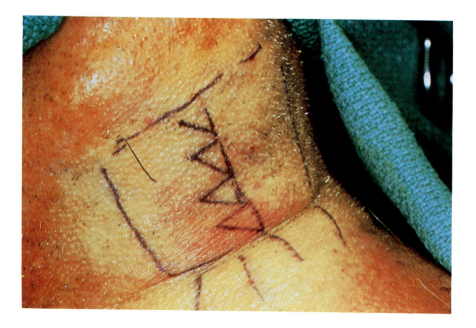

Figure 13–24
The submental crease, the suprahyoid crease, and the estimated amount of undermining and resection are marked.

area that is well below the usual arc of the marginal mandibular nerve (Fig 13-25). The plane of dissection is maintained in the subcutaneous layer superficial to the platysma.

Excess submental fat, if present, is then resected by direct scissors removal (Fig 13-26). If fat is removed, several millimeters is left on the inferior surface of the platysma muscle to allow for uniform skin draping postoperatively. Platysma muscle may be plicated and tightened in the midline with 4-0 Vicryl to create a muscular sling.

The previously marked vertical strip of skin is then excised by using inferior and superior horizontal incisions in the aforementioned creases and extending them only the distance necessary to remove the wedge of skin itself. The W-plasty configuration is, of course, preserved. Hemostasis is achieved by using bipolar cautery, and wound closure is accomplished with 5-0 Vicryl subcutaneous sutures and 6-0 Prolene interrupted sutures on the skin (Fig 13-27). The procedure is performed on an outpatient basis, and the patient returns in 5 to 7 days for suture removal.

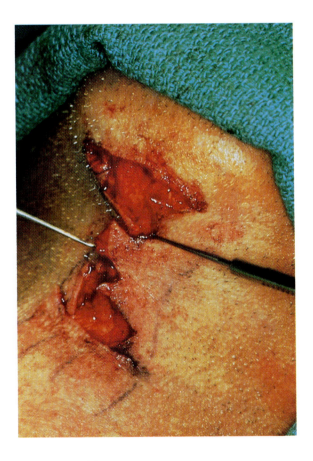

Figure 13-25
The wound edges are undermined in the subcutaneous plane, and excess skin is resected in a W-plasty configuration.

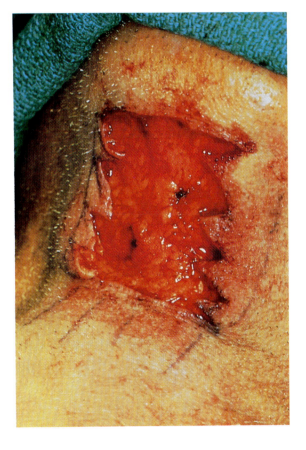

Figure 13-26
Excess fat is resected and the platysma plicated in the midline to form a muscular support sling.

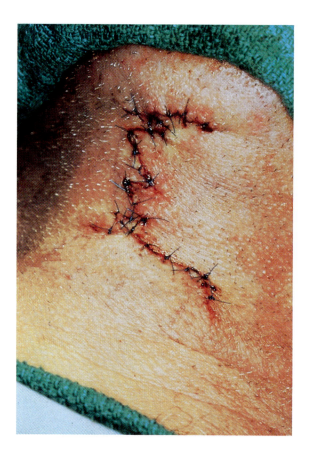

Figure 13-27
The incision is closed in multiple layers. The incision does not extend beyond the suprahyoid crease.

Results and Outcome

Following the procedure, the neck skin is quite snug. In older individuals especially, the W-plasty heals with minimal scarring. This procedure eliminates a lengthy vertical scar that is subject to banding or contraction. Instead it uses an interrupted W-plasty that lies closer to resting skin tension lines to provide a superior cosmetic result. When the incisions can be confined to an area above the suprahyoid crease, added camouflaging is achieved by the shadow of the chin and the fact that the scar lies in a plane parallel to the floor. The incision is not easily visible when looking at the patient face to face. Rarely, in patients with very excessive skin redundancy, the W-plasty is carried below the level of the suprahyoid crease. It is our opinion and that of our patients that in these instances the W-plasty provides adequate camouflage and that a small portion of visible scar is a definite improvement over the preoperative "turkey gobbler" appearance (Figs 13-28 to 13-31).

CHAPTER 13   Aesthetic Surgery of the Aging Neck

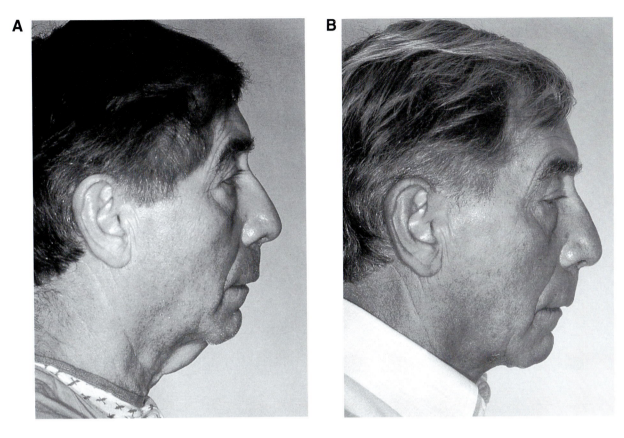

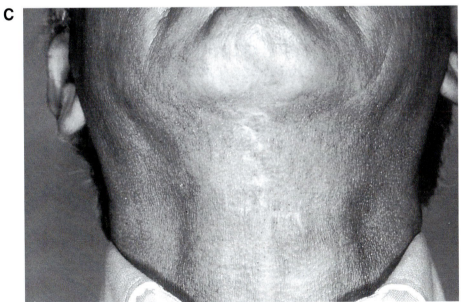

Figure 13-28
A, a typical midline "turkey gobbler" deformity. **B**, the patient's appearance 2 years postoperatively. **C**, submental W-plasty scar at 1 year.

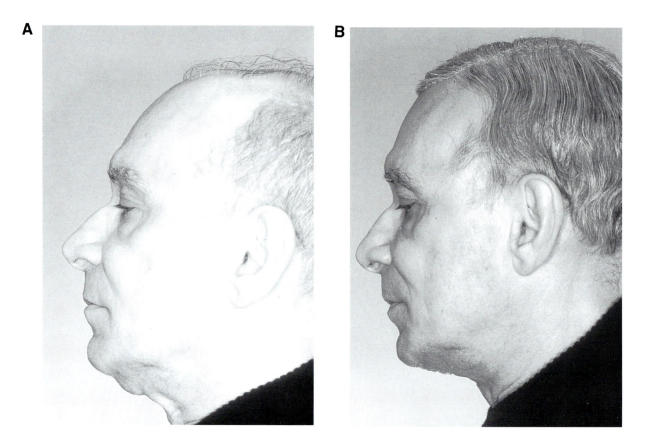

Figure 13-29
A and **B,** a midline submental deformity in one patient who does not otherwise require a rhytidectomy was corrected with the midline submental running W-plasty technique.

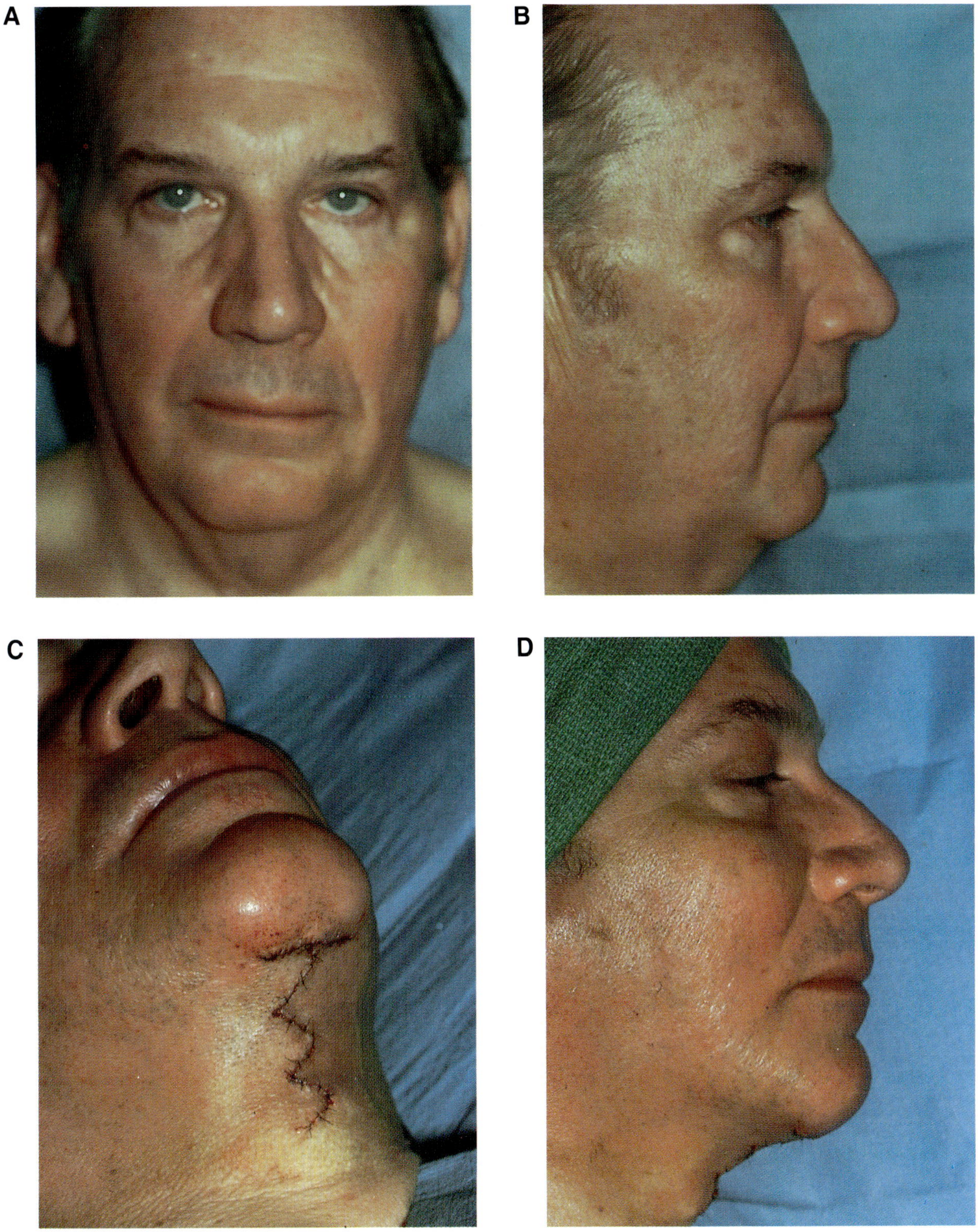

CHAPTER 13   Aesthetic Surgery of the Aging Neck

Figure 13–30
A–D, flaccid submental skin with associated fat in an older male was corrected with the multiple Z-plasty technique.

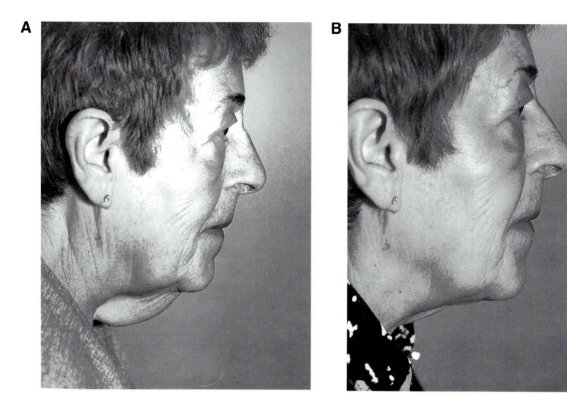

Figure 13-31

A and **B,** submental wattles corrected by multiple Z-plasty repair after large cervical skin resection. The result is shown at 3 months.

Complications and Sequelae

The usual sequelae are not unlike those of scar excision or other incisional procedures of the skin. An expected period of postoperative erythema and induration will be experienced while the incision is healing. Because of hair-bearing skin, a male patient may have difficulty with folliculitis or "ingrown" hair at the wound edge. This typically responds to cleansing with antiseptic soap and topical antibiotic ointment.

Complications have been rare. Hematoma or seroma formation is possible and treated by aspiration and evacuation depending on the degree. Wound infection has been suggested but has not been experienced by the authors. The running W-plasty configuration prevents significant scar contracture problems.

CHAPTER 13   Aesthetic Surgery of the Aging Neck

Suggested Reading

- Thomas JR: Facial plastic surgery applications for liposuction, in Cummings C, et al (eds): *Otolaryngology—Head and Neck Surgery, Update I.* St Louis, Mosby–Year Book, 1990, pp 160–165.
- Ehlert TK, Thomas JR, Becker FF: Submental W-plasty for correction of turkey gobbler deformities. *Arch Otolaryngol* 1990;116:714–717.
- Grazer FM: *Atlas of Suction Assisted Lipectomy in Body Contouring.* New York, Churchill Livingstone, 1992.
- Lambros V: Fat contouring in the face and neck. *Clin Plast Surg* 1992;19:401–414.

PART III

AESTHETIC AUGMENTATION PROCEDURES

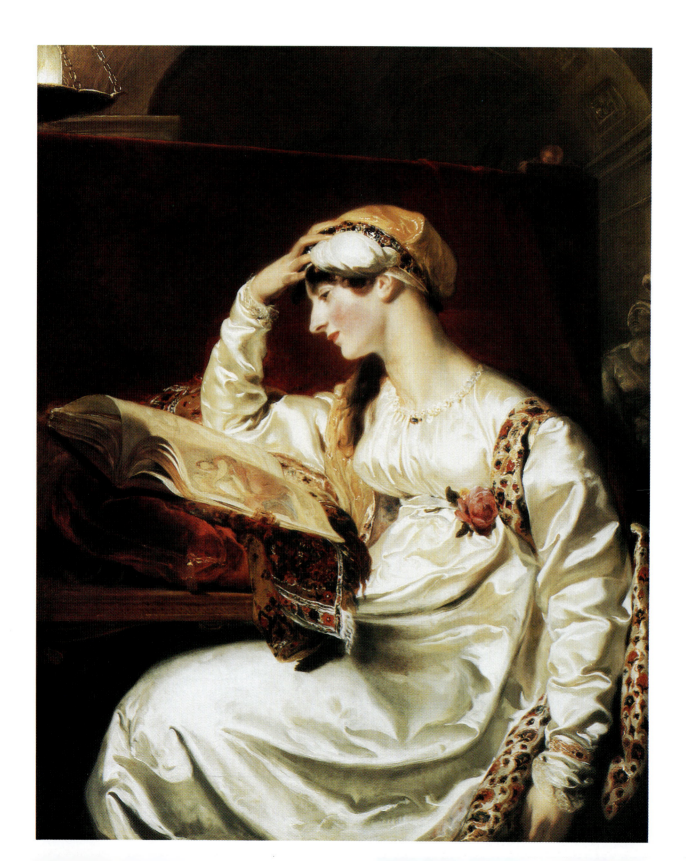

CHAPTER 14

Chin Augmentation

*Tis not the lip or eye we beauty call,
But the joint force and full result of all.*

Alexander Pope

Diagnosis and Candidate Selection

A long sweeping elegant jawline is a most desirable feature in an attractive face and neck (Fig 14-1). Retrognathia, manifested by bony mandibular deficiency and/or loss of muscular skin pad posture, creates facial disharmony and proportion imbalance (Fig 14-2). Inadequate chin projection is commonly encountered in patients seeking aesthetic facial surgery. Although chin augmentation may be performed as an isolated procedure, it is frequently performed as an adjunct to rhinoplasty or rhytidectomy (Fig 14-3). Submental lipectomy associated with chin augmentation adds a further refinement to the mandibulocervical definition (Fig 14-4).

Malocclusion and significant facial skeletal abnormalities are of course not corrected by chin augmentation alone. Patients with major mandibular deficiencies and asymmetries are best treated by orthognathic and orthodontic correction.

Patients most commonly are acutely aware of their facial features and proportions visualized in the frontal appearance. Experience teaches, however, that chin projection is poorly appreciated by most patients and only rarely do they accurately evaluate that component of the facial anatomy. The requirements of chin augmentation to establish facial or cervico facial balance typically must be introduced to the patient by the surgeon as an optional method of enhancing the overall facial appearance. Accurate lateral and oblique photographs play a helpful role in educating individuals about mandibular deficiencies. Computerized videoimaging, if demonstrated in a clinically accurate and realistic manner, is useful in this particular instance for underscoring the significant improvements possible with chin augmentation or reconstruction.

In the rhinoplasty patient, augmentation of the chin brings the lower third of the face into improved alignment and harmony with the middle third (see Fig 14-4). The degree of apparent nasal projection is often dramatically changed in appearance by relative changes in chin projection.

CHAPTER 14   Chin Augmentation

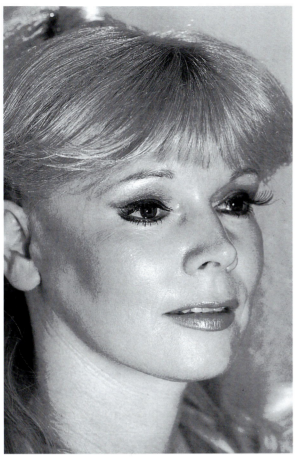

Figure 14–1
A long, sweeping, clean, and well-defined mandibular line ending in a normally projected chin is a highly desirable component of facial beauty.

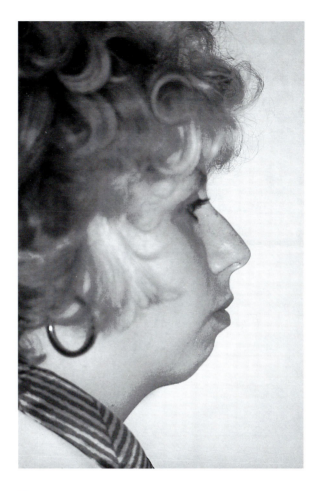

Figure 14–2
Retrognathia, particularly if associated with excess submental fat and a low position of the hyoid, results in significant imbalance and disharmony in the lower part of the face and the neck regions.

The rhytidectomy patient, as a consequence of aging, commonly exhibits poor chin projection associated with an obtuse cervicomandibular angle. Conservative augmentation with a chin implant establishes better projection and increased differentiation of the mandibular horizontal and cervical vertical planes. The implant may also serve to augment the ptotic chin soft-tissue structures frequently found in the aging chin; significant chin pad sagging, however, requires cephalic repositioning of the ptotic muscle pad to correct an inferior malposition of these tissues.

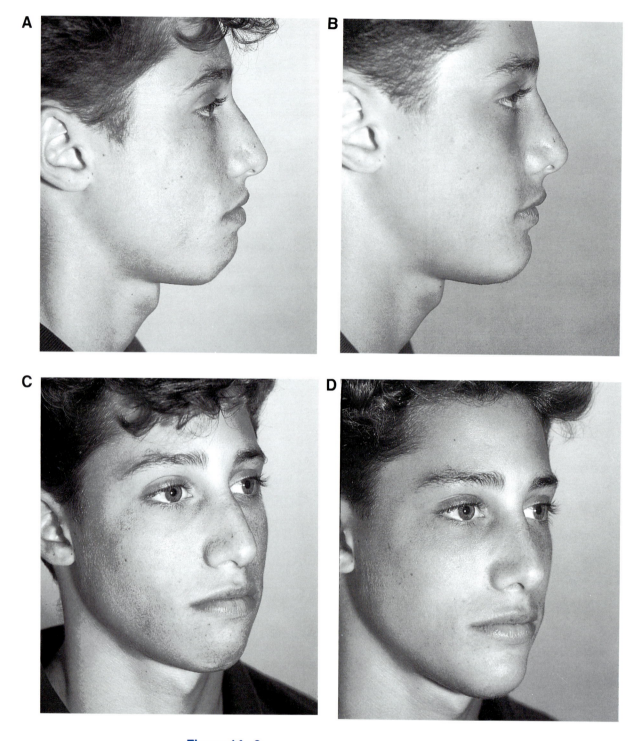

Figure 14–3
A and B, an inadequately developed chin robs the masculine face of a strong feature essential for facial balance. Chin augmentation (here combined with rhinoplasty) restores balance and strength to the facial appearance.

CHAPTER 14   Chin Augmentation

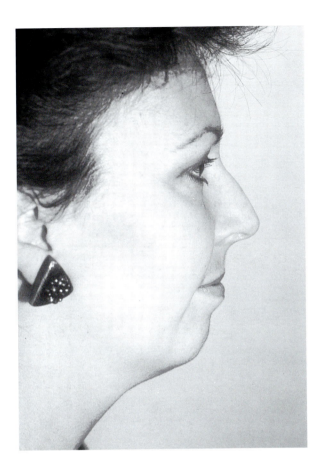
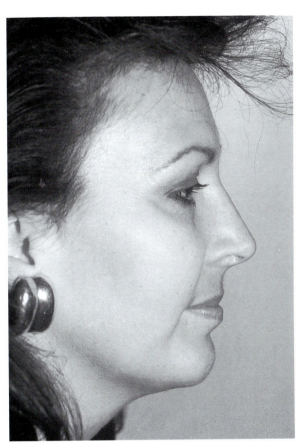

Figure 14–4
Significantly improved facial balance following chin augmentation combined with submental lipectomy and rhinoplasty.

Surgical Goals and Planned Outcomes

Restoration of a normal, natural, and pleasing position and projection of the chin in proportion with the remaining facial features is the primary goal of augmentation mentoplasty. The ideal anatomy and normal proportions of the chin in relationship to the remaining facial features are demonstrated in Figure 14–5.

We prefer to approach the chin augmentation operation through an external submental incision. The intraoral approach avoids an external scar but is technically slightly more difficult and creates a greater tendency of the implant or its lateral edges to migrate superiorly away from the inferior mandibular edge. In addition, the labial-gingival sulcus can be blunted by scar tissue or the cephalic edge of the implant. Potentially, the possibility of operative implant contamination is greater with the intraoral approach.

Incisions placed in the submental area can be strategically placed and well camouflaged. Through a single small incision, both chin augmentation and submental lipectomy, if indicated, can be carried out. A submental approach allows for direct-vision positioning of the implant in a highly accurate fashion relative to the mandibular margin and the lateral aspect of the mentum. Migration of the implant superiorly is resisted by retaining muscle attachments, which preserves the labial sulcus and mental crease. Implant materials should not only have a natural appearance following augmentation but should also be minimally palpable or completely impalpable. Stabilization to the mandible and within the surrounding soft

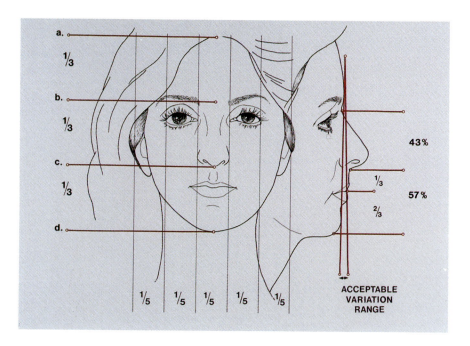

Figure 14–5

Parameters of proportion considered to be normal in the chin region.

CHAPTER 14 Chin Augmentation

tissues is important; the implant should not exist as a free-floating foreign body with excessive mobility. We prefer a solid soft Silastic implant that can be carved or modified to specific patient anatomic requirements. Such implants are soft and pliable and within a few weeks after implantation take on essentially the same palpable resistance and consistency as the remaining soft tissues of the skin. The midline for stability and accurate symmetry of positioning. When laterally extended implants are required, we prefer the soft silicone mittelman chin implant.

Surgical Technique

Retrognathia significantly detracts from even the finest of outcomes of aesthetic rhinoplasty. As a prominent feature in the overall facial profile, the chin and the submental neck configuration must not be neglected when considering appearance surgery. Patients with significant retrognathia who request rhinoplasty or rhytidectomy are routinely advised of the benefits of chin augmentation upon the ultimate favorable facial appearances; the final decision to add mentoplasty to the primary rejuvenative procedures is then left entirely up to the judgment of the patient.

If augmentation mentoplasty is elected, we prefer to complete this procedure at the outset of the operation in order that this sterile procedure be completed prior to less-sterile aspects of the operation.

Our preference of implants, from the plethora of choices available, remains the solid soft Silastic prosthesis (Fig 14–6). The advantages of this implant include ready availability, ease of insertion through a small inci-

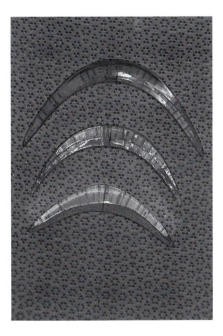

Figure 14–6
The soft, solid silastic chin implant.

sion, complete tissue acceptability, and little or no palpable evidence of the implant following healing. Prior to the current unresolved controversy surrounding silicone gel implants, we utilized exclusively the dacron-backed Gel-chin implant. To our knowledge, no implant of this type utilized in our institution over the past 20 years has undergone immediate or delayed host rejection, occasioned any episode of infection, or required removal. This safety record reinforces our preference for this chin prosthesis as the primary mentoplasty implant device. Until government regulatory bodies establish a definite policy, Gel-chin implants should probably not be employed, despite their exceptional safety record. Oral antibiotic coverage, not deemed necessary when septorhinoplasty alone is carried out, routinely ensues for 5 days after augmentation mentoplasty.

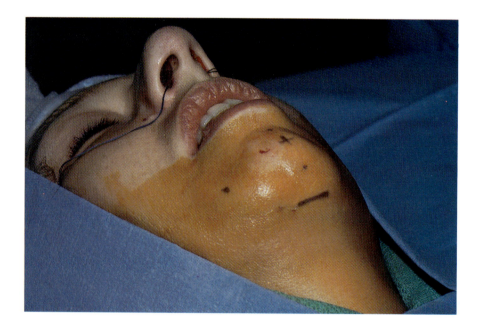

Figure 14–7
Following infiltration of 1% lidocaine with 1:100,000 epinephrine solution into the soft tissues of the chin and submental incision site, landmarks (the chin midline and lateral extent of the planned augmentation, incision site, and extent) are sited with a sterile marking pen. Povidone-iodine (Betadine) solution renders the operative field surgically clean.

CHAPTER 14   Chin Augmentation

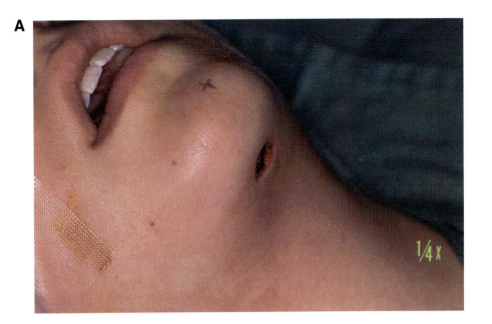

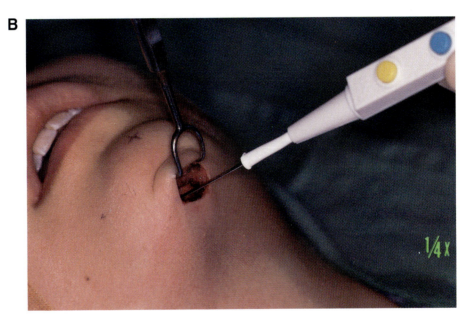

Figure 14-8
A, the entry incision, 1.5 cm long, exposes the submental fat for trimming to facilitate visualization of the muscle layer. To avoid the submental crease the incision is properly sited 2 to 3 mm posterior to the crease. This small but vital nuance avoids potential accentuation of the depth of the crease and aids in more accurate effacement closure of the skin incision. (If submental lipoplasty is to be combined with augmentation mentoplasty, this complementary procedure follows and is completed before continuing with the dissection necessary for positioning of the chin implant.) **B,** division of the muscular layer is performed with the cutting Bovie cautery unit to facilitate complete hemostasis and expose the periosteum overlying the chin.

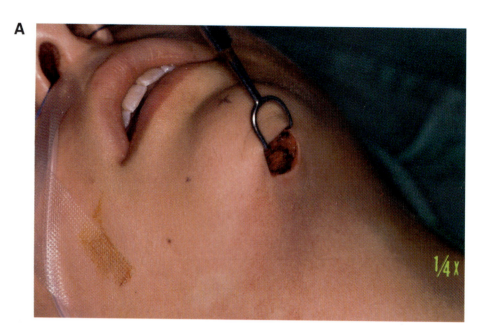

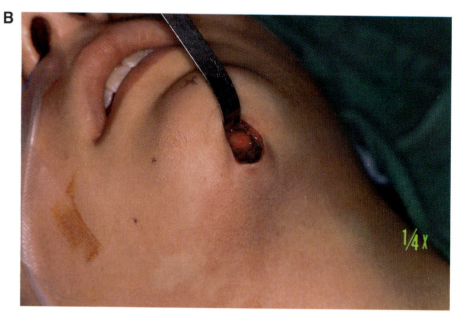

Figure 14–9
A, a wide double-pronged skin hook positioned in the superior flap of the incision lifts the incision site slightly cephalically in order to site the overlying muscle incision at a level slightly higher than the skin incision, thus allowing a staggered, layered suture closure of the tissues at different levels. **B,** exposure of the periosteum.

CHAPTER 14 Chin Augmentation

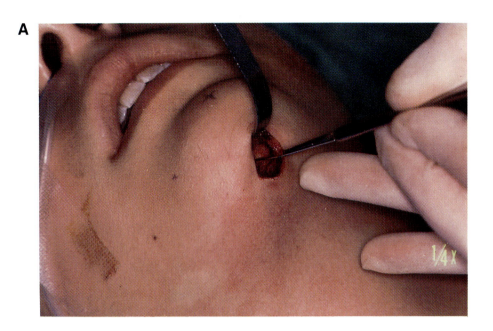

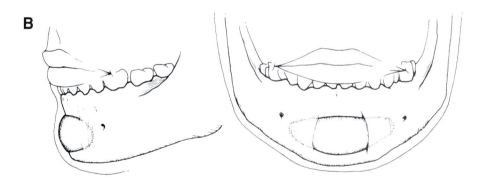

Figure 14–10
A, the horizontal periosteum incision, created at the inferior margin of the anterior portion of the chin, extends for a distance of 2 to 3 cm, depending upon the size of the required implant. At the lateral borders of this horizontal incision, a *vertical* cut in the periosteum **(B)** is positioned for ultimate periosteal undermining to accommodate the lateral margins of the implant. Meticulous hemostasis utilizing electrocautery follows. No step in the chin augmentation procedure should ensue until absolute hemostasis exists.

Figure 14-10 (cont.).
Elevation of the midline periosteum, attached throughout to the overlying soft tissues, follows with upward sweeping rotary motions of a Joseph periosteal elevator. Sufficiently large subperiosteal elevation should be developed in the up-down direction to allow the implant to sit exactly above the lower border of the mentum.

Development of the lateral subperiosteal pockets with the Joseph elevator extends the implant pocket sufficiently laterally to comfortably accommodate the chosen implant size and embrace it firmly without allowing excessive implant mobility following insertion. To discourage any intraoperative swelling, firm pressure is now maintained over the chin and submental area by the surgical assistant while the desired implant is selected and prepared for insertion.

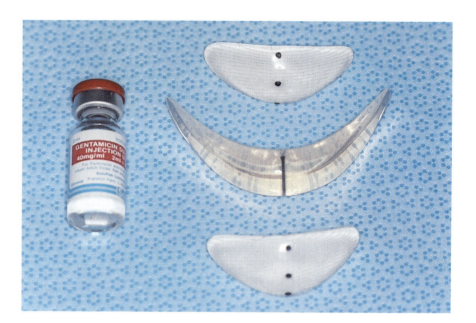

Figure 14–11
After coordinating the appearance of the exposed chin with the greater-than-life-size preoperative lateral slide photograph projected on the operating room wall, selection of the appropriately sized chin implant follows. As an additional safeguard, the implant undergoes immersion in gentamicin sulfate (Garamycin) antibiotic solution prior to insertion.

CHAPTER 14   Chin Augmentation

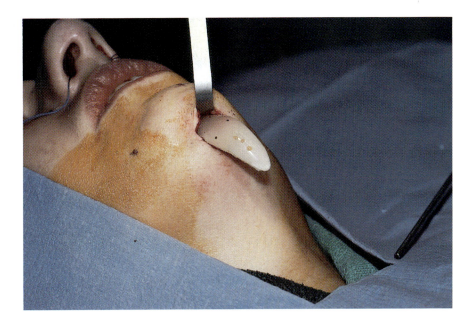

Figure 14–12
By employing the thin Siegal retractor to expose the lateral subperiosteal pockets, exact positioning of the lateral edges of the implant is facilitated by "shoe-horning," in turn, each lateral border of the prosthesis in place. A black dot centered on the implant assists in ensuring its midline position before closure.

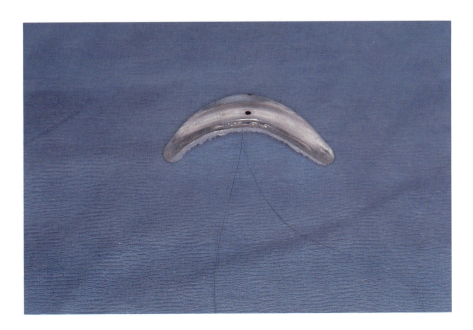

Figure 14–13
Securing the V-shaped midline Dacron tag of the implant to the inferior periosteum flap with a 5-0 polydioxane suture provides additional midline stabilization and discourages any tendency of the prosthesis to be distorted during the contractual healing process.

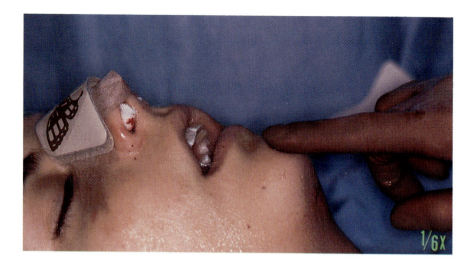

Figure 14-14
Visual and palpable assessment of the effect of augmentation is assisted by a hydrogen peroxide–moistened finger, which provides more sensitive tactile evaluation through the overlying epithelial chin canopy. Suture closure of the operative wound layers is accomplished in *staggered fashion* with buried 5-0 PDS interrupted sutures and cutaneous 7-0 nylon reinforced with Histoacryl glue. Slight eversion of the skin edges should result from proper closure.

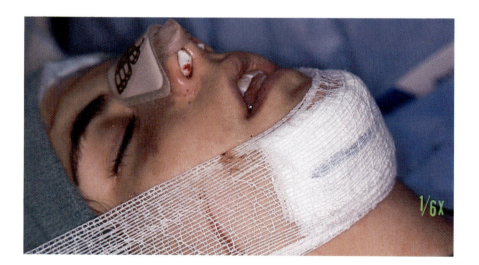

Figure 14-15
During the period of time devoted to the ensuing rhinoplasty or rhytidectomy, maintaining constant firm pressure on the chin and submental dissection areas with a 4-in. Conform dressing further limits operative site swelling while surgery is being carried out elsewhere. This small detail significantly speeds the healing process. The circumferential dressing remains in place for 24 to 48 hours following surgery.

Without question, conservative chin augmentation is preferable to even slight overaugmentation, particularly upon the frontal view. Because of the soft, flexible nature of the implant, within just a few weeks the chin achieves a natural, soft, and often palpably undetectable consistency that persists long-term.

Results and Outcomes

Overall facial balance and harmony of proportions result from appropriate augmentation mentoplasty, which often provides aesthetic improvement well out of proportion to the degree of difficulty of the operation. Mentoplasty ordinarily accompanies other facial rejuvenation procedures and adds significant improvement in patients exhibiting congenital retrognathia as well as retrognathia resulting from the aging process. Mentoplasty combined with submental lipectomy and cervical-lifting procedures restores a youthful, graceful mandibulocervical angle and provides a striking rejuvenation appearance.

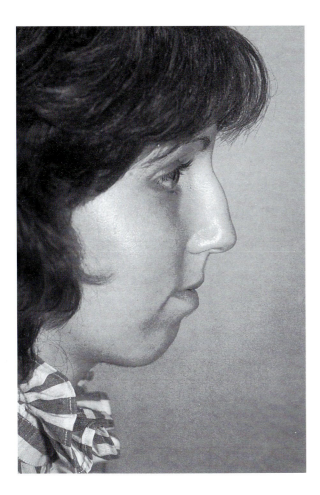
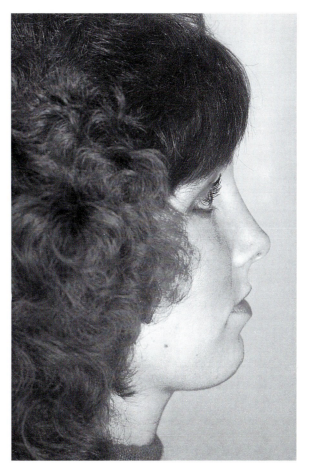

Figure 14–16
Major improvement in facial balance and aesthetics following augmentation mentoplasty combined with rhinoplasty.

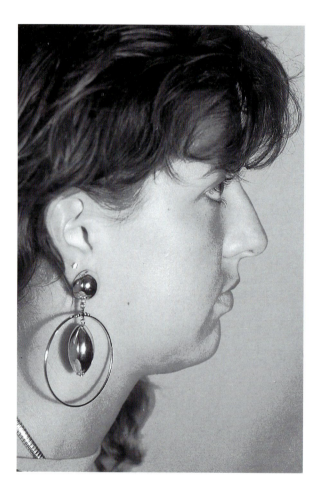
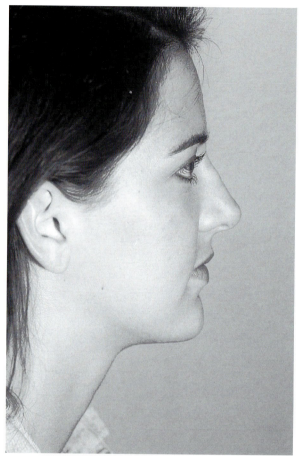

Figure 14–17
Submental lipectomy combined with chin augmentation in both younger as well as older patients refines the mandibular line and cervicomental angle.

CHAPTER 14 Chin Augmentation

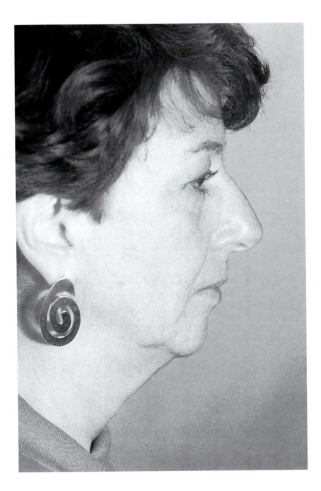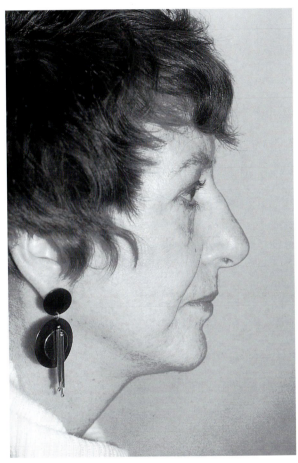

Figure 14–18
Chin augmentation significantly enhances the improvement in appearance provided by a facelift with submental lipectomy.

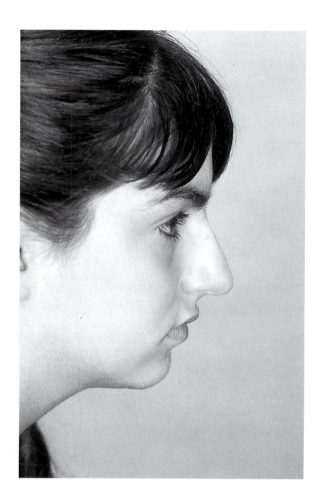
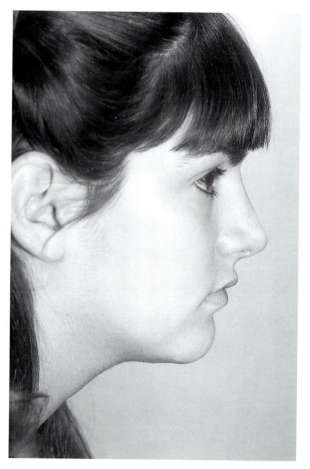

Figure 14–19
Improved facial balance following chin augmentation combined with rhinoplasty.

Complications and Sequelae

In the experience of the author, complications are rare and tend to be caused by the implant shifting its position rather than infection or extrusion. Oral broad-spectrum antibiotics administered for 5 days postoperatively provide essential protection against infection following chin augmentation.

Rarely, initial antibiotics fail to control infection, and removal of the implant is required (Fig 14–20, A and B). Because of the excellent soft-tissue protection and good vascularity of the region the possibility of extrusion is remote and limited still further by careful layered closure of the muscle and skin incision.

Erosion or resorption of the anterior table of the mandible has been reported as an incidental radiologic finding, although any related clinical sequelae appear to be rare. Clearly, soft implants reduce the constant mandibular pressure exerted by hard implants, apparently reducing or negating any significant bone resorption.

CHAPTER 14 Chin Augmentation

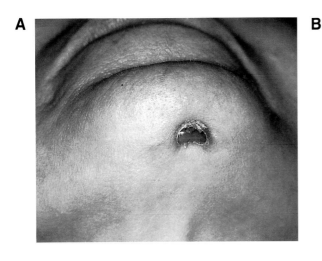
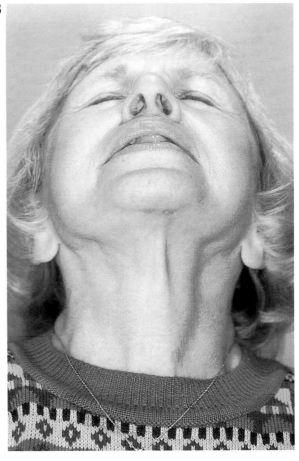

Figure 14-20
A, fistula surrounded by granulomatous tissue from chin implant infection in an older patient operated elsewhere. **B,** appearance following removal of the implant and granuloma.

The submental incision is well camouflaged when sited as demonstrated. In patients where extensive anterior chin projection is accomplished with augmentation it is helpful to position the incision a few millimeters more posteriorly. As the skin is advanced anteriorly because of the projection of the implant, this prevents the incision from being pulled anteriorly to a point that may be more visible.

The choice of a properly sized implant plays the most important role in the ultimate favorable outcome. In addition to proper size in the anteroposterior dimension, the implant must have sufficient lateral extension to properly augment the entire lower anterior portion of the mandible (where indicated) and not just the more limited midline segment. Lateral augmentation with layered rolls of Mersilene mesh or use of an extended Silastic implant are both excellent alternatives in these situations (Fig 14–21, A and B).

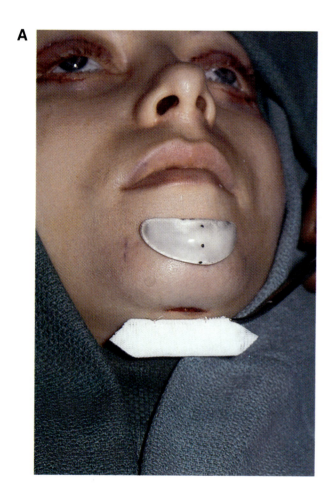
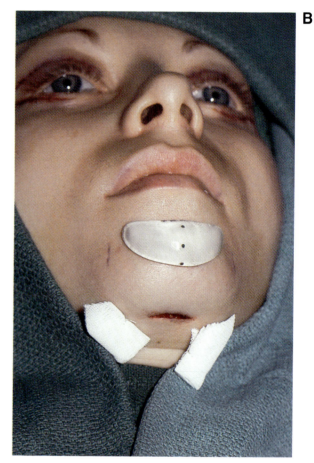

Figure 14–21
A, custom-contoured layered implants of Mersilene mesh are valuable in augmenting prefabricated implants to provide more lateral extension or to differentially augment asymmetrical chins. **B,** the custom-designed implant may be cut in half to facilitate insertion. The lateral margins are feathered as necessary to conform to the individual characteristics of each patient.

Suggested Reading

- Powell N, Humphreys B: *Proportions of the Aesthetic Face.* New York, Thieme Stratton, 1984.
- Thomas JR, et al: *Analysis of patient response to preoperative computerized video imaging.* Arch Otolaryngol Head Neck Surg 1989; 115:793–796.

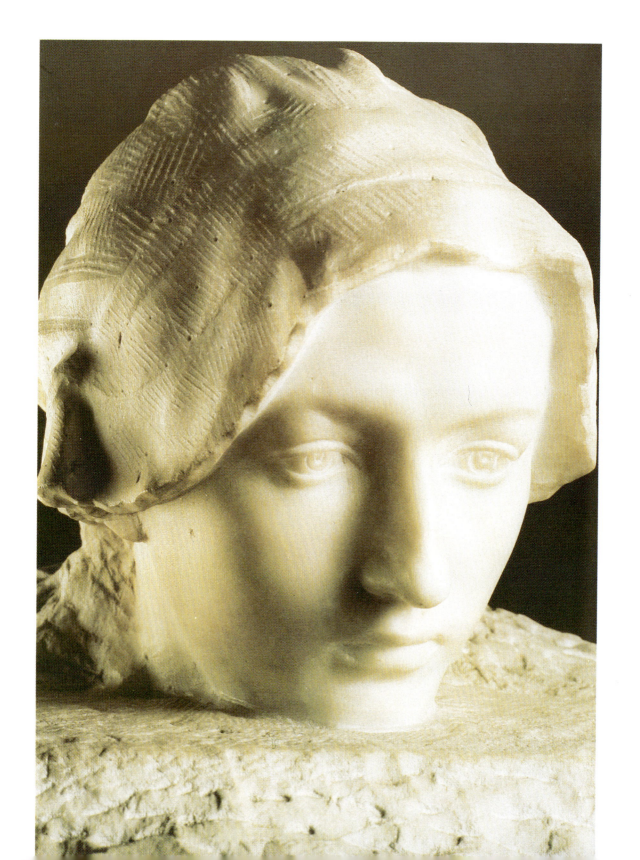

CHAPTER
15

 # Injectable Fillers

PART III AESTHETIC AUGMENTATION PROCEDURES

Age has a good mind and sorry shanks.

Pietro Aretino

Injectable collagen (Zyderm, Zyplast) was developed in the 1970s, and patient treatment series were begun in 1976. The medical collagen material is produced by enzymatic degradation of bovine collagen from calf hide. This process effectively removes the majority of antigenic potential from the telopeptide structure of the collagen molecule.

When injected the suspended material undergoes transformation to a firm mass of orderly fibrous collagen that may augment soft dermal skin depressions. Collagen remains localized and becomes vascularized, and a surrounding capsule does not develop within the tissue. The material is slowly but variably absorbed to result in a gradual loss of corrective augmentation. This typically occurs over a 6- to 12-month period for facial wrinkles.

Other types of collagen injection include the porcine derivative Fibrel. This product has been used satisfactorily by some practitioners, who mix the product with autogenous serum from the patient. It has not offered clinically significant advantages in terms of longevity for the authors; our experience has thus been primarily with the bovine Zyderm/Zyplast product.

Three bovine collagen products are presently available: Zyderm I, Zyderm II, and Zyplast (Collagen Corp., Palo Alto, Calif).

Zyderm I contains the basic purified bovine collagen molecule in a concentration of 35 mg/mL (all the products are dispersed in buffered physiologic saline plus 0.3% lidocaine). It is generally used for small intradermal depression defects more superficial in nature. It may also be used as a secondary superficial layer over deeper augmentation effected by Zyderm II or Zyplast.

Zyderm II, a more concentrated form of collagen containing 65 mg/mL, is preferred for use in deeper depressions. It is presently the recommended collagen type for augmentation in the glabellar region, where Zyplast should be avoided because of reported instances of tissue necrosis.

Zyplast has the helical collagen molecules cross-linked with glutaraldehyde in a suspension of 35 mg/mL. Theoretically it therefore provides longer-lasting augmentation. It is intended for deep dermal infiltration since nodular irregularities and tissue infarction may result if used too superficially.

CHAPTER 15 Injectable Fillers

Diagnosis and Candidate Selection

Collagen injection has proved to be an effective dermal skin augmentation for many depressed scars or facial depressions, especially facial rhytids. Depressions with sharp, defined edges and narrow "ice pack" acne scars do not usually respond well.

Patients with a personal history of lupus erythematosus, polymyositis, rheumatoid or psoriatic arthritis, scleroderma, or other autoimmune diseases and patients with a history of anaphylactoid reactions or known history of lidocaine hypersensitivity or hypersensitivity to the injectable collagen are not candidates for collagen injections. The material is only useful for dermal skin augmentation and should not be used for injection into bone, tendon, ligaments, or muscle.

All patients are skin-tested at least once prior to treatment. The test site is observed for 4 weeks before declaring reactions to collagen negative. Recently recommendations have been published by some for double-testing (at intervening 4-week intervals) to more intensively screen for positive reactions.

In addition to augmenting facial rhytids and depressed scars, injectable collagen has recently been used to augment and enhance the definition near the lips. The material is injected in the skin dermis near the lip margin and the subnasal vertical ridges of the philtrum. Since lip definition and fullness tend to diminish with aging, this process attempts to temporarily counter those changes.

Over the past decade most practitioners' experience with injectable collagen in the fine lines of the thin-skinned periorbital region is unsatisfactory. Not infrequently small "lumps" and "beads" of collagen are visible beneath the skin. A new form of collagen specifically designed for this region is undergoing its clinical investigation stages at the time of this publication. However, presently we avoid the use of injectable fillers around the orbit.

Goals and Planned Outcomes

The augmentation goals are to improve and efface skin depressions and rhytids. Depending on the nature and size of the area to be treated, adequate augmentation can usually be obtained in one to three sessions (typically 2 weeks apart). The patient should be aware that the correction attained is not permanent and that reaugmentation will need to be accomplished as the injected collagen is absorbed. This step is typically required in 6 to 15 months. Once the patient stops the follow-up treatment, the skin will gradually return to its pretreatment appearance.

Patients are able to resume work or other normal activities immediately following treatment. There is usually some erythema and swelling at the injection site. Occasionally localized bruising develops. Normal skin care and makeup may be resumed immediately following a treatment session. The redness and mild swelling subside within a few days.

The injected collagen is not generally visually distinguishable from the surrounding skin. Most patients will, however, be able to palpate the injection sites when they touch the outline of the injected material.

Patients are usually advised to return at 2-week intervals for "touch-up" sessions until definitive correction is obtained. The injected collagen will not only undergo resorption gradually but will also respond to the same mechanical forces from smiling or other muscle activity and biochemical processes that caused the original rhytids and skin depressions. There is marked variation from one patient to another in how much time will elapse before repeat augmentation is indicated. There are also differences within the same patient for different regions or locations of the face. Usually (unless the patient waits for a prolonged period) the amount of collagen required to restore full augmentation will be considerably less than that used in the initial correction injections.

Technique

Treatment with injectable collagen can be divided into three basic steps: a skin test, the treatment series, and periodic touch-ups. The technique for injection tends to exhibit a personal technical learning curve (as in most surgical and manual skill activities), with results improving as the physician gains more experience. A more difficult task to learn (or teach) is a critical, "aesthetic eye" for the result. Not unlike other aesthetic surgical procedures, the tissue relationships are crucial to gaining optimum results with injectable collagen.

Test Dose Injection

The skin test is identical for Zyderm I, Zyderm II, and Zyplast. Zyderm 1, 0.1 mL, supplied in the test-dose syringe is injected intradermally into the volar surface of the forearm. About 70% of reactions occur within 72 hours. The remaining 30% occur up to 4 weeks, and the arm is examined at this time. In the interim, the patient is instructed to notify the physician of any untoward response. For test results that are equivocal, a second test implantation is administered in the postauricular skin overlying the mastoid.

A positive test reaction is defined as erythema, induration, tenderness, and swelling at the test site, with or without pruritus, and the possible onset of rash, arthralgia, or myalgia. A positive reaction within the 4-week test period contraindicates treatment.

Treatment Injection Technique

For Zyderm I and Zyderm II the needle is inserted into the dermis at a 30- to 45-degree angle. The bevel of the needle may be directed downward or upward as a matter of individual preference. The authors prefer the lat-

CHAPTER 15   Injectable Fillers

ter. The site is stabilized by finger pressure, often by pinching the skin upward. Placement of Zyderm within the superficial dermis appears to offer the best results. When the bevel is within the dermis, the needle tip is rocked upward so that the skin surface is tented up. This helps to ensure superficial placement of the implant. If collagen extrudes from skin pores, the injection is stopped and the needle repositioned. Depressions are overcorrected 1.5 to 2 times with Zyderm I and 1.25 times with Zyderm II.

One may continue injecting the implant in this fashion with multiple punctures every one eighth of an inch or less along the depression. This method was originally described as the "serial puncture" method and provides the operator with a precise implantation technique. One may also continue injecting ahead of a horizontally advancing needle, along the axis of a linear scar, referred to as the "threading" technique.

A double-layer injection technique has also been described. With this method, Zyderm is first placed into the deep dermis or dermal-subdermal plane. Second, the superficial dermis is augmented in a second layer above the first. This method attempts to provide maximal dermal augmentation. We employ Zyplast for the deep injection and Zyderm I for the superficial injection.

For Zyplast injection, the needle is inserted into the deep dermal plane, and the skin is tented upward when the needle is rocked. This confirms accurate placement of the needle within the dermis. The skin is then allowed to rest normally, and the implant is injected with minimal overcorrection.

A 30-gauge needle is preferred for all three forms of collagen. The material for fine-line augmentation in the periorbital region that is presently under investigation utilizes a 32-gauge needle.

Magnification with loupes or an operating microscope is helpful and may assist with more accurate implantation. The authors do not use magnification routinely but certainly would not argue with its use by others. It is helpful to have an assistant view from another perspective and position to verify symmetry.

The injections may be initially somewhat uncomfortable, particularly around the lips or the nose. The collagen suspension contains small amounts of lidocaine to reduce discomfort as the injection proceeds. Additional local anesthetic injection is usually unwarranted and not required. Likewise, local injection distorts tissues and makes accurate collagen placement impossible. Some prefer the topical use of ice to the skin prior to injection.

The elevation of depressed dermal scars has been traditionally centered on excising the depression or planing down the surrounding normal tissue with dermabrasion (or chemical peeling for facial wrinkles). Use of the injectable collagens, however, is an attempt to elevate the depressed scar to the level of the surrounding normal skin by augmentation of the dermal or subdermal levels. Therefore injectable collagen and dermabrasion are often used together to approach the problem from both sides. Injection may in addition be added to direct surgical revision to produce a fine-line scar. When a satisfactory result may be obtained with surgery and dermabrasion alone, these methods are preferred over collagen because of lasting results.

A soft, mature scar is more amenable to implantation than a hard fibrous scar. In these latter cases, the "softening" effect of the implant allows improvement with later injections. A pretest injection with saline has been described to allow better assessment of the potential usefulness of collagen implantation for a given scar. Scars with sharply marginated edges respond less well than gently sloping depressions. Given their limitations, the injectable collagens provide an important adjunct in scar revision for selected patients.

Results and Outcomes

A patient with treatable fine rhytids will observe improvement immediately following the treatment session. Variable amounts of swelling, erythema, and ecchymosis will be present, but they subside within a few days. Most patients are able to easily cover the areas with makeup.

Frequent areas treated include perioral areas. Figure 15–1 shows treatment of radiating vertical rhytids of the lips. The patient demonstrated also had the small depressions at the area of the lateral commissures treated (Fig 15–1).

Other depressions may be corrected with injectable collagen. Figure 15–2 demonstrates improvement of buccal depressions in a patient with atrophy of facial adipose tissue. The patient must, of course, periodically return for reaugmentation.

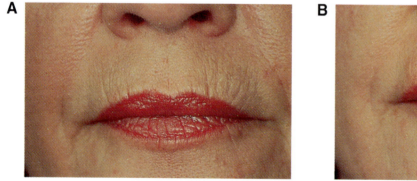
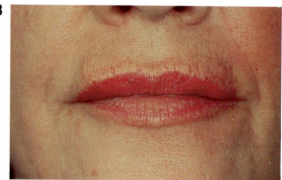

Figure 15–1
A, a common picture of perioral rhytids radiating from the vermilion border. **B,** post-treatment appearance following two treatment sessions.

CHAPTER 15   Injectable Fillers

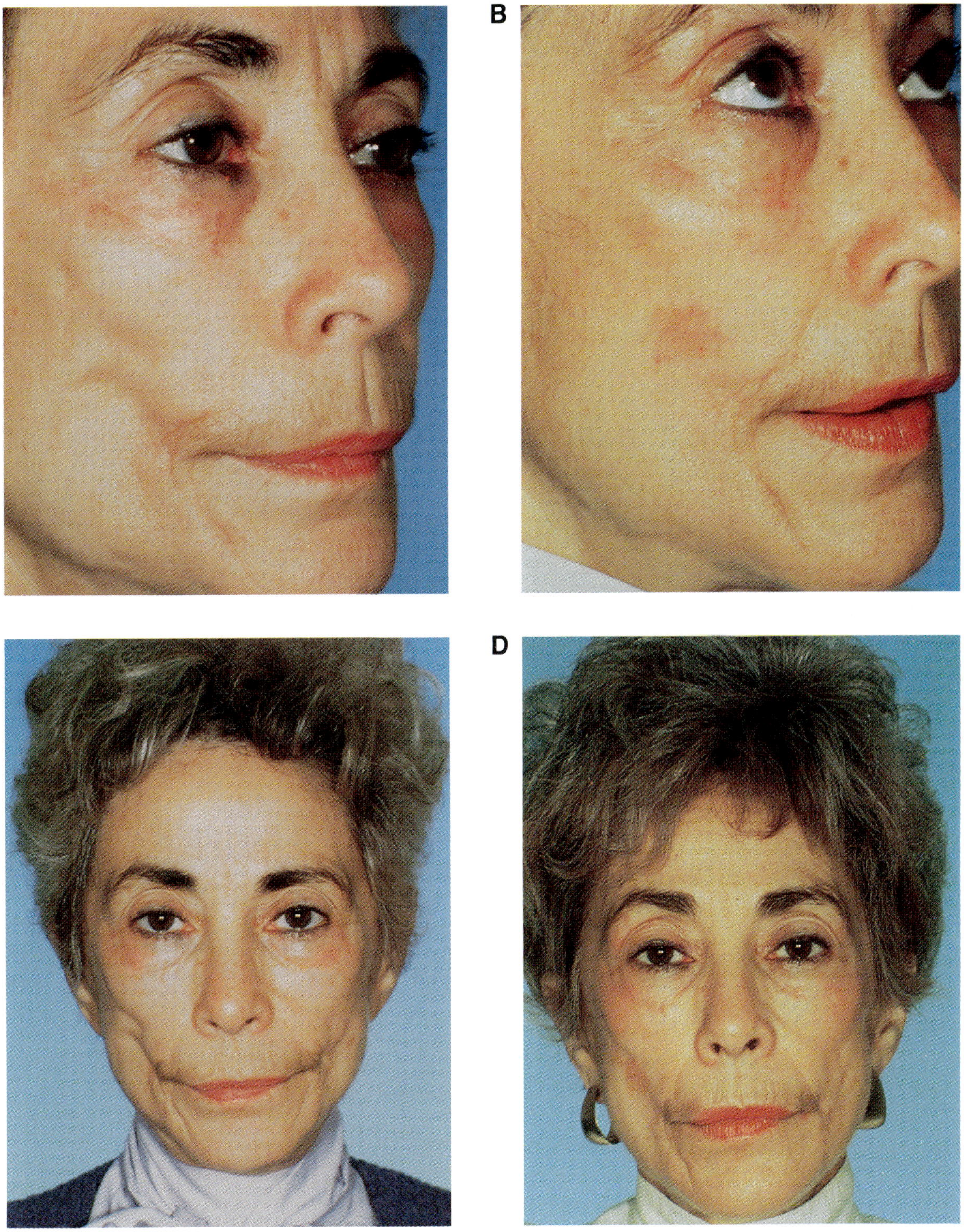

Figure 15-2
A, the facial appearance of a patient with adipose atrophy prior to treatment. **B,** post-treatment appearance of the buccal-cheek region. **C,** pretreatment appearance of the same patient. **D,** after treatment there is improvement of the cheek regions.

A new material is presently under investigation at the time of this publication for correcting the fine lines of the periorbital region. This injectable collagen is infiltrated through a 32-gauge needle (Fig 15–3). This material appears to have the ability to be injected through a fine needle in areas of thin skin. Even in very thin-skinned patients, there does not appear to be the problems of "beading" or clumps of collagen showing through at the injection site (Fig 15–4).

Enhanced definition near the lip line employs Zyplast collagen in the same manner as described for facial rhytids (Fig 15–5). In this region an

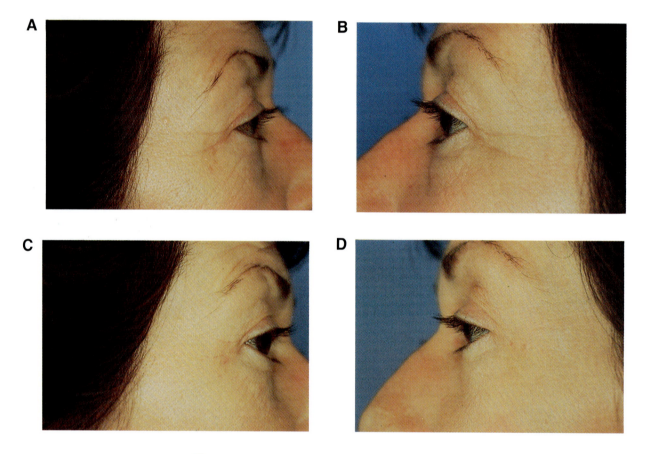

Figure 15–3
A and **B,** Lateral periorbital lines in the "crow's-foot" region in a patient with moderate to thick skin. **C** and **D,** good improvement is seen in these lateral lines following a single session of treatment.

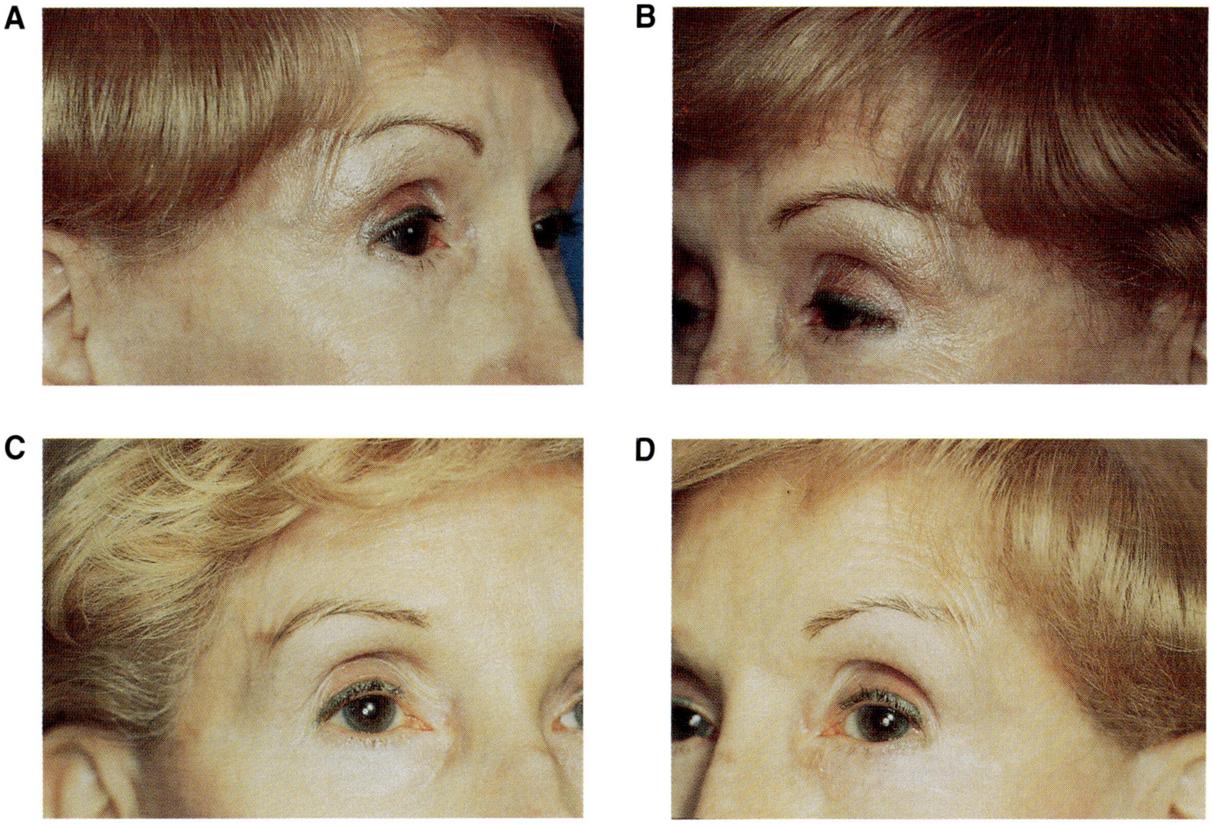

CHAPTER 15 Injectable Fillers

Figure 15–4
A and **B,** lateral periorbital rhytids in a patient with very thin, translucent skin. **C** and **D,** the appearance after a single session. There is no evidence of "beading" or visible collagen clumping in the treated areas.

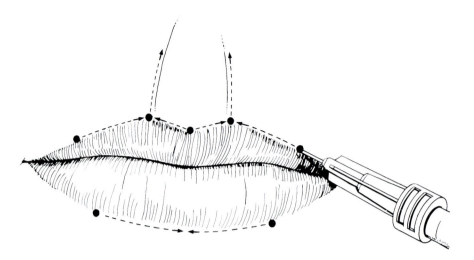

Figure 15–5
Lip margin enhancement with collagen injection.

initial injection pattern using the "threading" technique tends to give a smoother effect. Individual areas or vertical lip rhytids may then be treated with individual puncture technique injections as required.

The medial two thirds of each side above the upper lip are first injected into the dermis from the philtrum ridge above the vermilion border. Care is taken to maintain the injection with the dermal level as the collagen is injected above the lip on each side of the philtrum. Next, the "Cupid's bow" area, at the philtrum's junction with the midportion of the vermilion border, is injected in similar fashion (Fig 15–6, A and B).

Collagen is then injected vertically along the philtrum ridge on each side and extended about two thirds of the distance to the base of the nose (Fig 15–6, C). This adds definition to the natural philtral ridge and complements the enhanced lip line. The lower lip below the vermilion margin is injected similarly, beginning one third of the distance from the corner of the mouth and continuing to the center on each side. The patient returns in about 2 weeks for any touch-up that may be required. The "maintenance" retreatments are required three or four times each year as long as the patient wants to continue the lip enhancement (Figs 15–7 and 15–8).

CHAPTER 15 Injectable Fillers

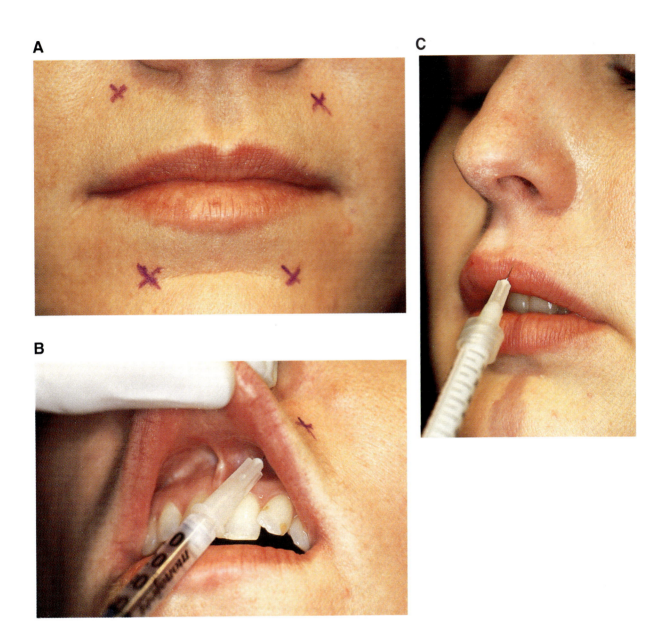

Figure 15-6
A, sites for local anesthesia block prior to collagen lip margin augmentation. **B,** the local injection is given through the sublabial mucosa. **C,** collagen injection is now painless (the left philtral ridge being injected).

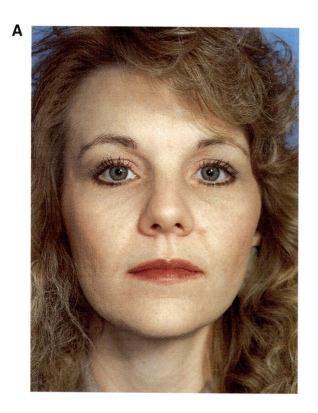
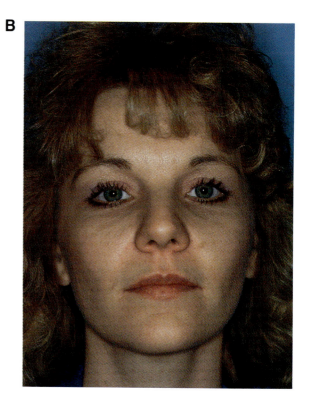
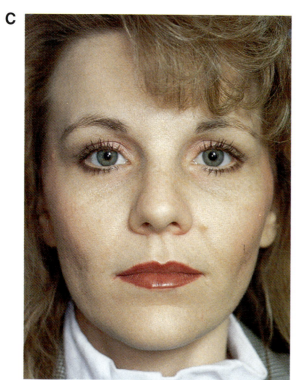

Figure 15-7
A, appearance before lip margin augmentation. **B,** immediately after augmentation. **C,** 2 weeks after augmentation and wearing makeup.

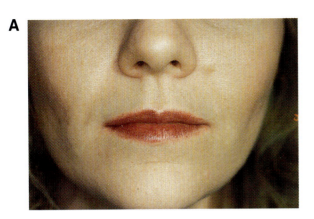 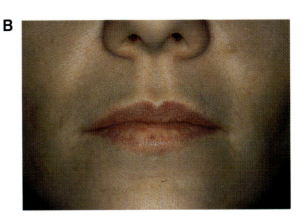

Figure 15–8
A, the same patient as in Figure 15–7 prior to augmentation. **B,** lip margin appearance after collagen augmentation.

Complications and Sequelae

As with any injection, there is always a possibility of ecchymosis or bruising at the treatment site (Fig 15–9). This should clear over the next 5 to 10 days as would any similar bruising. Likewise, localized tenderness, blushing, erythema, and puffiness are considered typical sequelae and will resolve in a matter of days.

Previously experienced facial herpes simplex may recur at the injection site and is a possible result of collagen or any other injection to the region. Antiviral medications such as acyclovir may be used to minimize this response.

The collagen may occasionally be visible through the skin at the injection site. This is usually in the form of small whitish lumps or "beads." These will slowly resolve through resorption of the material but may take several months to do so.

Actual complications with injectable collagen have been rare. Since its introduction in the 1970s, Zyderm and later Zyplast have been used in over 500,000 patients and have proven to be quite safe.

Only about 1% of patients who have had negative skin test results later show an allergic reaction at some point during treatment (Fig 15–10, A and B). These reactions are localized to the injection sites and consist of prolonged redness, swelling, itching, and/or firmness. There have been reports of a few of these reactions proceeding to a cyst-like reaction that may drain and eventually cause a scar. It is felt that perhaps 50% of these reactions have been in patients where a positive response to the initial skin test was unreported or unrecognized (Fig 15–11).

Fewer than 1 in 1,000 patients may have a systemic response to the injected collagen. These responses include nausea, rash, headache, joint

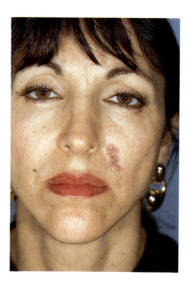

Figure 15-9
Bruising immediately following intradermal implantation of Zyderm II.

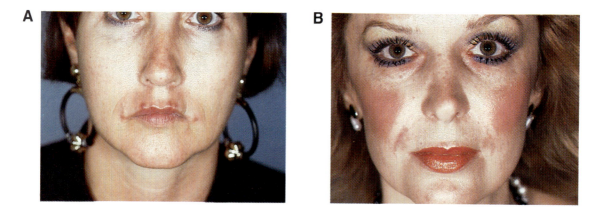

Figure 15-10
A, persistent erythema of the lip 7 weeks after Zyderm II implantation. **B,** persistent erythema of the nasolabial crease several months after Zyderm injection.

aches, or breathing difficulty. Finally, a small percentage of patients have been reported who have periodic recurrent symptoms similar to an allergic reaction. It is speculated that these patients may be allergic to bovine collagen. Most of the above allergic reactions have persisted between 3 and 4 months, but some cases have persisted for over 1 year.

There have been reports of skin slough, particularly in the glabellar area. It is felt that this was related to vascular compression or occlusion. It is recommended that Zyplast not be used in this region, only Zyderm I and II.

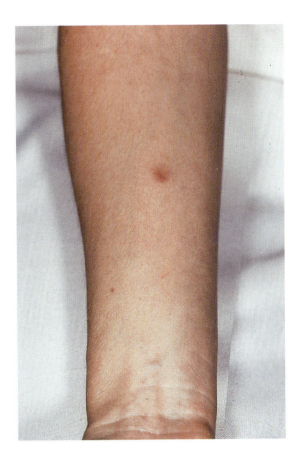

Figure 15-11
Positive Zyderm skin test result.

There is one reported case of vascular occlusion resulting in partial loss of vision in one eye.

Overall, when one considers that over 3 million injections of Zyderm or Zyplast collagen have been administered at this time, the material has proved to be very safe. Injectable collagen is a useful adjunct to other modalities in the treatment of facial irregularities.

Suggested Reading

- Goode RL, Burgess LPA: Injectable collagen materials, in Thomas JR, Holt GR (eds): *Scar Revision: Incision, Revision and Camouflage.* St Louis, Mosby–Year Book, 1989, pp 337–347.
- Stegman SJ, Tromovitch TA: Implantation of collagen for depressed scars. *J Dermatol Surg Oncol* 1980: 6:450–453.
- Swanson NA, et al: Treatment site reactions to Zyderm collagen implantation. *J Dermatol Surg Oncol* 1983; 9:377–380.

PART IV
RHINOPLASTY IN MIDLIFE AND AGING PATIENTS

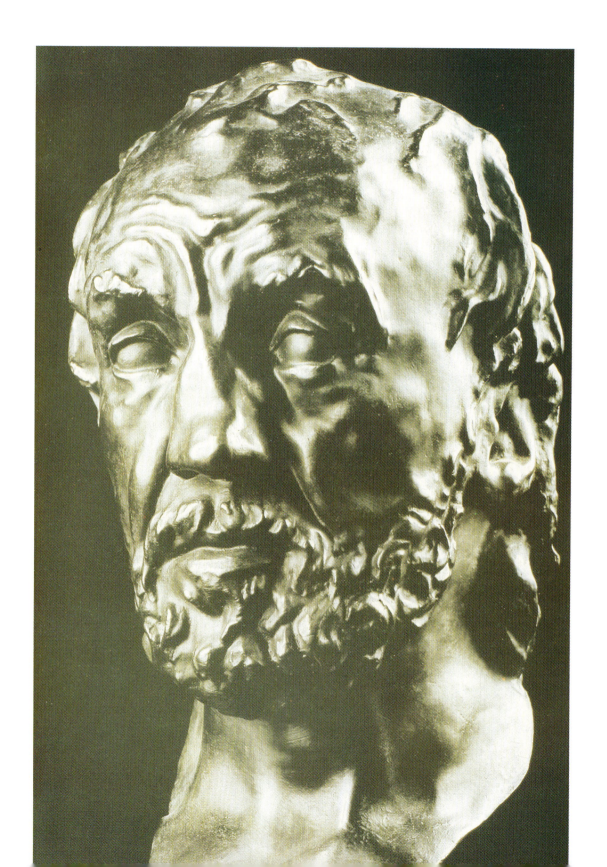

CHAPTER 16

Rhinoplasty in Midlife and Aging Patients

PART IV RHINOPLASTY IN MIDLIFE AND AGING PATIENTS

> *A thing of beauty is a joy for ever;*
> *Its loveliness increases; it will never*
> *pass into nothingness; but still will keep*
> *a bower quiet for us, and a sleep*
> *full of sweet dreams, and health, and quiet breathing....*
>
> **John Keats**

Diagnosis and Candidate Selection

Rhinoplasty in the older patient occupies an important niche in the overall comprehensive plan to surgically diminish the effects of facial aging. Accordingly, partial or complete rhinoplasty regularly accompanies other traditional and more profound facial rejuvenation operations and adds to the youthful and natural appearance of the face. Even subtle and minimal nasal refinement and lifting maneuvers produce substantial appearance benefits.

Further justification for midlife rhinoplasty revolves around the fulfillment of a lifelong wish, a request less identified with an overall rejuvenation regimen.

Finally, functional nasal disorders, tolerated but consistently troublesome in earlier life, commonly evolve into major health problems at this stage of life. The obstruction created by a long-term deviated septum eventually becomes intolerable, often heralded by increasingly frequent rhinosinusitis. Early alar collapse and/or insufficiency may become manifest. Ptosis and elongation of the nasal tip may so restrict the normal nasal airflow patterns that quiet, comfortable nasal breathing no longer exists.

The past two decades have witnessed an increasing incidence of rhinoplasty in middle-aged and older individuals. The reasons for this trend are diverse and variable but not unexplainable. Both prospective patients and surgeons have become more sophisticated about the benefits of rhinoplasty in complementing the overall facial rejuvenation management plan.

Patients requesting rhinoplasty in midlife (in the fourth to sixth decades) present clearly different challenges, both psychological and physical, from those of the traditional young adult or teenage patient. Segmental or "partial" rhinoplasty clearly occupies an important role in older patients, often furnishing the "finishing touches" so important to the overall improvement in appearance (Fig 16–1).

CHAPTER 16   Rhinoplasty in Midlife and Aging Patients

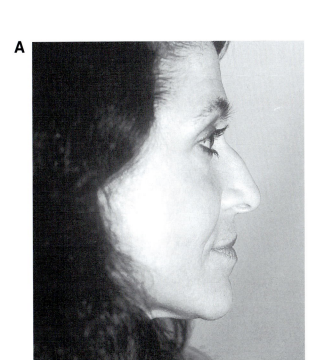
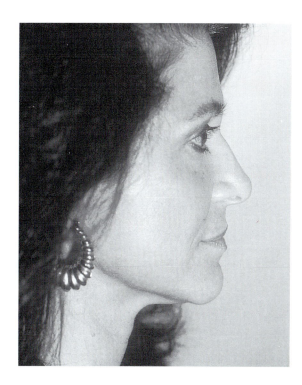
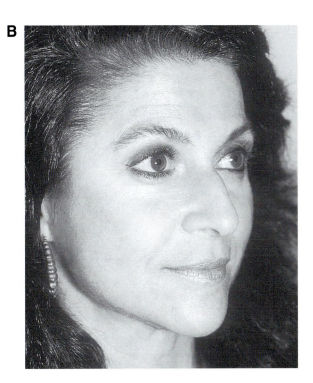
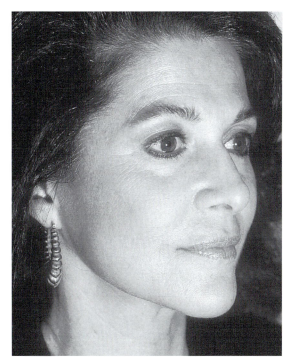

Figure 16–1
A and **B,** late postoperative outcome (15 months) in a patient in whom partial rhinoplasty only achieves a pleasing result. The tip, inadequately projected, has been elevated with a generous tip graft combined with a supportive strut. A strong bridge has been maintained by cartilage graft augmentation of the nasofrontal angle.

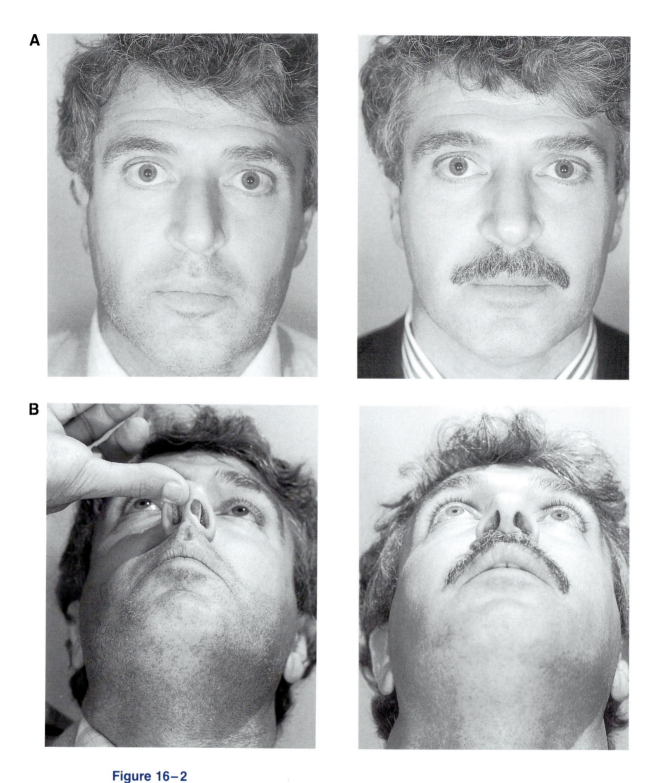

Figure 16–2
A–D, two year outcome of conservative total rhinoplasty in a midlife patient with an emphasis on subtlety of changes of all major anatomic components of the nose along with septal reconstruction.

CHAPTER 16   Rhinoplasty in Midlife and Aging Patients

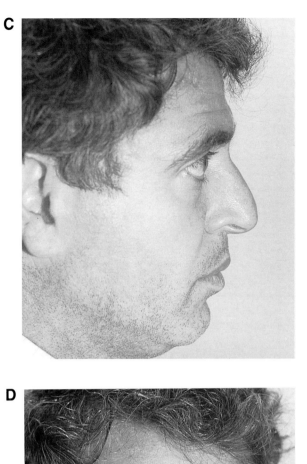
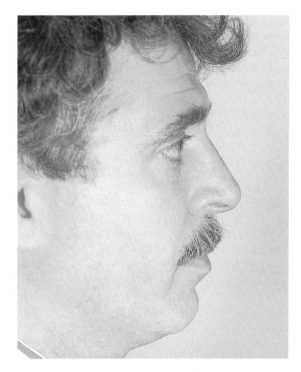
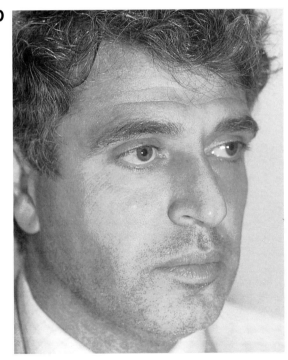
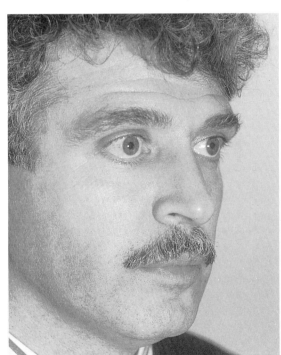

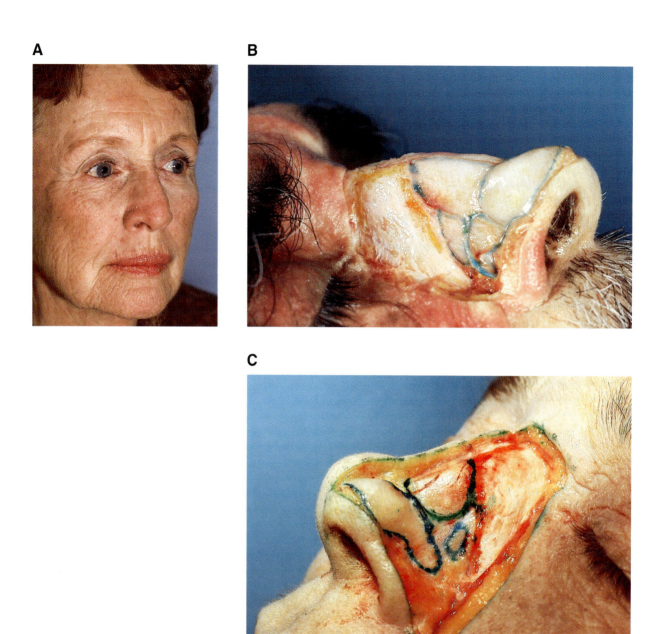

Figure 16–3

A, The characteristic changes wrought by aging on the unoperated nose. The skin often thickens in the distal two fifths of the nose while thinning and attenuation develop in the upper three fifths. Telangiectasis become more apparent as the skin sleeve becomes too large for the supportive nasal skeleton. Horizontal rhytids develop at the nasal root, and the nose elongates as the supportive tissues lose integrity. The tip becomes more dependent, even ptotic, as bony and fatty tissue absorption occurs in the midface and columellar-labial interface. A more acute nasolabial angle often ensues. Normal support of the nasal tip is reduced, and the nose loses much of its delicacy and definition. **B,** dissected aging cadaver specimen demonstrating thinning of the epithelial cushion over the rhinion, distraction of the upper lateral–lower lateral interface, and a developing acuteness of the nasolabial angle. **C,** cadaver specimen with an unusually thick skin–subcutaneous tissue covering. The skin is thickened and redundant. Distraction of the upper lateral–lower lateral interface is apparent.

CHAPTER 16 Rhinoplasty in Midlife and Aging Patients

Psychologically, patients in midlife commonly possess a well-imprinted body image and may therefore find anything other than a conservative change in nasal features undesirable and even highly stressful. Generally, mature adults have developed a firm conception about the ideal (and less-than-ideal) appearance; consequently, added responsibility falls on the rhinoplasty surgeon to clearly extract from patients their exact wishes regarding facial appearance modifications. Although specific exceptions exist, *conservative and subtle changes in the aesthetic appearance of the nose are generally best for the patient in midlife,* with a natural nonoperated appearance preserved (Fig 16–2). Surgical efforts should be directed toward creating improved facial balance and proportion and avoiding profound nasal appearance changes readily acceptable in a young patient eager for major changes. Whether performed as an isolated procedure or in concert with other aesthetic facial operations, the desired outcome is a natural, nonoperated appearance designed to complement and enhance the face.

To achieve this laudable goal, an understanding of and appreciation for the inevitable aging changes that affect the nose must be incorporated into the operative plan (Fig 16–3). Surgical modifications designed to accommodate the altered physical constitution of the aging nose are essential. Diminished skin elasticity, reduced skin and subcutaneous tissue thickness, fragile bones, potentially calcified septal cartilage, and increasingly rigid blood vessels suggest an alteration in traditional surgical techniques. It is well documented that the aging nose exhibits functional as well as structural changes. Not only does the nasal appearance change, but alterations in respiration and olfaction also frequently occur. Skin texture and elasticity deteriorate as atrophy and thinning of the epidermis, dermis, and subcutaneous tissues develop. Redundancy and wrinkling of skin, especially near the nasal root, appear. A decrease in body water contributes to drying of the skin in general. Telangiectasis appear and worsen with advancing age. Sebaceous glands enlarge and appear prominent; they make the nasal tip more bulbous and at times result in substantial tip enlargement and dependency. Tip ptosis may occur as a consequence of the loss of tip support as the upper lateral cartilage loses its close attachment to the alar cartilage; cartilage softening and weakening of the medial crura further contribute to the loss of tip support. The medial crural footplates spread laterally, retreat posteriorly, and thereby contribute to a more acute nasolabial angle. Thus the aging nose typically elongates and the lobule rotates inferiorly, ultimately resulting in a symptomatic diminution of normal airflow patterns through the nasal chambers. Progressive mucus membrane dryness coupled with thickening and reduced viscosity of nasal secretions exacerbates symptoms of nasal stuffiness.

In light of these changes wrought by aging, the best surgical modifications are usually subtle and nondramatic, ideally preserving the patient's tissues and established self-image.

This discussion centers on rhinoplasty patients, both female and male, who fall generally between the ages of 35 and 60 years, a group that is increasingly desiring and requesting rhinoplasty (Table 16-1). Clearly, a considerable cultural aesthetic awareness currently exists, perhaps to a greater extent in this midlife group than in any other. Social affluence often heightens the desire for improved appearance; and the media, both print and electronic, influences and crystallizes this awareness. Commonly the older patient has just realized the economic means to afford the corrective surgery desired since childhood; often the decision is reached after observation of a rewarding surgical experience of a younger family member or close friend. Surgery may be sought as the outgrowth, whether conscious or unconscious, of a midlife change (in current terms, a "passage"), whether in career, marital status, or renewed optimism and enthusiasm.

Table 16–1

Requests for Midlife Rhinoplasty: Precipitating Causes

- Trauma
- Ageing Nasal Changes
- Increasing Nasal Obstruction
- Improved Economics
- Rejuvenation Concerns
- Revision Rhinoplasty
- Critical Comment-Friends/Family
- Midlife Career Changes

Increasingly, as women, in particular, enter the athletic arena, often with possibly less preparation and physical endowment than men, nasal trauma assumes a major role in creating a need for nasal reconstruction (Fig 16–4).

Patients in this age group are more likely to request other facial rejuvenation procedures like a facelift or blepharoplasty, and clearly rhinoplasty can play a profound and valuable role in total facial rejuvenation. Airway obstruction along with nasal deformity, experienced and tolerated for years, may become sufficiently symptomatic in midlife (combined with a drooping, aging nose) to prompt a request for nasal surgery. The unintentionally critical comment of a family member, often a child or grandchild, may spawn a desire for appearance improvement in older patients as they seek to please those whom they respect and care for deeply. Finally, patients who have undergone rhinoplasty at a much earlier age may choose the midlife period to request revisional improvement, either from their original surgeon or, more commonly, from a surgeon in whom renewed confidence is placed. Individuals are regularly encountered who have tolerated less-than-perfect rhinoplasty outcomes in their youth (youngsters tend to be less critical of small imperfections) but with advancing age and heightened expectations in all aspects of life feel that they deserve further improvements. Alar collapse symptoms are not uncommon in patients operated on as teenagers with excessive sacrifice of the nasal tip and alar support mechanisms; this annoying airway blockade may take years to become sufficiently symptomatic to elicit airway discomfort during sleep, while exercising, and even at rest.

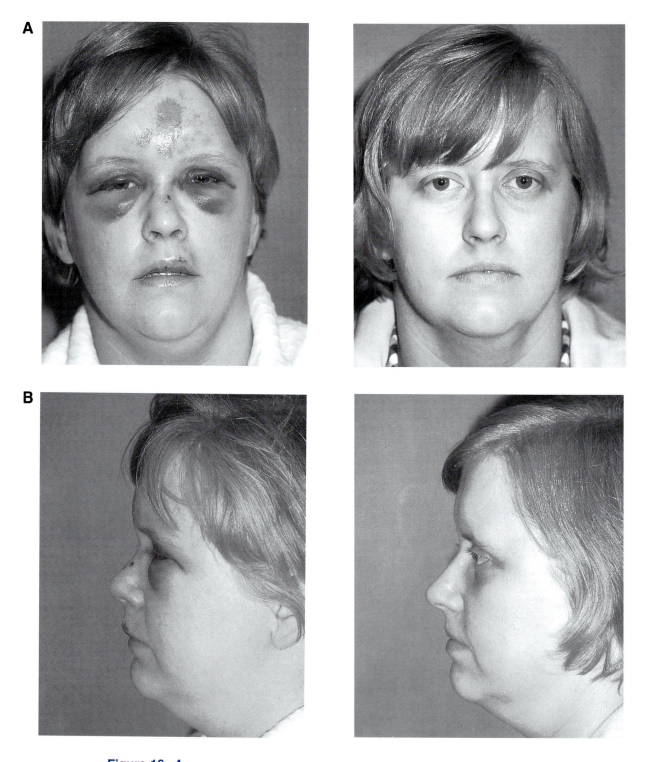

Figure 16-4
Nasal trauma in older patients must be managed carefully. Unsuspected injuries to the ethmoid perpendicular plate and cribriform region must be presumed and treated with gentle care during dissection and manipulation to avoid more severe surgical injury. The result of open reduction of nasal fractures is shown at 6 months.

Evaluating Midlife Patients: Assessing Needs

Positive communicative interaction with midlife patients is the key to producing a happy and content patient. Seasoned by life's experiences both positive and negative, they most commonly express exactly and clearly the anatomic changes desired. When compared with teenage patients, older individuals often tend to have higher expectations. Since they are usually paying the costs themselves, "good value" is expected and demanded of the chosen surgeon.

These heightened and at times unrealistic expectations often contrast sharply with young patients, who have difficulty in expressing desired changes, especially those that may be necessarily subtle. To avoid potential misunderstandings about what can be surgically achieved and what is realistically possible, more time must ordinarily be expended with older patients to ensure an effective communication process and avoid later disappointment and disenchantment.

Beneficial structuring of the patient's attitudinal approach can be favorably influenced in advance of the initial doctor-patient interview and examination. A new patient requesting an office appointment whose stated interest is in rhinoplasty receives by mail a personalized informational packet containing a confirmatory appointment letter, general brochures describing the operation of rhinoplasty, and a relatively detailed monograph discussing the general indications, limitations, ramifications, and potential complications of facial plastic surgery. Patients (especially mature adults) appreciate this professional courtesy and arrive for the initial office evaluation with increased confidence and more specific knowledge of the questions that need resolution and further discussion. It is absolutely astonishing how much misinformation and misunderstanding exist among lay people as regards rhinoplasty. This proven form of patient pre-education often catalyzes communication with patients, an absolute prerequisite in aesthetic surgery. The occasional patient who for whatever reason reacts negatively to this preinterview approach and fails to arrive for consultation more than likely is motivationally suspect. Experience confirms the truism that an educated patient stands a much greater chance for postoperative satisfaction and contentment with the surgical outcome.

The initial office interview and examination of the head and neck are conducted in two parts by the surgeon and a skilled office nurse. Many of the routine concerns regarding the length of hospital stay, management of insurance forms, length of work absenteeism, and approximate cost are personally handled by nursing personnel and reinforced, when needed, by the surgeon.

The surgeon's primary role is to determine and convey an accurate diagnosis of obvious and subtle abnormalities, factually and thoroughly communicating to the patient this information in a convincing and understandable manner. This communication process is usually facilitated early in the doctor-patient encounter by the use of a combination of "open-ended" and more detailed and specific queries. Useful questions include "How can I help you?" "What brings you in to see me today?" "Let's begin by having you ask any questions of me you would like—I am sure you have quite a few." Such simple openers provide the patient, enhanced and guided by the knowledge gained through a review of the preinterview materials, an opportunity to come directly to his desires and needs. The intent, of course, is not to confine the patient to preconceived questions but rather to open communication channels rapidly and freely. The surgeon's role initially must be that of a good *listener* providing meaningful prompts. Motivational factors, both realistic and inappropriate, emerge during this process and are assimilated, correlated, and analyzed by the surgeon, who should be sensitive to the patient's desires and needs.

More specific and incisive questions can then ensue: "What don't you like about your nose?" How would you like your nose changed?" "Show me exactly (by use of the three-way mirror) what you would ideally like to correct or change." Ideal and less-than-ideal features are then pointed out and emphasized to the patient (and family if present) while underscoring the limitations inherent in the patient's anatomy. Major and minor feature disproportions are painstakingly discussed. The ultimate intent is to diagnose, inform, and educate—not to "sell" an operation. A thoughtful, concerned, sensitive surgeon will have no difficulty in finding patients eager for his services. Strong emphasis is placed throughout the initial interview on *limitations* imposed upon the desired surgery by anatomy that is not ideal. The surgical problem inherent in patients with overly thick or alabaster-thin skin, large hooded alae, sebaceous and telangiectatic tip skin, inelastic skin, and associated facial asymmetries is emphasized, demonstrated in a three-way mirror, and documented.

Multiple-view photographs are then taken by the surgeon. Accurate, uniform photographic records are as important as the operative procedure itself (Fig 16–5). The photography session conducted by the surgeon affords an opportunity for continued dialogue and evaluation since defects and disproportions overlooked or minimized during the physical examination are commonly revealed through the camera lens. An uncooperative patient during the photographic sequence—inappropriate behavior, inability to strike and hold an accurate head position for even a few seconds, hyperactivity—may signal the lone clue to an uncooperative and therefore inappropriate surgical candidate. Less than 90 seconds of the surgeon's time is required to photographically record two of each of the six standard views required for rhinoplasty evaluation—a valuable investment of personal effort. Importantly, this complete control of the standardization and uniformity is critical in plastic surgery photography (Fig 16–6 and 16–7).

The majority of patients seeking nasal plastic surgery are fortunately realistic and appropriately motivated. These individuals are accepted, and the process for surgical scheduling is carried out by the office staff. We believe that no guarantee of results should be made, that overwhelming promises and assurances should be avoided, and that all patients should be apprised that occasionally more than one surgical procedure may be necessary to effect the most ideal outcome (fewer than 5% to 7% of the patients). Patients requesting a review of the surgeon's past surgical rhi-

CHAPTER 16 Rhinoplasty in Midlife and Aging Patients

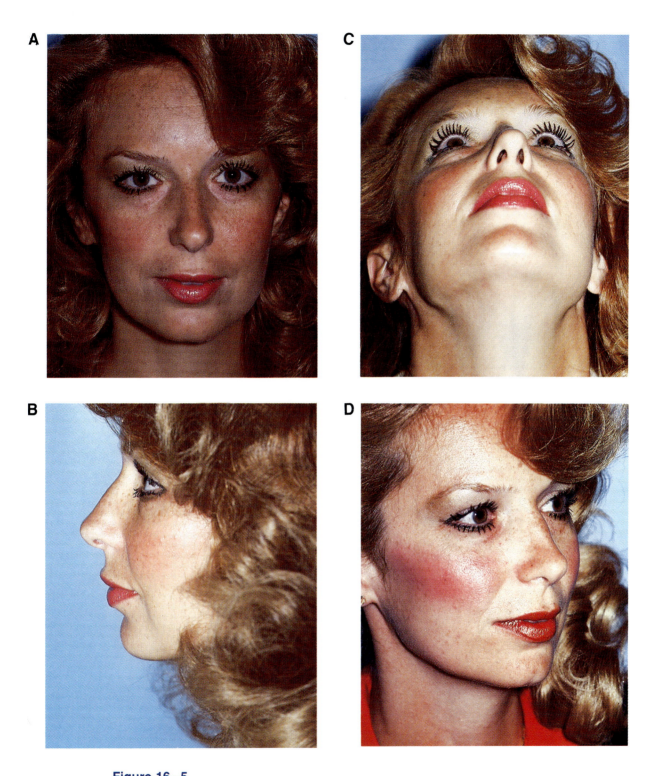

Figure 16–5
A–D, standardized uniform photodocumentation is essential for accurate preoperative and postoperative evaluation, proper record keeping, teaching and medicolegal documentation, and technical self-evaluation. When judged helpful in unique situations, additional close-up views are recorded.

PART IV   RHINOPLASTY IN MIDLIFE AND AGING PATIENTS

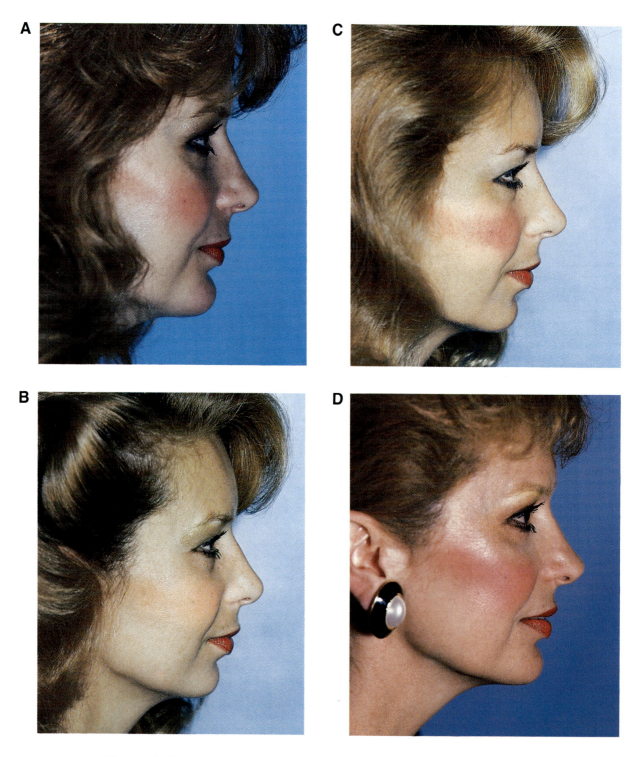

Figure 16–6
A–D, standardization of photographic views from sitting to sitting allows accurate visual assessment of evolving healing changes and provides a vital unsurpassed form of surgical self-education and feedback. Views are shown at 2, 3, 11, and 120 (10 years) months postoperatively.

CHAPTER 16   Rhinoplasty in Midlife and Aging Patients

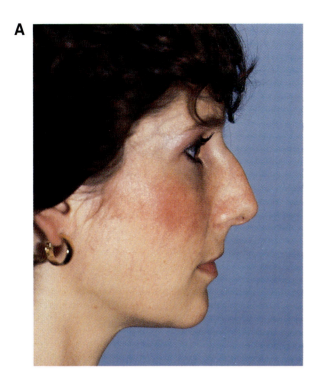

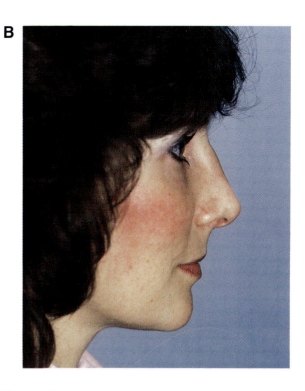

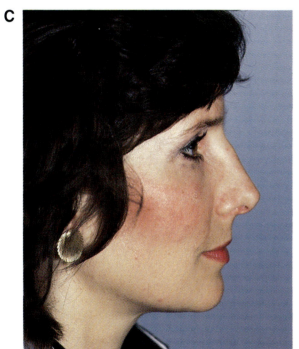

Figure 16–7
Long-term standardized photographs following surgery are indispensable for final assessment of outcome. Result shown at two months and three years.

noplasty results are gently refused by pointing out that in our practice patients' medical records are private and confidential and that except for teaching and publishing purposes we will not be showing future patients the photographs just completed. We find this explanation quite satisfactory and reassuring to all reasonable rhinoplasty candidates. An exception to this rule of patient photographic privacy is made for patients with significant retrognathia whose overall facial balance and ultimate rhinoplasty result will clearly be enhanced by chin augmentation. Since patients have difficulty viewing their profile accurately, demonstration of the merits of mentoplasty during rhinoplasty is nicely achieved by a review of photographs of several patients who have benefited from the dual procedures. The surgical recommendation is made in the form of a suggestion for enhancement of the overall result, but in all cases the decision for chin augmentation in an aging patient is left entirely to the patient.

Specific and detailed permission slips are obtained for photographic and operative procedures, and informational booklets reviewing postoperative care, instructions, and practices are provided, with specific topics highlighted that may be peculiar to the individual's problem.

A mature individual seeking rhinoplasty uniformly responds positively and enthusiastically to this approach, which is reinforced by both the sensitive experienced surgical nurse's discussion and a short slide-tape audiovisual presentation. If for any reason the response is not definitively positive, an additional office consultation is mandatory, and additional opinions with competent colleagues (often in various overlapping surgical specialties) are recommended. We encourage all patients to return for a second preoperative visit if they so desire. No charge is made for a second (or even a third) preoperative visit, during which time the patient's photographs are reviewed, specific surgical plans are documented, and the patient is in general reassured (usually the patient's most vital need).

A hesitant patient who repeatedly returns and finds it difficult to decide either for or against surgery is likely so insecure that any surgery may best be avoided.

The majority of patients seeking rhinoplasty alone require and desire only one office consultation to plan their surgical event, especially when their previsit educational process has been thorough and they are realistically motivated. By contrast, for patients seeking rejuvenation surgery for an aging face, more than one preoperative visit is desirable and even mandatory to elicit true motivation and expectations. The visits provide comforting reassurance, solidify realistic expectations, and cement a trusting, enthusiastic surgeon-patient relationship.

Patients commonly leave the consultation suite with a quiet excitement and reassurance regarding surgery. Careful preoperative conditioning pays welcome dividends in the overall management of patients seeking a favorable appearance change who yet consciously or subconsciously fear self-image dissatisfaction.

CHAPTER 16 Rhinoplasty in Midlife and Aging Patients

Surgical Goals and Planned Outcomes

General and Specific Principles

The surgical goals in midlife patients undergoing rhinoplasty are not unlike those sought and identified in young patients, but the operative means of achieving those intended goals and results vary in certain important areas. Conservative, nondramatic appearance changes are generally the most appropriate. A totally "natural" appearance in which the final result draws no attention to itself as an individual feature serves the patient and surgeon best.

This may be best achieved by approaching the rhinoplasty operation as one in which the various components of the nose are basically rearranged, reoriented, and restructured in their relationship to one another and major resections and removal or weakening of cartilage and bony support elements avoided (Fig 16–8). Commonly, however, partial or segmental rhinoplasty, targeted to correct specifically identified nasal deficits, fulfills the needs of the aging patient superbly.

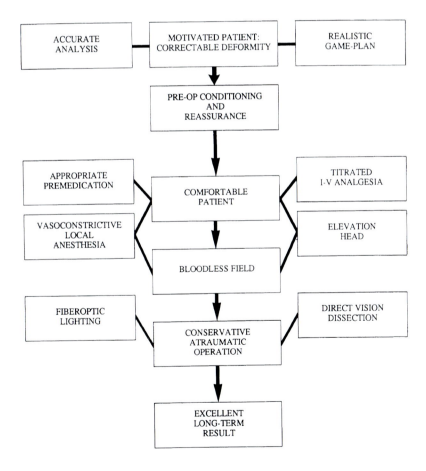

Figure 16–8
Flow chart depicting the components of a successful rhinoplasty.

469

The nose in midlife, especially if the unintended target of repeated trauma, may in fact require tissue *augmentation* with autogenous cartilage, bone, dermis, fascia, or soft tissue in order to reconstitute the nasal structure and lend support and form while improving appearance (Fig 16–9). It is our conviction that the nose fulfills very few if any of the essential requirements for long-term acceptance of nonautogenous synthetic implants, so these are assiduously avoided in all patients requiring augmentation.

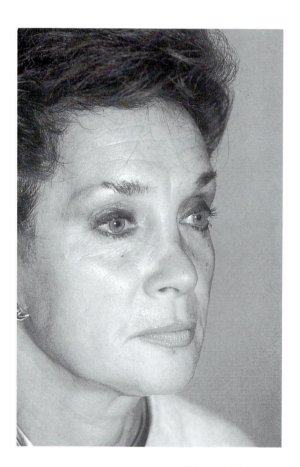
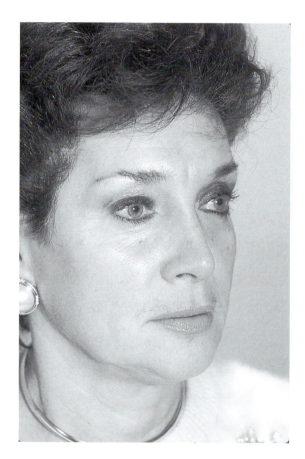

Figure 16–9
Augmentation rhinoplasty with autogenous cartilage grafts in an older patient with saddle nose deformity.

CHAPTER 16   Rhinoplasty in Midlife and Aging Patients

Specific surgical principles are followed in most procedures in older patients, including a somewhat wider undermining of nasal skin and soft tissue to accommodate a lessened skin elasticity (and therefore less rapid shrinkage) and promote adequate skin redraping, more conservative sculpture of the tip cartilage, conservative hump removal and profile alignment, and minimalization of the extent of osteotomy and trauma with micro-osteotomies. In older patients "greenstick" or incomplete osteotomy fractures, unpredictable and generally best avoided in young patients, may be created in older patients with the anticipation of permanent favorable results. To this end micro-osteotomies accomplished with 2- or 3-mm sharp osteotomes impart extremely minimal trauma (Fig 16–10).

Older patients exhibit a greater redundancy of mucosa and vestibular skin that uniformly fails to "be taken up" during the healing process. This redundancy is witnessed to a greater extent when tip rotation and nasal shortening become necessary to elevate an aging nose. Proper excision to bring the internal mucosa/skin sleeve into proportion with the new nasal skeleton is mandatory to avoid lining redundancies after overall healing.

The lax, increasingly flaccid alar sidewalls common in older patients require careful assessment to ensure that aesthetic reduction of lower lateral cartilage volume does not result in alar support weakening with inspiratory collapse. Cartilaginous alar battens, when indicated, provide substantial structural support to weak sidewalls (Fig 16–11).

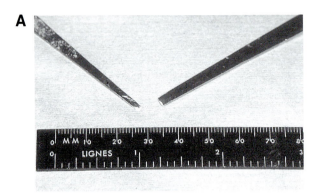
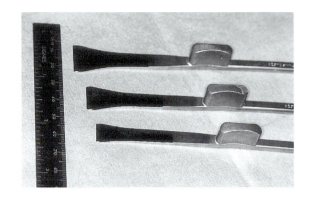
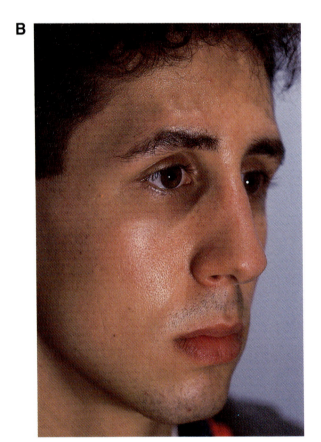
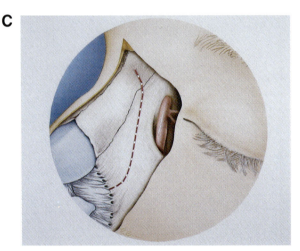

Figure 16-10
A, 2- and 3-mm sharp micro-osteotomes impart minimal tissue trauma during nasal osteotomy techniques. The 2-mm osteotome serves particularly well at the nasofrontal angle and for transcutaneous osteotomies of the lateral nasal wall, if indicated. Razor-sharp Rubin osteotomies preferred for bony hump removal (Fig. 10-A, right). **B,** the resulting cutaneous scar, particularly in aging skin, is essentially no more traumatic or visible than an 18-gauge needle penetration and heals without obvious identifiable scarring. **C,** typical site of lateral and medial-oblique osteotomies performed with micro-osteotomes.

CHAPTER 16 Rhinoplasty in Midlife and Aging Patients

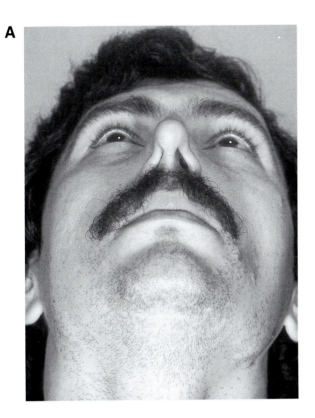
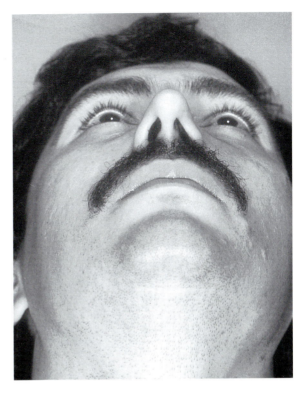
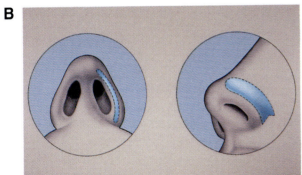
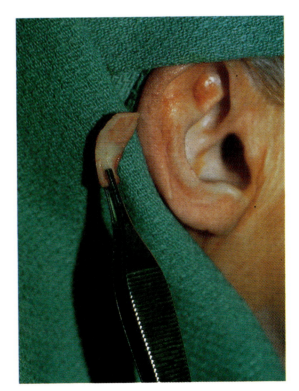

Figure 16–11
A, iatrogenic alar collapse in an older patient was corrected by a curved cartilage batten implant from auricular cavum concha. **B,** typical supra-alar lobule site of alar batten in correction of alar collapse. The exact site of the cartilage graft will depend upon where the lateral sidewall is weakest and collapses most readily.

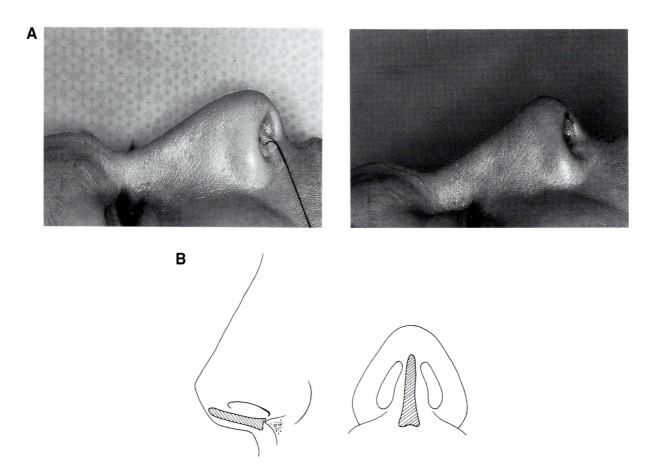

Figure 16–12
A, custom-contoured cartilage tip grafts, usually sutured in place to the intermediate crura, can impart essential projection, contour, and support to the nasal tip. Onlay tip grafts are less suitable for exacting contouring but may be useful in thick or scarred (previously operated) skin. **B,** strong cartilaginous struts (harvested from the floor of the septum, residual cartilaginous hump, or the auricle) are useful in providing support and contour to tips weakened by aging tissues. They are less useful for increasing tip projection, however, and are thus employed to provide a supportive base upon which cartilage tip grafts are positioned.

Enhancement or augmentation of tip support in the aging nose, a common requirement, may be realized with supportive cartilage columellar struts as well as onlay or infratip lobule tip grafts (Fig 16–12, A and B).

Aging tends to render the columella-labial angle more acute and therefore less ideal. In conjunction with tip elevation, augmentation of the angle with "plumping" cartilage grafts restores a more normal configuration to this confluence of the nose and lip and diminishes the aged characteristics (Fig 16–13).

The thinning, dry skin of older patients commonly exhibits unsightly telangiectasia formation. Microcautery applied in pinpoint fashion to the central feeding vessel transcutaneously effectively diminishes or eliminates the majority of these unsightly microvascular formations (Fig 16–14). In more severe cases, superficial laser treatments may be employed effectively.

Finally, the tendency in older patients for less subcutaneous scarring to occur (particularly the dreaded supratip fullness) influences the surgical approach favorably, with the ultimate surgical outcome developing more quickly than in young patients.

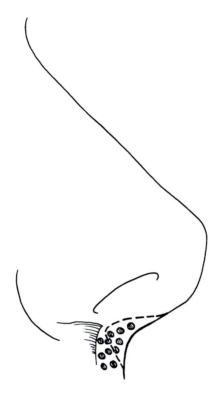

Figure 16–13
Cartilage plumping and contouring grafts in the columellar-labial regions correct excessive angle acuteness as a consequence of aging tissue absorption and subsequent nasal elongation. Even the illusion of nasal shortening and tip elevation may be achieved with contouring grafts, which are usually placed through a lateral paracolumellar medial-crural splitting incision.

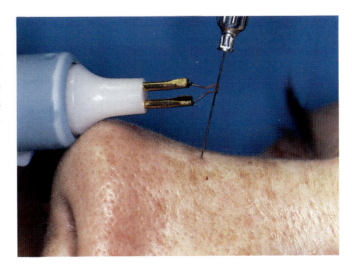

Figure 16–14
Microcautery of superficial nasal telangiectasia with a 30-gauge needle thrust into the vessel transcutaneously to seal vessels with heat from a disposable Concept cautery.

Surgical Techniques

Specific Anatomic Considerations

Aesthetic septorhinoplasty, in all age groups, must be planned and executed with proven approaches and techniques *based entirely on the individual, unique anatomy encountered.* The quality and thickness of the skin–subcutaneous tissue layer is vital to appropriate camouflage of the altered structure. The strength, shape, and inherent support of the nasal tip structures commonly dictate the tip-sculpturing approach and technique chosen (Fig 16–15). The skeletal substructure of the cartilaginous and bony pyramids is best largely preserved to achieve a strong and elegant appearance consistent with the older patient's bearing and overall facial appearance.

Significant anatomic factors influencing midlife rhinoplasty are detailed in Figures 16–16 through 16–21.

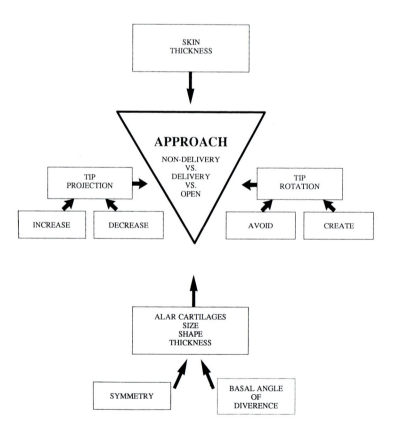

Figure 16–15
Flow chart depicting decision making in nasal tip surgery.

CHAPTER 16   Rhinoplasty in Midlife and Aging Patients

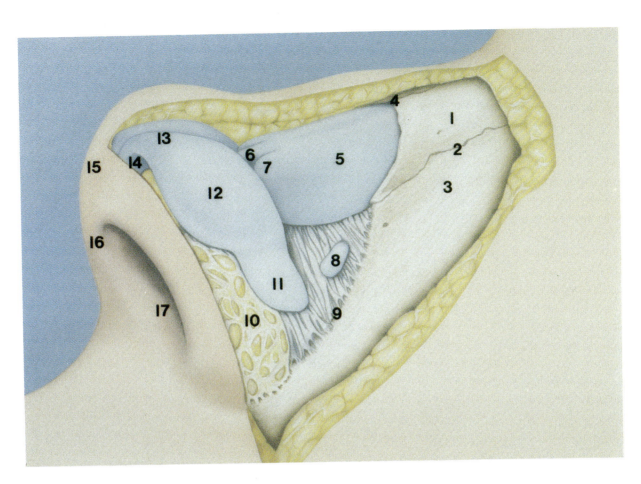

Figure 16–16
Key anatomic landmarks and standard terminology useful in nasal anatomy and surgery and easily identified in fresh cadaver dissection.

1, nasal bone;
2, nasomaxillary suture line;
3, ascending process of the maxilla;
4, osseocartilaginous junction (rhinion);
5, upper lateral cartilage;
6, anterior septal angle;
7, caudal free edge of the upper lateral cartilage;
8, sesamoid cartilage;
9, pyriform margin;
10, alar lobule;
11, lateral crus of the alar cartilage—lateral portion;
12, lateral crus of the alar cartilage—central portion;
13, tip-defining point;
14, transitional segment of the alar cartilage (intermediate crus);
15, infratip lobule;
16, columella;
17, medial crural footplate.

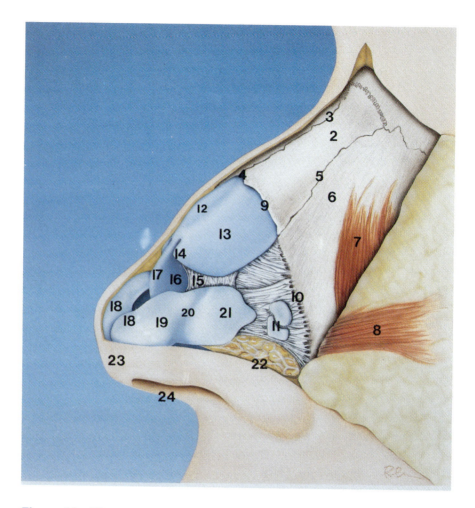

Figure 16–17

Additional anatomic landmarks and standard terminology.

1, nasofrontal suture line;
2, nasal bone;
3, internasal suture line;
4, osseocartilaginous junction (rhinion);
5, nasomaxillary suture line;
6, ascending process of the maxilla;
7, levator labii superioris muscle;
8, transverse nasalis muscle;
9, cephalic portion of the upper lateral cartilage (articulates to the undersurface of the nasal bone;
10, pyriform margin;
11, sesamoid cartilages;
12, cartilaginous dorsum;
13, upper lateral cartilage;
14, caudal free margin of the upper lateral cartilage;
15, intercartilaginous ligament;
16, quadrangular cartilage;
17, anterior septal angle;
18, tip-defining point of the alar cartilage;
19, lateral crus of the alar cartilage;
20, concavity ("hinge") of the lateral crus;
21, lateral aspect of the lateral crus;
22, alar lobule;
23, infratip lobule;
24, columella.

CHAPTER 16 Rhinoplasty in Midlife and Aging Patients

1a, transverse nasalis;
1b, alar nasalis;
2a, medial fascicle procerus;
2b, lateral fascicle procerus;
3, anomalous nasi;
4, dilator naris anterior;
5, compressor naris minor;
6, levator labii superioris alaeque nasi;
7, depressor septi nasi;
8, orbicularis oris.

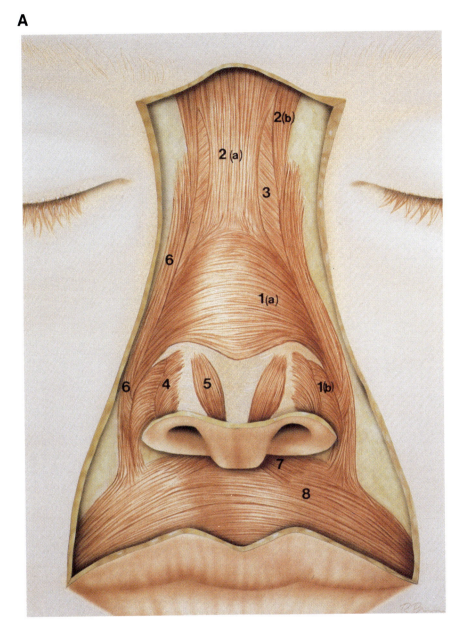

Figure 16–18

A, the mimetic muscles of expression influencing the nose exist in a continuous sheet interconnected by a thin tendon-like aponeurosis. The individual muscles are inconstant in their development and degree of action from patient to patient but are clearly contributory to the extensive layer of the superficial musculoaponeurotic system (SMAS) of tissue that distributes and counterbalances motion forces impacting upon the nose. The SMAS layer is largely ignored in standard descriptions of rhinoplasty technique when, in reality, it plays a vital role in achieving favorable long-term healing results. Specifically, the SMAS layer provides a continuous, although variably thick layer of "cushioning" over the nasal skeleton that aids in smooth contouring and appearance of the nasal epithelial surface (if cut or torn during surgery, the edges may retract and create bulges, irregularities, and depressions because during healing the dermis adheres directly to the nasal skeleton with no intervening musculoaponeurotic layer).

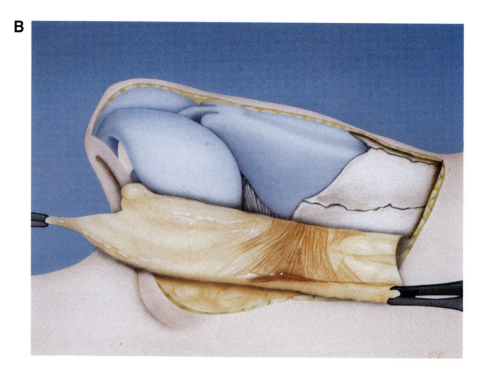

Figure 16-18 (cont.)
B, the SMAS plane provides an important surgical landmark for the surgeon during primary rhinoplasty. Anesthetic infiltration, surgical dissection, and elevation of the nasal soft tissues should be carefully confined to the favorable tissue dissection plane just deep to the SMAS layer, intimate to the perichondrium of the cartilaginous dorsum, and beneath the periosteum of the nasal bones. During primary rhinoplasty, dissection proceeds easily and largely bloodlessly in this important tissue dissection plane, while in secondary rhinoplasty, scar obliteration and disruption of the valuable plane (and the overlying SMAS layer) frequently result in poor spreading and dissemination of infiltrated local anesthetic (requiring a greater volume of anesthetic), difficulty in elevation of the scarred soft tissues, and inevitably increased surgical bleeding. Surgeons who achieve the highest degree of finesse in rhinoplasty respect the SMAS layer and take pains to disturb it as little as possible. Since the SMAS ordinarily increases in its thickness in the supratip region, retraction and bunching up of its torn edges may be one important etiology for the dreaded soft-tissue "pollybeak" deformity in susceptible patients postrhinoplasty.

CHAPTER 16 Rhinoplasty in Midlife and Aging Patients

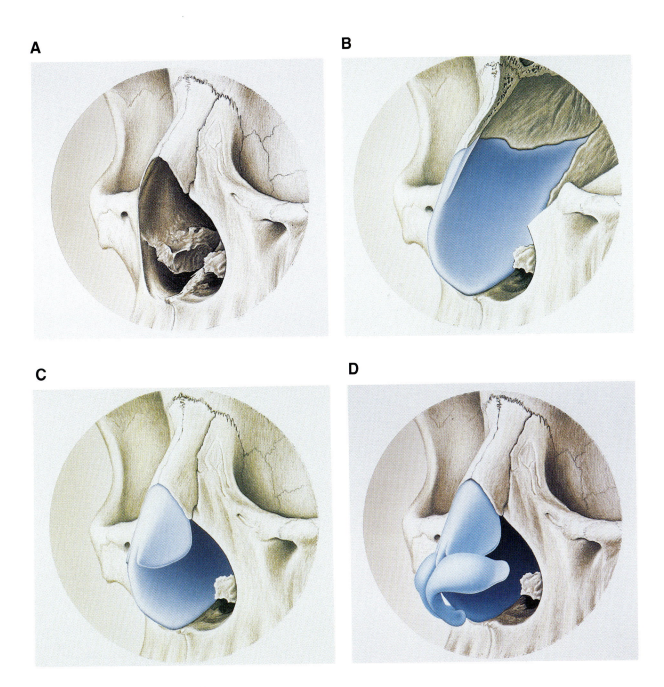

Figure 16–19
The principal anatomic components of the nose. **A**, bony pyramid. **B**, cartilaginous pyramid added. **C**, upper lateral cartilages added. **D**, alar cartilages added to complete the nasal structure.

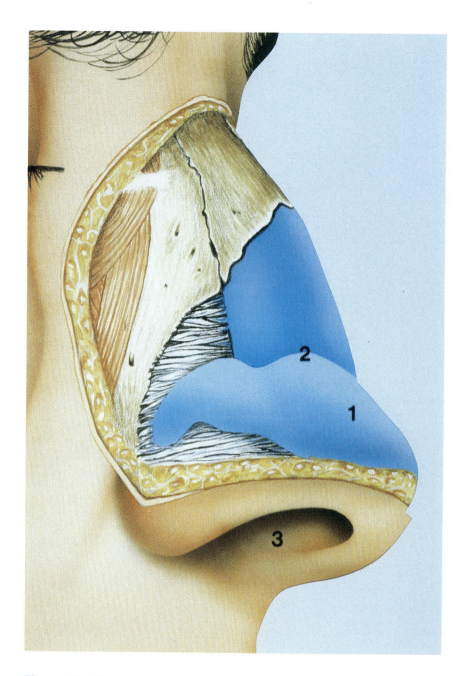

Figure 16-20

The three major tip supports of the nasal tip:

1, the alar cartilages
2, upper lateral-alar cartilage attachment
3, medial crural footplate attachment to caudal septum

CHAPTER 16   Rhinoplasty in Midlife and Aging Patients

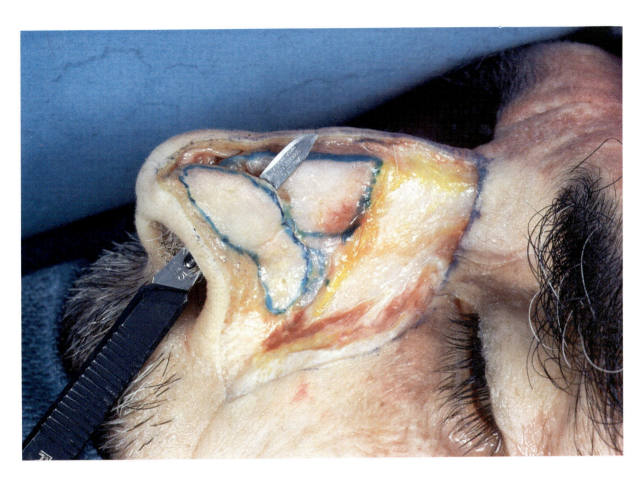

Figure 16–21
Alar cartilage being delivered via a bipedicle chondrocutaneous flap to expose the lateral crus with its tip-defining point, which connects through the more narrow intermediate crural segment to become the medial crus, usually half as wide as the lateral crus.

Operative Sequence

In this most sophisticated and dynamic of all aesthetic and reconstructive operations, the operative sequence develops in essentially the same manner in midlife patients as in younger patients. Specific or segmental rhinoplasty, however, when associated with other rejuvenation operations, possesses important value in older patients. An effective and common sequence of events flowing and blending in dynamic fashion is often as follows:

1. Induction of continuously monitored intravenous anesthesia
2. Minimal Infiltration of local anesthetic (3.5 to 5 cc) into tissue planes
3. Reconstructive septoplasty (if required)
4. Tip surgery (conservative sculpture, reorientation, or augmentation) with appropriate support, contour correction, rotation, and supportive struts and tip grafts if required

5. Correction of caudal septal abnormalities, nasolabial angle deficiencies, and medial crural correction
6. Periosteal elevation of the bony pyramid (conservative)
7. Incremental cartilaginous profile alignment
8. Bony profile alignment
9. Angled medial and curved low lateral osteotomies
10. Incision repair
11. Application of the dressing and splint

Although this general sequence of steps is followed in the majority of patients, one must be prepared to alter or interrupt this flexible schedule of events whenever nasal dynamics are changed or anatomic features demand a change in schedule. For example, partial rhinoplasty, a useful operation in the older patient, will require fewer steps to correct a specifically targeted outcome. Isolated tip sculpture, nasal tip elevation, cephalic rotation, and even minimal bony hump removal may be performed as partial procedures with pleasing results (see Fig 16–1). *Total rhinoplasty is not always required for correction of less-than-major abnormalities to achieve natural results.*

Anesthesia

Middle-aged patients undergoing rhinoplasty are premedicated with a single drug, ordinarily a reversible narcotic only. Combinations of drugs, particularly when intermingled with intravenous medication given during surgery, are often unpredictable in their effectiveness; more importantly, the actions of narcotics are reversible, whereas any potential drug reaction from the use of multiple families of pharmacologic agents is confusing to treat and may be impossible to intelligently counteract.

A state of relaxed sedation is then induced by an experienced anesthesiologist in the operating room who infuses titrated increments of droperidol and fentanyl (see Chapter 4). We have undertaken thousands of procedures over the past 20 years with no serious operative or postoperative anesthesia complications when using this regimen. In the past several years the addition of midazolam (Versed) in small titrated doses has been helpful in smoothing the intravenous anesthetic course and has provided significant anterograde amnesia for surgical events.

Nasal local anesthesia is next effected with 1% lidocaine (Xylocaine) with epinephrine (a 1:100,000 dilution if the patient is older and a 1:50,000 dilution in younger patients). No attempt is made to block specific sensory nerves, but rather to diffuse a plane of anesthesia solution in the nasal area to be incised and operated upon, principally in the immediate supraperichondrial and supraperiosteal planes (Fig 16–22). Minimal quantities are infused, commonly between 3.5 and 5 cc only. Five cubic centimeter of 4% cocaine solution delivered via intranasal cottonoids shrinks and numbs the nasal mucosa (Fig 16–23).

CHAPTER 16 Rhinoplasty in Midlife and Aging Patients

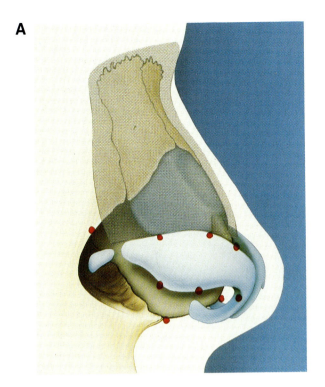
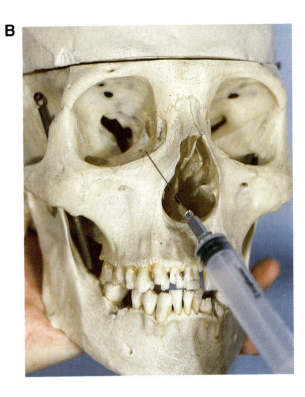
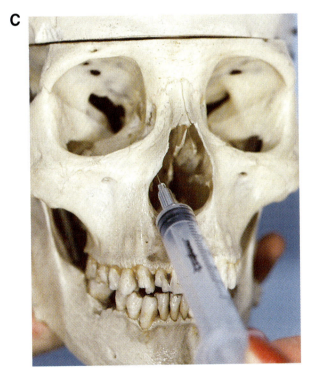

Figure 16–22
A, regions of nasal dorsum and lateral sidewalls. Variable injection sites depicted at red dots infiltrated with local anesthesia. **B**, local anesthetic infiltrated *medially* as well as *laterally* along the ascending process of the maxilla produces a vasoconstricted pathway for lateral osteotomies, thereby minimizing or eliminating osteotomy bleeding. **C**, deposit of local anesthetic *internal* to the ascending process of the maxilla.

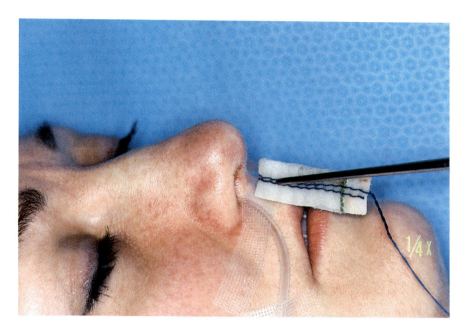

Figure 16-23
One cubic centimeter of 4% colored-coded cocaine delivered to the nasal mucus membranes via a neurosurgical cottonoid.

Exploitation of the important potential planes, first with anesthetic infusion and later with surgical knife dissection, is a critical factor in our trauma-reduction concepts of rhinoplasty; there is uniformly minimal bleeding, reduced disturbance of normal and aesthetically favorable nasal areas, and thus less scarring. Improved surgical control over the vagaries of healing is thus maximized.

Preferred and Alternative Techniques

If septoplasty is indicated, it is accomplished first in order to straighten and correct this most important aspect of the abnormal nose. Emphasis is placed on preservation and reconstruction of the septum by disarticulating the perpendicular plate from the ethmoid and freeing the quadrangular cartilage from the maxillary crest to create a "swinging door" effect. Septoplasty should be conservative in the older patient to minimize the possibilities of disturbing rigid sclerotic vessels and causing intraoperative or postoperative hemorrhage, a somewhat greater danger in these patients. Once the septal corrective and straightening procedures are complete, the septal flap(s) is reapproximated with a running through-and-through 4-0 chromic catgut suture, thereby eliminating dead space and negating the need for nasal packing. With few exceptions, the contralateral mucoperichondrial flap is left intact and unelevated to preserve support and blood supply.

CHAPTER 16 Rhinoplasty in Midlife and Aging Patients

Nasal tip sculpturing is ordinarily carried out next in sequence, the lower lateral cartilages approached through *cartilage splitting (nondelivery), retrograde (nondelivery), or intercartilaginous and marginal incision approaches (delivery)* (Figs 16–24 to 16–26). In specific anatomic tip variants, the *open approach* to rhinoplasty allows maximal diagnosis of unrevealed deformities, binocular visual surgery, and bimanual surgical correction. Thus a systematic, graduated approach to the nose prevails (Fig 16–27).

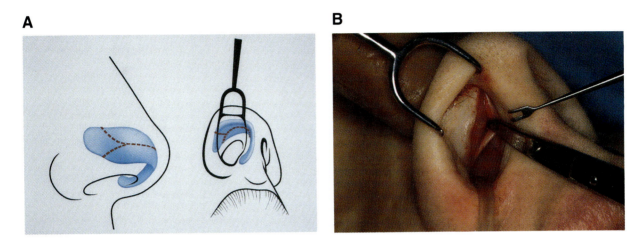

Figure 16–24
Transcartilaginous approach (nondelivery) to the tip. **A,** typical incisional alternatives. **B,** surgical incision site.

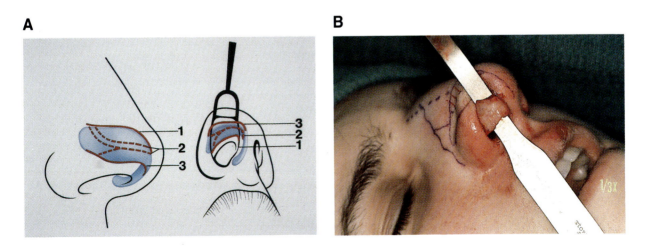

Figure 16–25
A, incisions 1 and 3 (intercartilaginous and marginal) employed for delivery of the alar cartilages. **B,** alar cartilages delivered for diagnosis and sculpture.

Figure 16–26
Transcolumellar irregularized incision for an open approach to the tip.

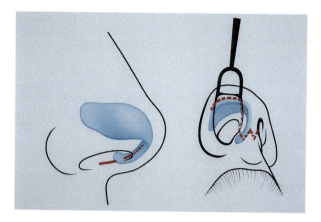

Figure 16–27
Algorithm depicting a graduated anatomic systematic approach to nasal deformities in which the *least traumatic* and invasive approach is applied to minimal to modest deformities while more extensive approaches are selected for major deformities. In every instance, the approach and subsequent technique are dictated by the anatomy encountered since no single surgical process will suffice to manage the wide range of anatomic variants encountered.

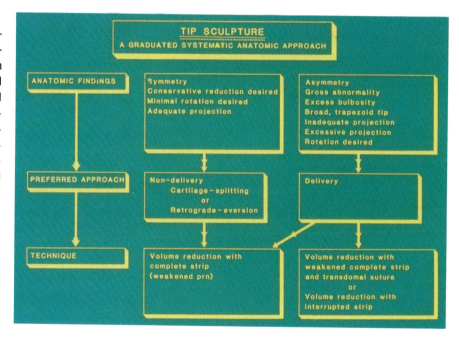

The chosen technique and the extent of sculpturing depend entirely on the anatomic features encountered. Seldom in older patients is the dome of the lower lateral cartilage interrupted; we attempt instead to preserve a complete continuous caudal segment of lower lateral cartilage for support and symmetry (Fig 16–28). Often a narrowing transdomal mattress suture is placed for added tip definition and refinement (Fig 16–29); this effectively reorients a broad, trapezoidal tip configuration to a more triangular, narrow appearance while preserving (and often improving) existing tip support (Figs 16–30 to 16–32). All cartilage cut edges are beveled and smoothed since the thinner skin of midlife patients may in time reveal the sharp cut edge of an abrupt cartilage offset. If severe anatomic or asymmetrical abnormalities of the alar cartilages require segmental cartilage excision or complete strip interruption, suture reconstitution with 6-0 clear nylon is always effected to restore integrity to the complete strip.

Figure 16–28
Volume reduction of alar cartilage in the medial cephalic region. A generous complete strip is preserved for symmetry and support whenever possible (the majority of cases).

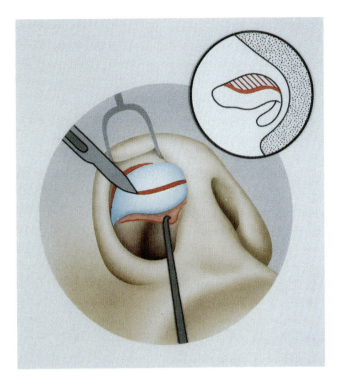

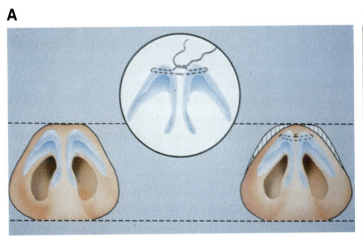

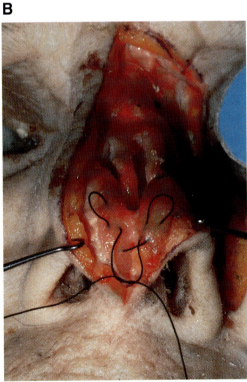

Figure 16–29
A and **B,** transdomal suture narrowing of a broad tip with 5-0 PDS clear suture, a reliable and effective tip refinement technique.

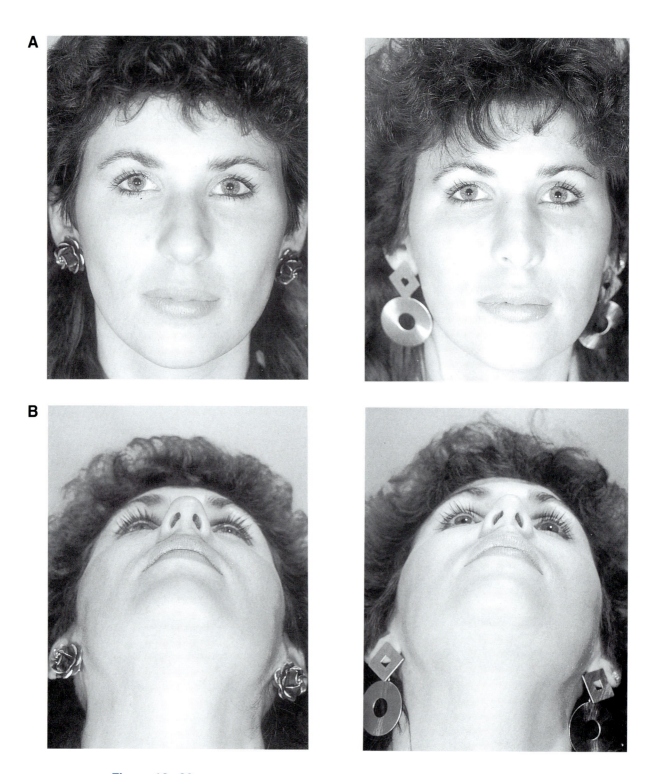

Figure 16–30
A–D, reduction refinement of the nasal tip by utilizing the transdomal suture technique.

CHAPTER 16 Rhinoplasty in Midlife and Aging Patients

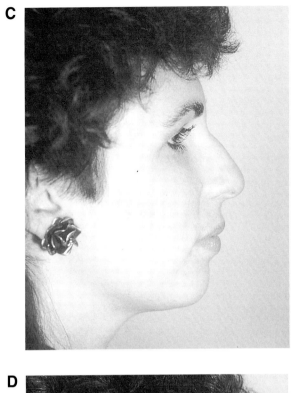

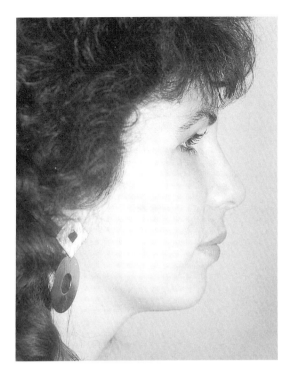

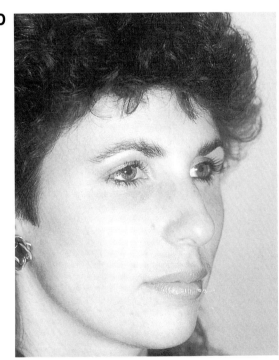

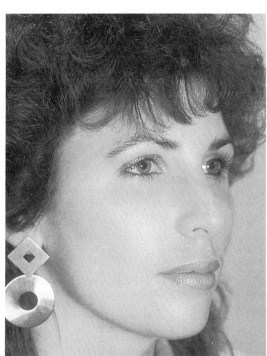

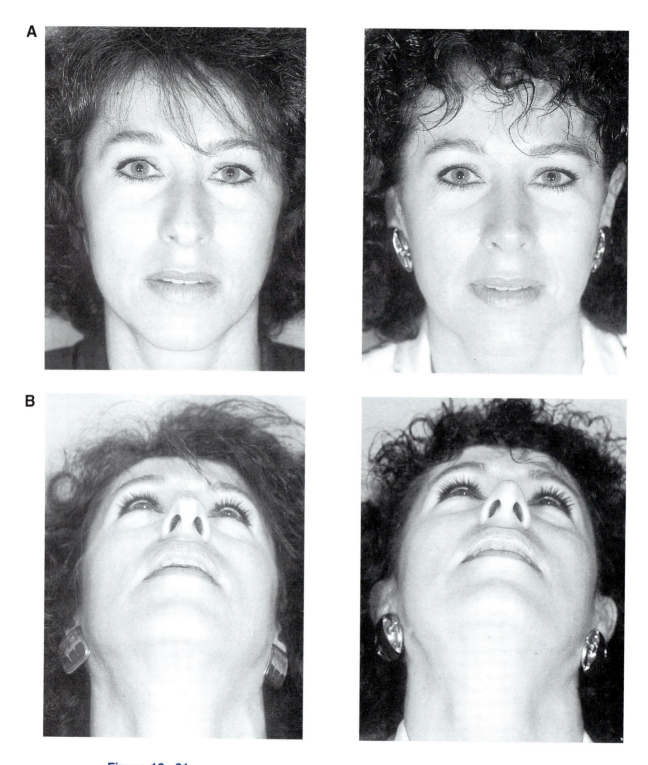

Figure 16–31
A–D, narrowing tip refinement following alar cartilage cephalic trim with the transdomal suture technique.

CHAPTER 16 Rhinoplasty in Midlife and Aging Patients

C

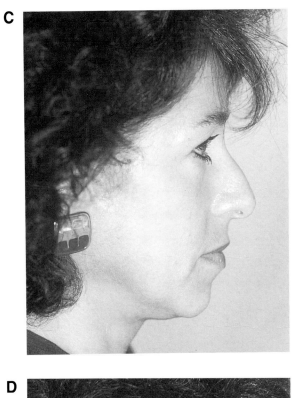 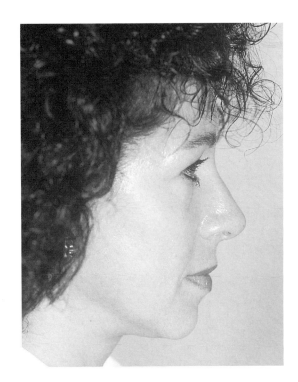

D

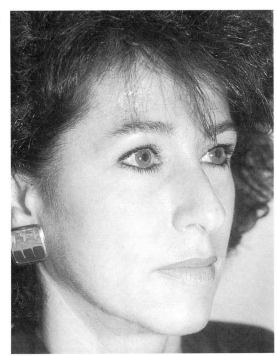 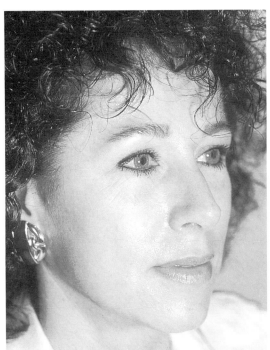

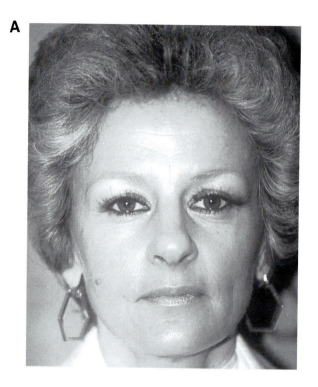

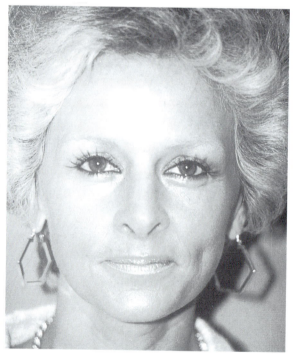

Figure 16–32
A and **B,** transdomal suture reorientation of broad alar cartilages. Thick cartilages, thin skin, and intercrural bifidity form a triad that when encountered, should suggest correction with transdomal sutures.

CHAPTER 16 Rhinoplasty in Midlife and Aging Patients

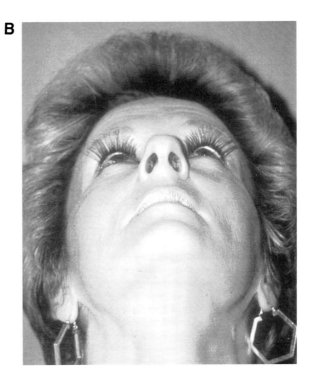

B

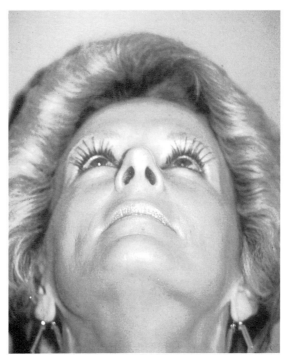

Cephalic rotation of the nasal tip may be accomplished primarily by calculated excision of the caudal septal margin, excision of redundant excessive vestibular skin and mucus membrane, reorientation of the alar cartilage inclination, and supportive columellar and nasolabial angle cartilage grafts (Fig 16–33, A to C).

Cartilage autograft augmentation of the tip cartilages, columella, or nasolabial angle, if indicated, is accomplished at this juncture in an attempt to stabilize the tip projection and attitude prior to operating on the remainder of the nose (Fig 16–34).

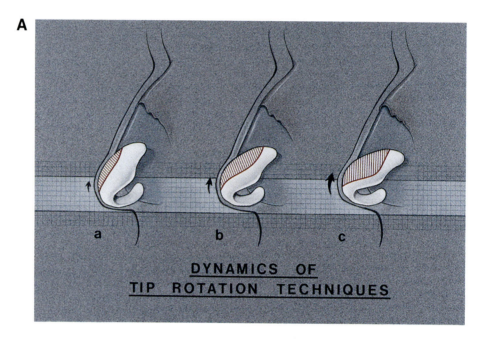

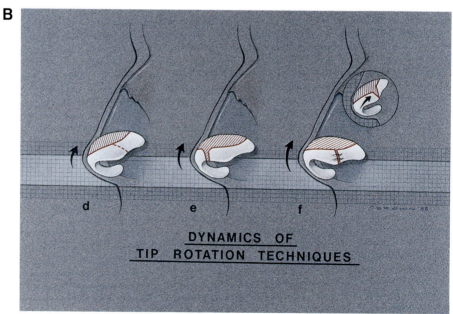

CHAPTER 16 Rhinoplasty in Midlife and Aging Patients

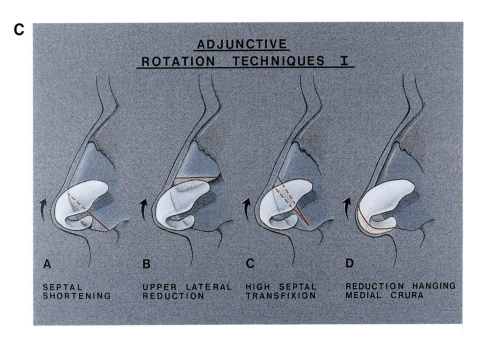

Figure 16–33
A–C, methods employed individually or in combination to intentionally effect cephalic tip rotation. Preservation of a strong complete alar cartilage residual strip results in very little tip rotation, while interrupted strip techniques tend to foster cephalic tip rotation.

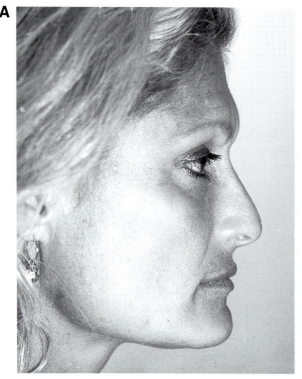
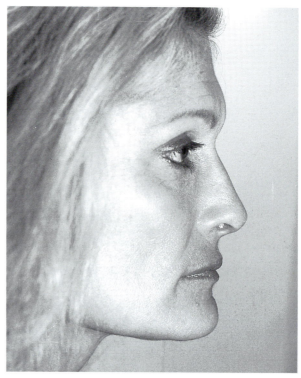

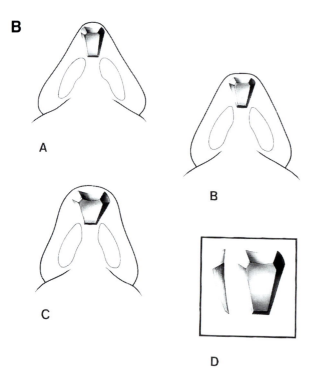

Figure 16-34

A, Structured reorientation of inadequately projecting nasal tip with cartilage tip grafts. **B,** varied sizes and shapes of tip grafts utilized.

CHAPTER 16 Rhinoplasty in Midlife and Aging Patients

Appropriate conservative profile alignment is next undertaken under direct vision, with the goal of developing a pleasing tip-supratip relationship and maintenance of a high, strong, "aristocratic" dorsum (Fig 16–35). In middle-aged and older aged patients excessive dorsal profile lowering is a dignity-diminishing maneuver that robs the nose and face of a stately appearance consistent with the patient's age and status. A sharp knife and thin osteotome are utilized to develop the appropriate profile alignment, initially on the septal cartilage under direct vision followed by osteotome shaving of the bony profile or more generous hump removal (Fig 16–36, A and B). On occasion the bony profile requires only minimal change with a sharp rasp, and the need for medial and lateral osteotomies is obviated by maintaining an narrow intact nasal roof. Precision radial sculpturing of the bony dorsum by shaving small slivers of bone may be accomplished atraumatically with the nasal osteoplane (Fig 16–37). In patients with exquisitely thin skin overlying the nasal bony dorsum, the approach of Skoog may occasionally be helpful: more bony-cartilaginous hump is resected than planned and then this bony-cartilaginous graft is replaced after removal of all mucosa (if present) and the size of the new dorsal graft reduced (Fig 16–38, A and B). This procedure finds particular usefulness in midlife and older patients since it reestablishes a closed, smooth, and natural dorsum, but absolute precision is required in removal, hump sculpturing, and replacement.

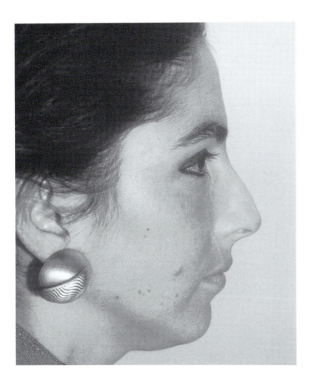
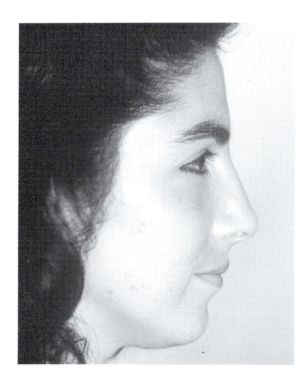

Figure 16–35
Strong, modestly reduced nasal profiles are preferable in older patients to avoid profound and dramatic changes in appearance.

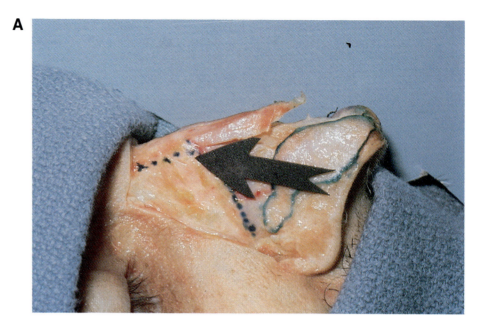

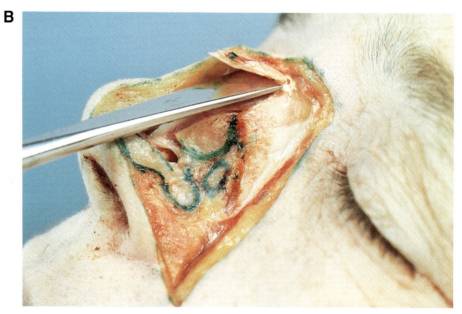

Figure 16-36
A, resection of the cartilaginous dorsum in preparation for bony hump excision in an en bloc fashion. **B,** sharp Rubin osteotome excision of a bony hump.

CHAPTER 16 Rhinoplasty in Midlife and Aging Patients

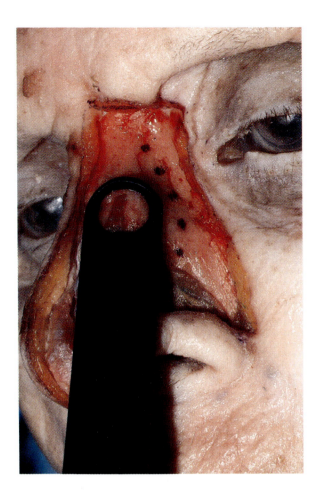

Figure 16–37
A sharp nasal osteoplane, useful in shaving bony prominences, produces less trauma than rasps.

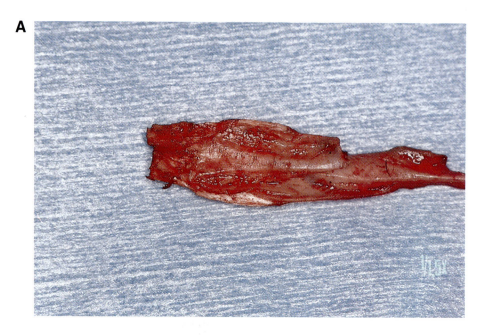

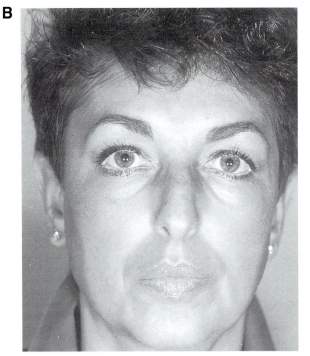 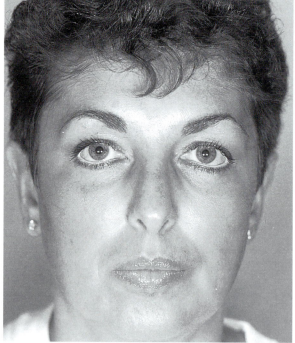

Figure 16–38
A, if a hump replacement procedure is contemplated, slightly more hump than normal is resected en bloc, trimmed of mucosa and required bulk, and reinserted into its previous anatomic bed. **B–D,** a patient with a remarkably thin skin–subcutaneous tissue covering was treated by the hump replacement method of Skoog.

CHAPTER 16 Rhinoplasty in Midlife and Aging Patients

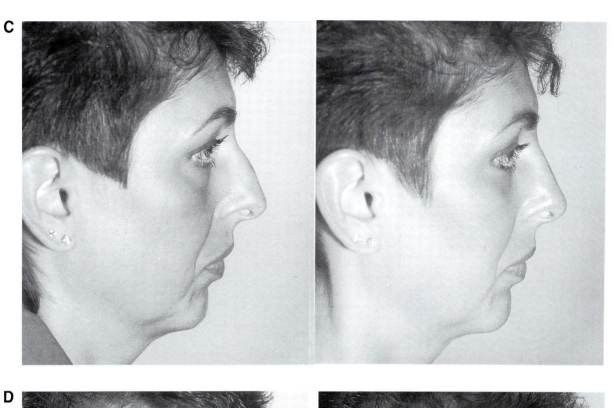

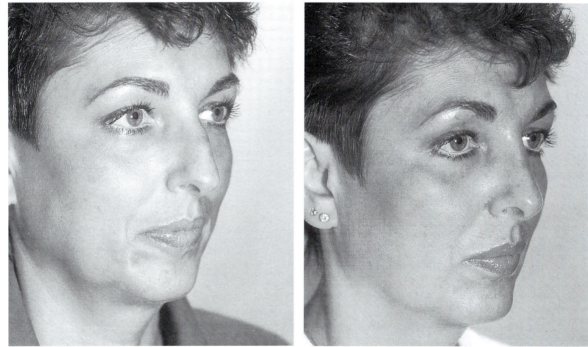

Figure 16–38 (cont.).

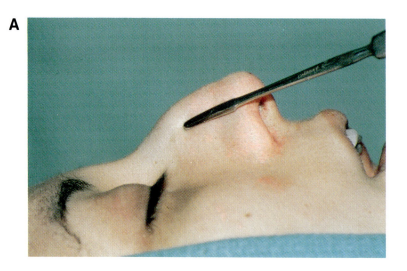

Figure 16-39
A, conservative undermining of the periosteum with a Joseph elevator to develop the thickest possible skin-subcutaneous tissue-periosteal overlying flap. Tiny irregularities develop in a certain percentage of patients as the nose changes over many years in even the best of hands. Since the overlying soft tissues are least thick at the rhinion, virtue exists in maintaining a thick overlying skin canopy. **B,** interdigitated muscular aponeurosis (nasal SMAS) covering the nasal skeleton. **C,** rendering of the nasal SMAS layer dissected away from the skeleton that reveals the ideal plane of tissue dissection during rhinoplasty.

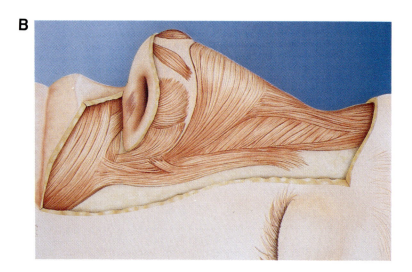

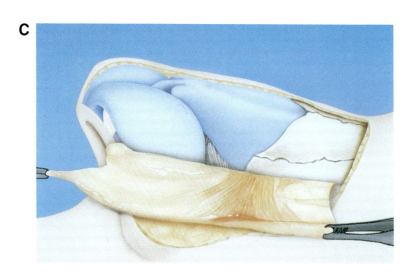

CHAPTER 16 Rhinoplasty in Midlife and Aging Patients

Somewhat wider skin and periosteal elevation may be indicated in an older patient to effect more satisfactory redraping, but periosteal elevation should never extend to or beyond the intended level of the lateral osteotomies lest the nasal bone fragments lose all periosteal support following osteotomy (Fig 16-39). The thickest possible skin-subcutaneous tissue-muscle-periosteal flap should be developed in order to permanently conceal any profile irregularities that may be unmasked months or years later as the skin shrinks and thins.

As a final operative step, angled medial-oblique and low curved lateral osteotomies are created when necessary (Fig 16-40). Because brittle bones in older patients may fragment easily, small (2 to 3 mm) sharp osteotomes are mandatory (see Fig 16-40, A and B). Greenstick fractures, undesirable in younger patients, can be tolerated in an older patient and in fact may be safer.

Finally, all incisions are sutured completely, and a Velcro-metal splint cushioned by a layer of Gelfoam placed directly over the nasal dorsum is positioned (Fig 16-41). If any intranasal dressing is used, it consists of ventilated nasal tampons, which are removed the morning following surgery.

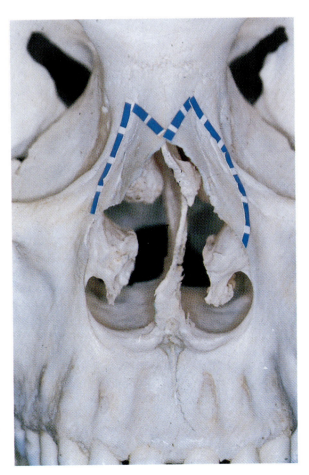

Figure 16-40
Skull with osteotomy sites marked.

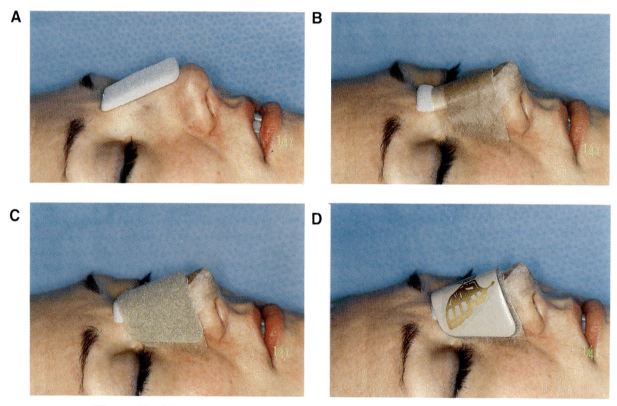

Figure 16-41
A, layer of Gelfoam creating additional pressure and cushion over the nasal skin. **B**, flesh-colored micropore taping. **C**, inner layer (Velcro) of the Denver splint. **D**, outer aluminum/velcro layer of splint.

Postoperative Care

The protective nasal splint is maintained for 5 to 7 days and then gently removed by teasing it away from the nasal skin while avoiding any traction upon the healing skin-skeleton complex.

Guidelines to patients regarding appropriate postoperative care principles are presented in Figure 16–42.

PATIENT INSTRUCTIONS FOLLOWING NASAL PLASTIC SURGERY

A. **INTRODUCTION**

Please read and familiarize yourself with these instructions both <u>BEFORE</u> and <u>AFTER</u> surgery. By following them carefully you will assist in obtaining the best possible result from your surgery. If questions arise, do not hesitate to communicate with me and discuss your questions at any time. Take this list to the hospital with you and begin observing these directions on the day of surgery.

B. **INSTRUCTIONS**
  1. Do not blow nose until instructed. Wipe or dab nose gently with Kleenex, if necessary.
  2. Change dressing under nose (if present) as needed.
  3. The nasal cast will remain in place for approximately one week and will be removed in the office. Do NOT disturb it; keep it dry.
  4. Avoid foods that require prolonged chewing. Otherwise, your diet has no restrictions.
  5. Avoid extreme physical activity. Obtain more rest than you usually get and avoid exertion, including athletic activities and intercourse.
  6. Brush teeth gently with a soft toothbrush only. Avoid manipulation of upper lip to keep nose at rest.
  7. Avoid excess or prolonged telephone conversations and social activities for at least 10–14 days.
  8. You may wash your face—carefully avoid the dressing. Take tub baths until the dressings are removed.
  9. Avoid smiling, grinning, and excess facial movements for one week.
  10. Do not wash hair for one week unless you have someone do it for you. <u>DO NOT GET NASAL DRESSINGS WET.</u>
  11. Wear clothing that fastens in front or back for one week. Avoid slipover sweaters, T-shirts, and turtlenecks.
  12. Absolutely avoid sun or sun lamps for 6 weeks after surgery. Heat may cause the nose to swell.
  13. Don't swim for one month since injuries are common during swimming.
  14. Don't be concerned if, following removal of dressing, the nose, eyes, and upper lip show some swelling and discoloration—this usually clears in 2–3 weeks. In certain patients it may require 6 months for all swelling to completely subside.
  15. Take only medications prescribed by your doctor(s).
  16. Do not wear regular glasses or sunglasses that rest on the bridge of the nose for at least 4 weeks. We will instruct you in the method of taping the glasses to your forehead to avoid pressure on the nose.
  17. Contact lenses may be worn within 2 to 3 days after surgery.
  18. After the doctor removes your nasal cast, the skin of the nose may be cleansed gently with a mild soap or Vaseline Intensive Care Lotion. <u>BE GENTLE.</u> Makeup may be used as soon as bandages are removed. To cover discoloration, you may use "ERASE" by Max Factor, "COVER AWAY" by Adrien Arpel, or "ON YOUR MARK" by Kenneth.
  19. <u>DON'T TAKE CHANCES!</u> If you are concerned about anything you consider significant, call me at 312-472-7559.

Figure 16–42
Instructions given to patients for postrhinoplasty care.

CHAPTER 16 Rhinoplasty in Midlife and Aging Patients

Evaluation of Results and Outcomes

The older patient undergoing rhinoplasty as a rule is among the most pleased and gratified of any group requesting nasal surgery. Conservative, subtle changes are appreciated by this more sophisticated group; major satisfaction is experienced when the results are natural and not overly dramatic (Figs 16–43 to 16–49). In addition, no other group is such a potent referral source for the skilled surgeon since midlife patients are quick to make their peers (and others) aware of the physical and psychological benefits of aesthetic surgery. Appearance is of exceeding importance to most patients at this stage of life.

Follow-up photographs are obtained 1 week and 2, 3, 6, 12, and 36 months following surgery. Every effort is expended to secure photographs even later since postoperative deformities of healing may be unveiled for several years following surgery. *There is no better postgraduate continuing educational experience than a critical review of one's long-term standardized photographs of patients.*

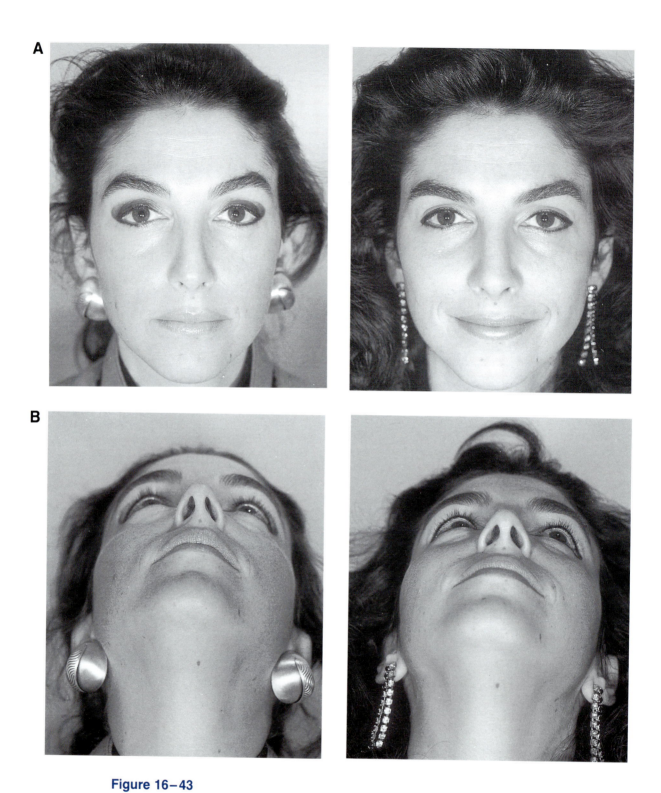

Figure 16–43
A–D, refinement rhinoplasty outcome in a midlife patient. A strong elegant profile is maintained along with favorable aesthetic lines on the frontal view.

CHAPTER 16   Rhinoplasty in Midlife and Aging Patients

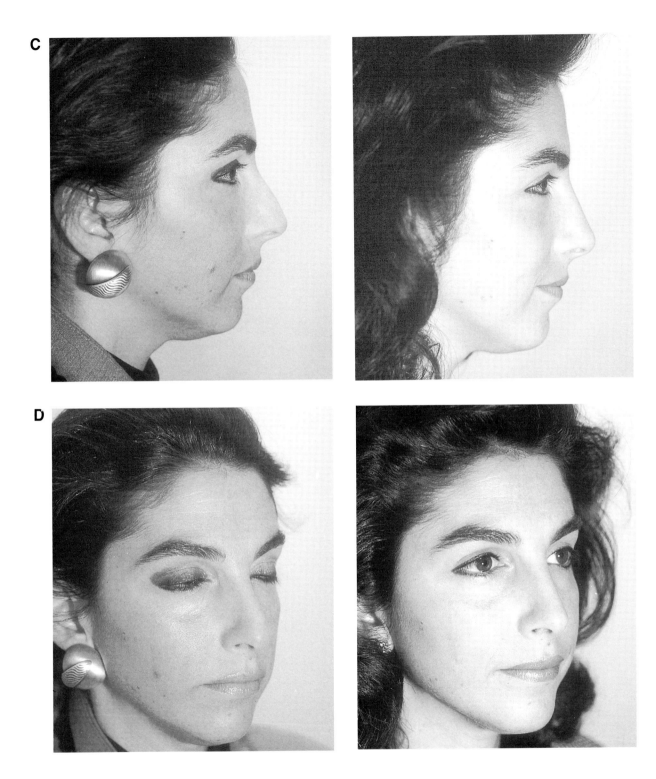

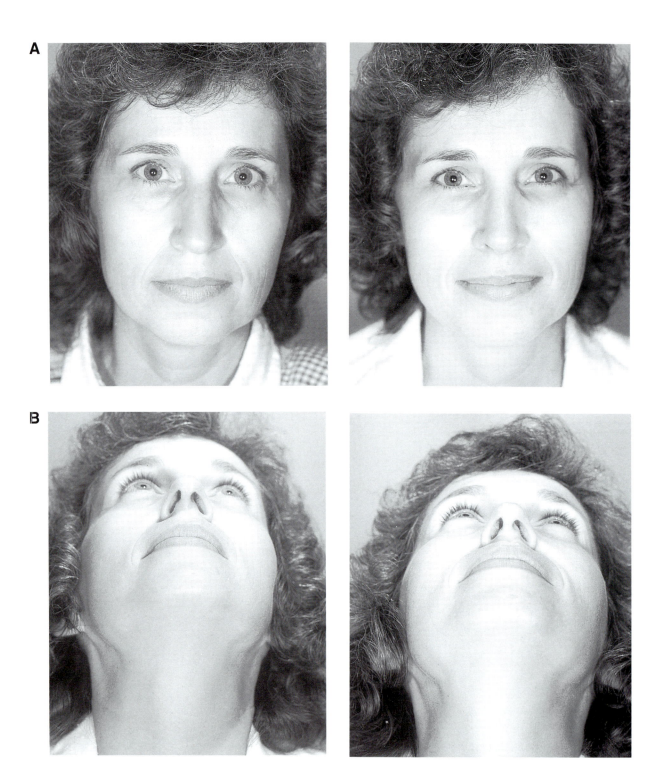

Figure 16-44
A-D, subtle rhinoplasty improvement in an older patient with extremely thin skin, bony pyramid ridging, and elongation of the nose. Changes have been made in all regions and components of the nose to effect a more youthful and natural appearance. Total septoplasty was required.

CHAPTER 16 Rhinoplasty in Midlife and Aging Patients

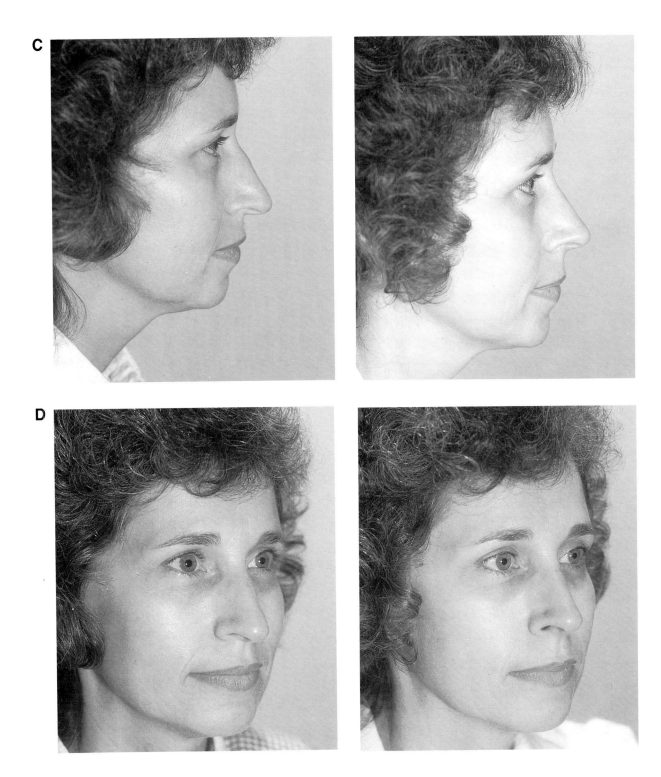

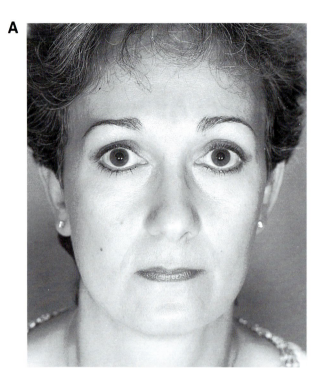
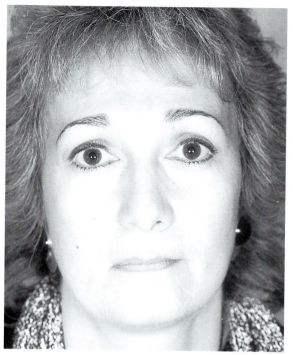
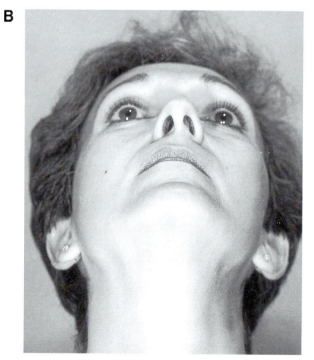
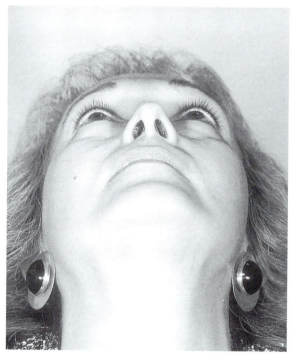

Figure 16–45
A–D, rhinoplasty outcome in an older patient with profile irregularities, septal subluxation, and an asymmetrical tip. Note the correction of the left medial crural footplate abnormality. Changes are natural and in keeping with the patient's age group and wishes. A strong profile is maintained.

CHAPTER 16 Rhinoplasty in Midlife and Aging Patients

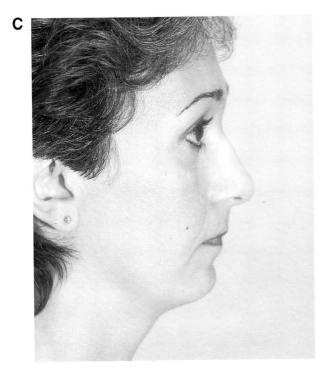
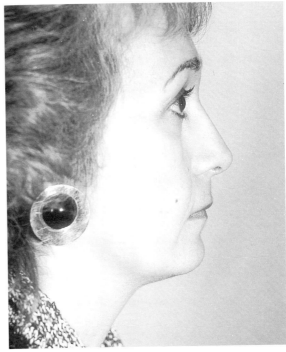
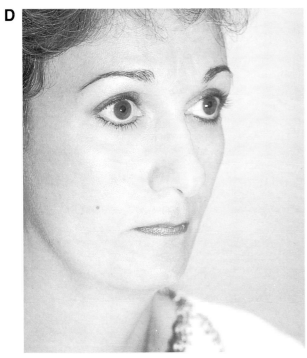
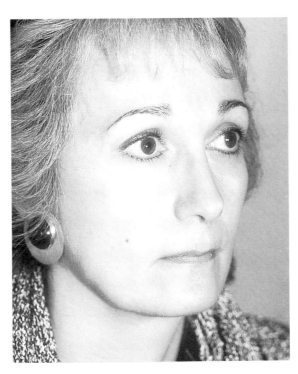

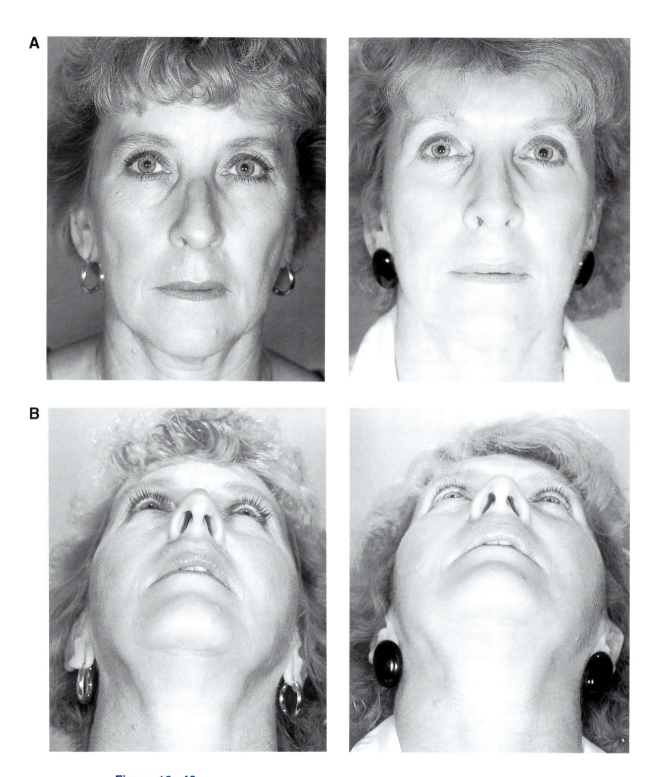

Figure 16–46
A–C, aging nose in need of better balance of the anatomic components and profile reduction. At 1 year the nose is better proportioned to itself and to the face.

CHAPTER 16 Rhinoplasty in Midlife and Aging Patients

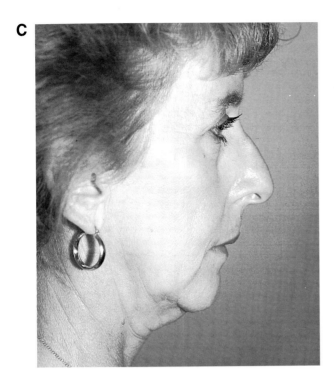
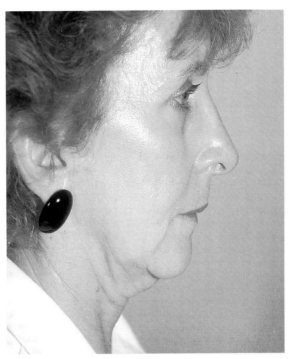

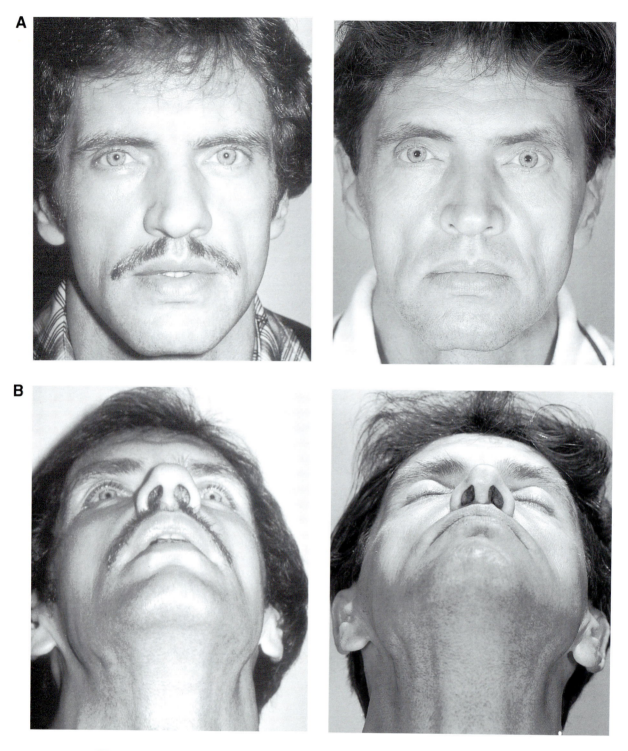

Figure 16–47

A–C, severely traumatized, deviated nose with marked tip asymmetry and airway obstruction. An improved result at 10 years demonstrates a straighter nose with improved appearance of the tip and profile.

CHAPTER 16   Rhinoplasty in Midlife and Aging Patients

C

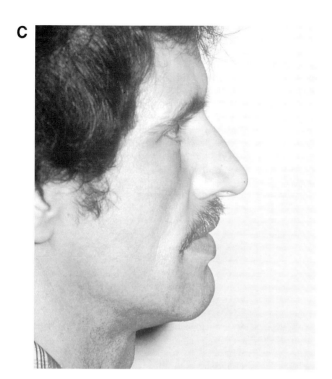
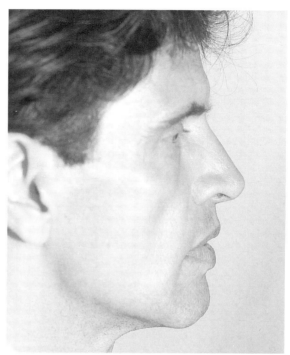

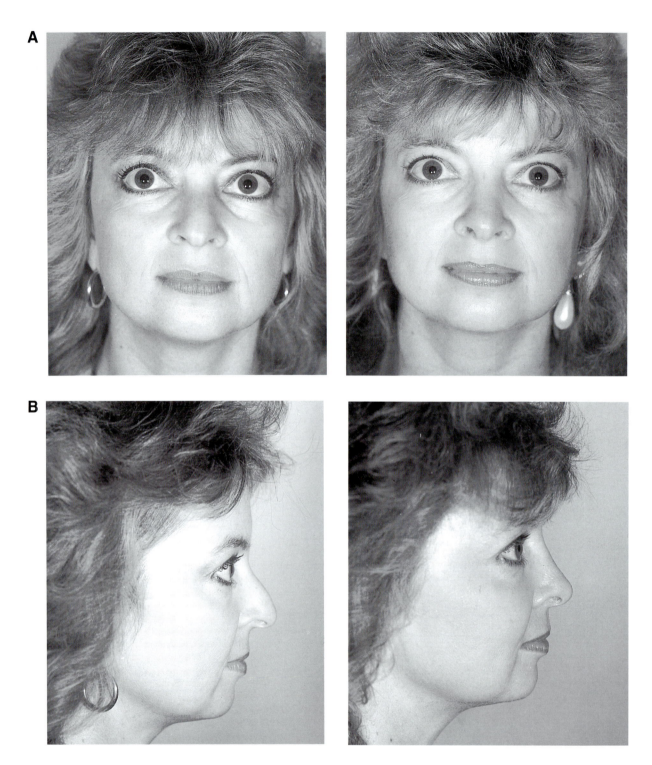

Figure 16–48
A–D, middle-aged patient exhibiting a small nose with a hump and tip-supratip disproportion. Refinement of the tip plus reduction of the prominent supratip profile provides an improved nasal appearance. Modest augmentation of the nasal tip with cartilage grafts improves tip projection.

CHAPTER 16   Rhinoplasty in Midlife and Aging Patients

C
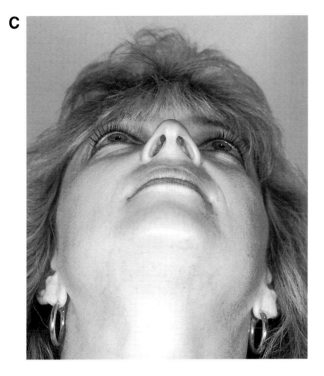
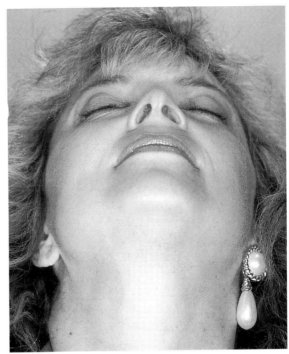

D
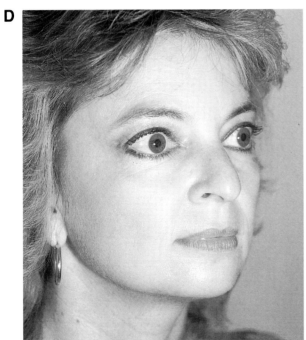
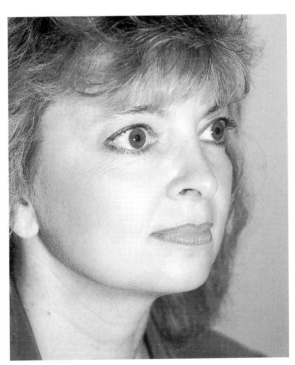

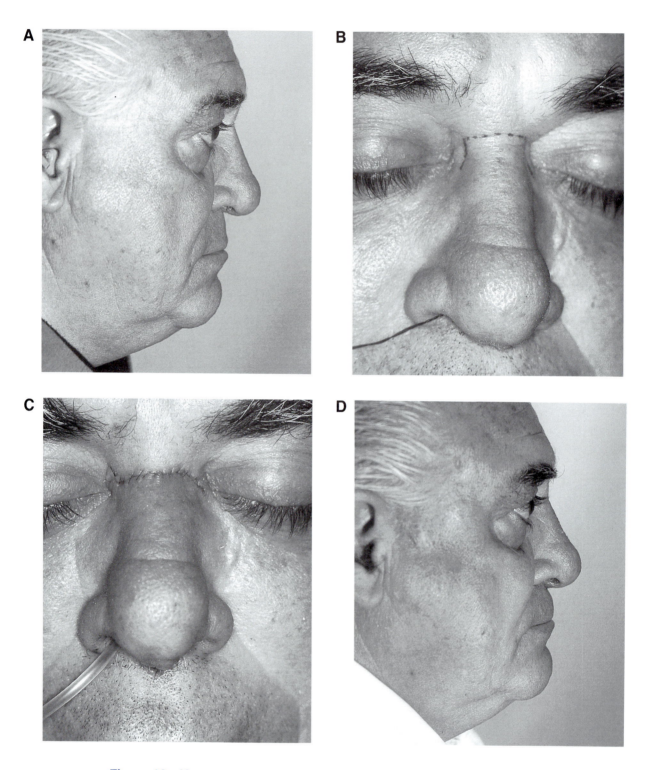

Figure 16–49
Aging nose characterized by tip ptosis, enlargement of the skin sleeve, and narrowing of the nasolabial angle—airway blockade results. Rhytidorhinoplasty improves the appearance and corrects the airway obstruction.

CHAPTER 16 Rhinoplasty in Midlife and Aging Patients

Comparative evaluation of a progressive series of postoperative photographs dispassionately viewed and critically assessed is of even greater personal educational value when coupled with an individualized graphic operative record (Fig 16-50) completed in a highly visual style immediately at the completion of each rhinoplasty; the graphic record provides an invaluable, infallible record of the accuracy of the surgeon's diagnostic and applied surgical capabilities. In addition, this personalized record lends itself well to computer storage of surgical technique and details when projected side by side with standardized preoperative and postoperative photographs—a valuable teaching device is graphically visualized that allows the observer a rapid assessment of the outcome of the chosen approach and technique.

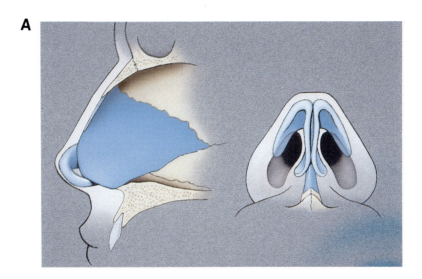

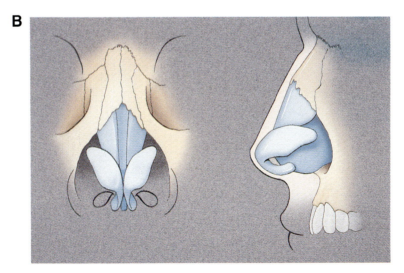

Figure 16-50
A and **B**, graphic record developed by Jack Gunter, M.D., highly instructive when utilized for graphic recording of surgical procedures.

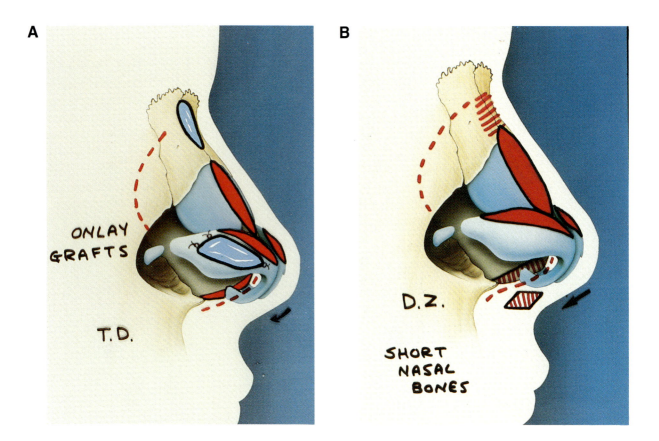

Figure 16-51
A and B, additional graphic records employed to record details of surgical refinements.

CHAPTER 16   Rhinoplasty in Midlife and Aging Patients

Sequelae and Complications

Older rhinoplasty patients differ substantially from young patients in that a much less exuberant healing response is evident, essentially eliminating problems with supratip soft-tissue polly-beak formation.

The thin, less elastic skin of older patients, however, requires a longer period to shrink and accommodate favorably to the new nasal skeleton. In a few carefully selected patients, rhytidorhinoplasty is indicated to directly excise redundant skin at the nasal root and camouflage incisions in existent wrinkle and contour lines (see Fig 16–49). The diminished subcutaneous layer contributes to a thinner epithelial covering in older patients; thus even minor irregularities of the bony pyramid are subject to visible or palpable exposure as the healing process unfolds over many months. It is essential that the surgeon ensure exacting smoothness of the surgically altered profile with sharp delicate tungsten carbide rasps.

Other possible complications following midlife rhinoplasty are similar to those experienced in younger individuals. Thus a small percentage of rhinoplasty patients will require minor revision procedures to correct slight but annoying healing irregularities, ensure total patient satisfaction, as well as satisfy the surgeon's quest for near perfection.

A favorable side effect of rhinoplasty results from the development of a "favorable" fibrosis layer of scar tissue beneath the skin–subcutaneous tissue layer; this provides a significant deterrent to the further aging elongation of the nose that is witnessed over time in nonoperated patients.

Summary

Because of altered physical changes and psychological patterns, patients requesting rhinoplasty in midlife and beyond must be managed and treated with specific goals and limitations in mind. Subtle and conservative nasal appearance changes generally suit this category of patient best, with a dramatic metamorphosis avoided in patients whose body image is firmly imprinted. When performed in conjunction with other age-diminishing operative procedures, rhinoplasty plays a critical role in overall facial appearance improvement. Breathing difficulties brought on by aging changes in the nose may be eliminated by septal reconstruction, nasal tip elevation, and when indicated, alar sidewall reinforcement support with cartilage autografts.

By observing the principles and limitations discussed in this chapter, the surgeon can find exceeding satisfaction in performing conservative rhinoplasty in patients who find themselves in the middle stages of life and beyond.

Suggested Reading

- Brennan HG, Parkes ML: Septal surgery: The high septal transfixion. *Int Surg* 1973; 58:732.
- Fry HJH: Nasal skeletal trauma and the interlocked stresses of the nasal septal cartilage. *Br J Plast Surg* 1967; 20:146.
- Gilbert JG, Felt LJ: The nasal aponeurosis and its role in rhinoplasty. *Arch Otolaryngol* 1955:61:433.
- Goin MK, Goin JM: Changing the Body. Baltimore, Williams & Wilkins, 1981.
- Goodman WS, Charles DA: Technique of external rhinoplasty. *Can J Otolaryngol* 1978; 7:13.
- Gunter JP: Anatomical observations of the lower lateral cartilages. *Arch Otolaryngol* 1969; 89:61.
- Janeke JB, Wright WK: Studies of the support of the nasal tip. *Arch Otolaryngol* 1971; 93:458.
- Natvig P, et al: Anatomical details of the osseous-cartilaginous framework of the nose. *Plast Reconstr Surg* 1971; 48:528.
- Ortiz-Monisterio F, Olmedo A, Oscoy LO: The use of cartilage grafts in primary aesthetic rhinoplasty. *Plast Reconstr Surg* 1981; 67:597.
- Padovan IF: External approach in rhinoplasty. *Surg ORL Lug* 1966; 3:354.
- Parkes ML, Brennan HG: High septal transfixion to shorten the nose. *Plast Reconstr Surg* 1970; 45:487.
- Smith TW: As clay in the potter's hand: A review of 221 rhinoplasties. *Ohio Med J* 1967; 63:1055.
- Sheen JH: Achieving more nasal tip projection by use of small autogenous vomer or septal cartilage grafts. *Plast Reconstr Surg* 1975; 56:35, 211.
- Sheen JH: *Aesthetic Rhinoplasty.* St Louis, Mosby–Year Book, 1985.
- Sheen JH: Secondary rhinoplasty. *Plast Reconstr Surg* 1975; 56:137.
- Skoog T: *Plastic Surgery.* Philadelphia, WB Saunders, 1975.
- Straatsma BR, Straatsma CR: The anatomical relationship of the lateral nasal cartilage to the nasal bone and the cartilaginous nasal septum. *Plast Reconstr Surg* 1951; 8:443.
- Tardy ME: Nasal reconstruction and rhinoplasty, in *Ballenger's Textbook of Otolaryngology,* ed 12. Philadelphia, Lea & Fibiger, 1977.
- Tardy ME: *Rhinoplasty.* Baltimore, Williams & Wilkins, 1984.
- Tardy ME: Rhinoplasty, in Cummings CW et al (eds): *Otolaryngology—Head and Neck Surgery,* vol I. St Louis, Mosby–Year Book, 1986.
- Tardy ME: *Rhinoplasty.* Memphis, Tenn, Richard's Medical Co, 1980.
- Tardy ME: Rhinoplasty in midlife. Symposium on the aging face. *Otolaryngo Clin North Am* 1980; 13:289–303.
- Tardy ME: Rhinoplasty tip ptosis: Etiology and prevention. *Laryngoscope* 1973; 83:923–929.
- Tardy ME: Septal perforations. *Otolaryngol Clin North Am* 1973; 6:711–714.

- Tardy ME: Surgical correction of facial deformities, in *Ballenger's Textbook of Otolaryngology*, ed 12. Philadelphia, Lea & Febiger, 1977.
- Tardy ME: Transdomal suture refinement of the nasal tip. *Facial Plast Surg* 1987; 4:000.
- Tardy ME, Broadway D: Graphic record-keeping in rhinoplasty: A valuable self-learning device. *Facial Plast Surg* 1989; 6:108–112.
- Tardy ME, Denneny JC: Micro-osteotomies in rhinoplasty—a technical refinement. *Facial Plast Surg* 1984; 1:137–145.
- Tardy ME, Denneny JC, Fritch MH: The versatile cartilage autograft in reconstruction of the nose and face. *Laryngoscope* 1985; 95:523–533.
- Tardy ME, et al: The cartilaginous pollybeak: Etiology, prevention and treatment. *Facial Plast Surg* 1989; 6:113–120.
- Tardy ME, et al: The over-projecting tip—anatomic variation and targeted solutions. *Facial Plast Surg* 1987; 4:327–350.
- Tardy ME, Hewell TS: Nasal tip refinement—reliable approaches and sculpture techniques. *Facial Plast Surg* 1984; 1:87–124.
- Tardy ME, Schwartz MS, Parras G: Saddle nose deformity: Autogenous graft repair. *Facial Plast Surg* 1989; 6:121–134.
- Tardy ME, Tom L: Anesthesia in rhinoplasty. *Facial Plast Surg* 1984; 1:146–156.
- Tardy ME, Toriumi D: Alar retraction: Composite graft correction. *Facial Plast Surg* 1989; 6:101–107.
- Thomas JR, McKinney J: Rhinoplasty: Clinical categorization as a practical preoperative guide. *South Med J* 1985;78:1470–1473.
- Webster RC: Advances in surgery of the tip: Intact rim cartilage techniques and the tip-columella-lip aesthetic complex. *Otolaryngol Clin North Am* 1975; 8:615.
- Webster RC, Smith RC: *Rhinoplasty*, in Goldwyn RM, (ed): *Long-Term Results in Plastic and Reconstructive Surgery*. Boston, Little, Brown, 1980.
- Wright MR, Wright WK: A psychological study of patients undergoing cosmetic surgery. *Arch Otolaryngol* 1975; 101:145.
- Wright WK: Study on hump removal in rhinoplasty. *Laryngoscope* 1967; 77:508.
- Wright WK: Surgery of the bony and cartilaginous dorsum. *Otolaryngol Clin North Am* 1975; 8:575.

PART V

LIPECTOMY OF THE FACE AND NECK

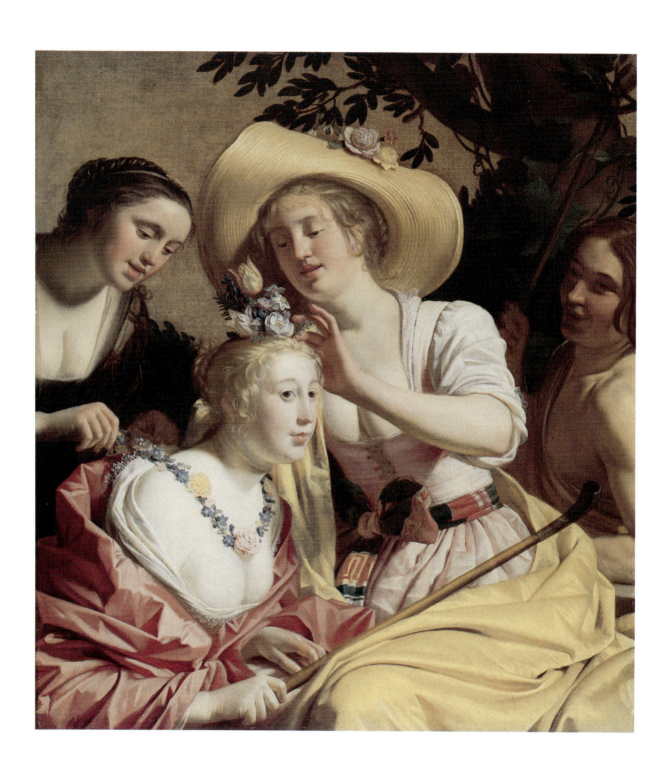

CHAPTER

17

 Lipectomy of the
Face and Neck

*There are two of me
and I am afraid...
I don't know the other me...
I know the young and eager girl
Just reaching out to life
But there is the other
She is looking at me
From the glass
In the windows that I pass
Who is this creature with graying hair
and skin no longer young and fair?
I cry out...I am not she!...I am Me
I want to hide...I want to run
But the creature that I fear
Ever close and ever near
Just follows...and
Lies in wait
To swallow me*

Fanny Gersten

Diagnosis and Candidate Selection

In recent years suction lipectomy (SL) has favorably complemented more traditional methods for removal of localized excess fatty tissue by direct sharp surgical resection. In the submental area in particular, SL has gained wide acceptance because it allows added refinement and contouring of the soft tissues with minimal risk and diminished morbidity. In selected patients SL may be used as an isolated procedure, while in other individuals it serves as an adjunctive technique to initial skin flap surgical elevation with direct fat excision (Fig 17–1).

When fat excess is localized in the immediate submental region, especially when subplatysmal accumulation spoils the submental cervical profile, direct surgical dissection and excision are often preferred and are more immediately effective. Concomitant SL may be employed as an effective adjunct. Direct fat excision with fastidious hemostasis possesses the virtue of being less traumatic than cannula SL and results in less swelling and bruising with more rapid shrinkage of the submental skin and soft tissues.

CHAPTER 17   Lipectomy of the Face and Neck

General agreement exists among the various pioneers of SL regarding its indications. The ideal patient demonstrates localized adipose tissue excess rather than generalized obesity, with the localized fat accumulation resistant to dieting and general weight loss. In addition, the ideal patient must possess sufficient skin elasticity and contractility to allow adequate shrinkage after liposuction and permit adherence to its new skeletal/subcutaneous contour without sagging.

As additional experience has accumulated in the use of SL in the head and neck region, its indications have broadened. Classically, cervicofacial rhytidectomy has been performed by sharp excision, excessive fat in the neck and facial regions being removed with direct sharp excision. Often, however, despite full skin flap elevation with excision and advancement of redundant skin combined with plication of the superficial muscular aponeurotic system (SMAS) and platysmal banding, results may be suboptimal because of submental, submandibular, and jowl region fat accumulations (Fig 17–2). Removal of fat by sharp dissection in these areas can be technically difficult as well as potentially dangerous. SL with small cannulas during facelift flap elevation offers potentially improved contouring of the soft tissues without adding significant risk.

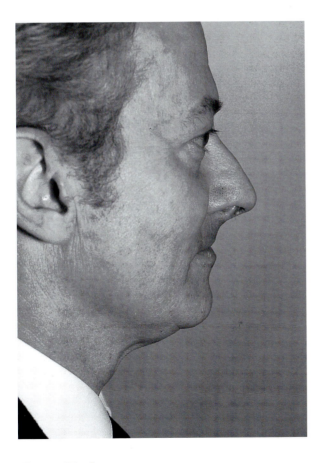
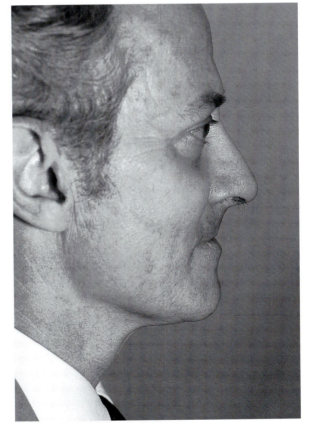

Figure 17–1
Rejuvenation of the ageing submental region by utilizing a combination of SL and direct submental fat excision.

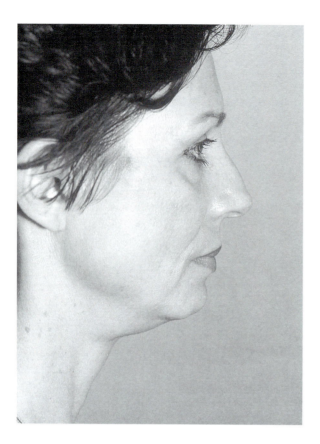
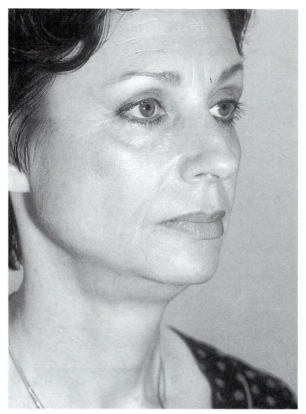

Figure 17–2
Isolated fat accumulation in the submental and submandibular regions.

Liposuction of the cheek–lip fold region has been advocated by some. The higher rate of complication from grooves and irregularities make this a less acceptable region for the authors.

Surgical Goals and Planned Outcome

Experience has taught a *vital principle* in SL procedures—removal of *less* rather than *more* fat produces an eventually more favorable outcome. The trauma of suction ruptures and fatally damages fat cells not immediately removed by the cannula. Thus fat necrosis and absorption in the suctioned region continue to occur in the postoperative period and progressively improve (or if overdone, diminish) the final outcome. *Attempts to sculpture the suctioned areas with near-complete removal of fat too often creates ultimate irregularities and ridging.* Children, after all, appear youthful and cherubic due to substantial facial fat contributing to smooth skin contours (Fig 17–3, A). Aging produces a loss of smooth contours as fat, muscle, and bone diminish through atrophy or redistribution (Fig 17–3, B). In relatively thin necks, excessive SL deprives the neck of sufficient cushioning fat to effectively hide the ridging and stringiness of the aging platysma and digastric

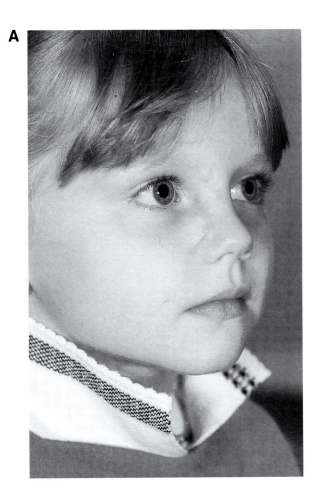 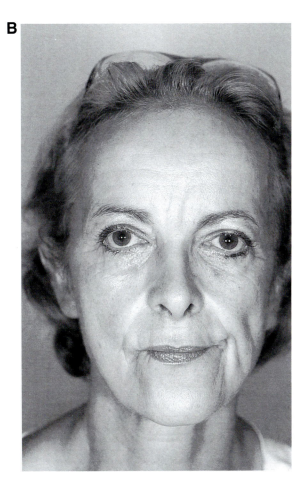

Figure 17–3
A, the cherubic facial appearance of a child as a consequence of abundant "baby" fat of the face, which produces a smooth and youthful contour. **B,** with aging, fat absorption in the face, often asymmetrical, produces an aged, even withered appearance.

muscles. Careful follow-up observation of patients confirms that faces and necks left slightly surgically *undercorrected* by SL will continue to improve for many months afterward.

The aesthetic surgeon must also shoulder the responsibility for *planning ahead* for the patient who may wish additional or secondary rejuvenation surgery in years to come. As more individuals seek appearance surgery earlier in the aging process—a "preventive maintenance" approach—it is reasonable to assume that additional operations may be considered as the years pass. Preserving a sufficiently uniform layer of fat to adequately separate newly lifted skin and the repositioned SMAS layer from the cervical facial skeleton always provides a better result. Thus while performing any rejuvenation procedure, thoughtful surgeons should be anticipating the next procedure, thereby setting the stage for continued natural appearance maintenance.

Since the late 1970s, SL has emerged as a prominent technical refinement and adjunct to cervical facial contouring techniques. The inevitable process of aging creates both excesses and deficiencies of localized fat, each of which detracts from desirable facial proportions and contours. Even teenagers benefit from localized fat removal (predominantly submental)—cervical SL not uncommonly accompanies and adds appearance refinement to rhinoplasty and chin augmentation. The latter results are immediate, significant, and lasting.

It is now clear that localized fat excesses are genetically predetermined adipose depots and do not respond to dietary control or weight loss as do general body fat distributions. Also, as the body ages, some degree of muscle mass is replaced by fat deposition.

The selection of candidates likely to realize an ideal outcome from SL is critical and is influenced by experience and seasoned surgical judgment. A decision must be made about whether each individual patient who demonstrates regional localized fat excesses can benefit from SL alone or in combination with traditional SMAS lifting and contouring procedures (see Chapter 13). An ideal candidate should possess elastic skin capable of rapid contractility following fat extraction and not be overweight. Chronologic age is of limited value in assessing these characteristics. Younger patients as a rule retain elasticity unless the skin has been compromised by excessive sun exposure damage or genetically determined inelasticity. Certain patients over 40 years of age continue to retain good elasticity because of fastidious skin care and favorable genetic influences. But in general, the

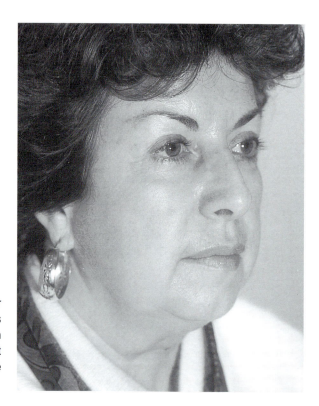

Figure 17–4
Less-than-ideal candidate for facial rejuvenation procedures because of abundant fat in an already heavy face. A short neck further compromises the potential improvement.

majority of Caucasian individuals in this age group begin to lose the capability to contract this fat-expanded skin after SL. In the latter group, SL followed by traditional lifting procedures remains essential to ensure favorable recontouring.

A fundamental error in surgical judgment is made, however, when significantly overweight patients undergo extensive cervical-facial SL in the vain attempt to convert a poor facelift candidate to a favorable candidate (Fig 17–4). Contour irregularities, facial asymmetries, and a less-than-ideal outcome commonly result from this ill-conceived approach.

The ideal candidate, then, demonstrates normal or near-normal body weight, elastic contractile skin, normal jaw length and hyoid position, localized fat excesses, a positive mental attitude, and reasonable informed expectations about the outcome (Fig 17–5).

In order to provide more definition to the cervical region, SL can be safely carried to both medial borders of the sternocleidomastoid muscle and down to the last cervical rhytid in a plane superficial to the platysma. The precise limits of cannula penetration depend upon the location and extent of regional adipose tissue. The intent of lipectomy is simply to uniformly reduce the volume of cervicofacial fat to allow favorable recontour-

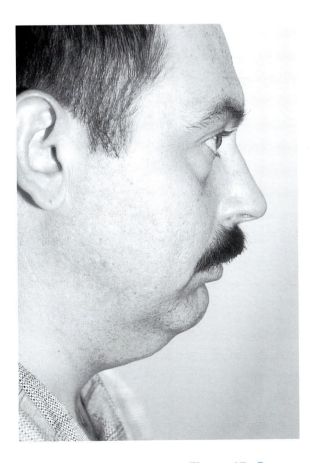
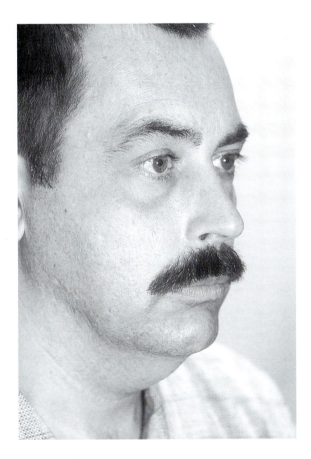

Figure 17–5
Localized cervical submental fat amenable to improvement by suction lipectomy.

ing of the skin envelope by either elastic skin shrinkage or skin flap repositioning. Submental liposuction helps to avoid the submental depression occasionally seen in the anterior part of the neck following excessive sharp dissection and midline removal of fat. If a low-positioned hyoid creates an obliquity to the anterior columellar neck, lipectomy is less satisfactory because it is limited by this common anatomic variant.

In selected patients SL may be combined with direct-excision submental lipectomy and chin augmentation to more favorably define a chin-neck profile, all carried out through the same 1.5- to 2.0-cm submental incision.

SL as an aid in elevating rhytidectomy flaps, as well as in removing excessive preparotid and SMAS levels of fat from the face and jowl, is a useful and frequent adjunct to facelifting. After partial elevation of the preauricular flap (less than 3 cm), SL directly in the preparotid fat and into the cheek and jowl fat assists in contouring the facial cushion. Once the entire flap has been fully elevated, residual adipose tissue may be suctioned by the open suction technique with a cannula of larger diameter. In some cases fat may appear to be encapsulated and not be removed easily with suction. In this circumstance crushing the fat with a forceps may enhance its suction extraction; direct scissors excision is another option. The surgeon may then continue with the routine rhytidectomy, including SMAS plication or imbrication.

Surgical Technique

Preoperative Evaluation

The preoperative evaluation of patients for SL parallels that for other facial procedures, including a review of general medical problems, medications being taken, relevant allergies, and an evaluation of the patient's relative skin tone and elasticity.

In both the sitting and reclining positions, the sites of localized and generalized fat should be delineated by palpating the extent and depth of excess fat with the educated thumb and forefinger (Fig 17–6). *Fat localization is commonly asymmetrically distributed;* patients must be made aware of this preoperative state and further admonished that perfect bilateral symmetry following SL is uncommon. Skin thickness plays a vital role in that thicker skin loses elasticity earlier in life and commonly has less fat cushion beneath it. Sun-damaged skin compromises elasticity, thus limiting the effectiveness of SL.

CHAPTER 17 Lipectomy of the Face and Neck

Care should be taken to not mistake a ptotic submaxillary gland for a localized fat bulge, since removing the local investing fat may result in further unwanted and unsightly gland ptosis. Since SL is commonly combined as an adjunct to traditional rhytidectomy or other aesthetic procedures, appropriate preoperative evaluation should be performed as required for the planned operative intervention. With the head turned in various positions—laterally, head up and down—the thickness of fat is palpated with the thumb and forefinger by rolling the fat on itself and upon the underlying muscular and bony skeleton. Accurate estimation of the varying quantities of excess fat is a skill refined by practice and experience (Fig 17-6).

Anatomy

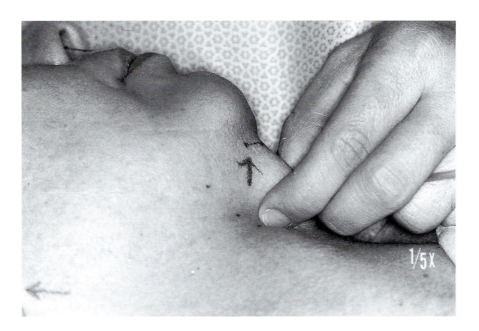

Figure 17-6
With experience, the degree of removable fat may be accurately estimated by palpating and rolling fat between the thumb and forefinger.

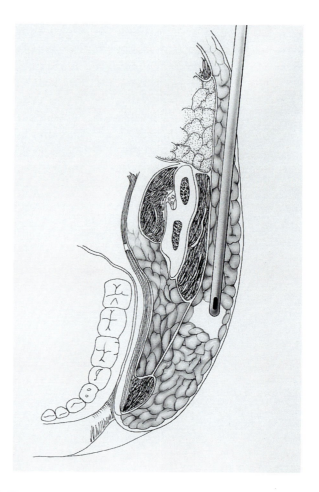

Figure 17–7
The superficial subcutaneous fat of the face and neck, particularly where localized in pockets of excess, may be successfully and relatively atraumatically removed with SL techniques. A thin layer of uniform fat must be maintained on the overlying skin flap to ensure continued smoothness of the ultimate skin appearance and thereby avoiding contour defects. Suction is essentially superficial to the mimetic facial musculature, thus avoiding danger to facial nerve branches.

CHAPTER 17 Lipectomy of the Face and Neck

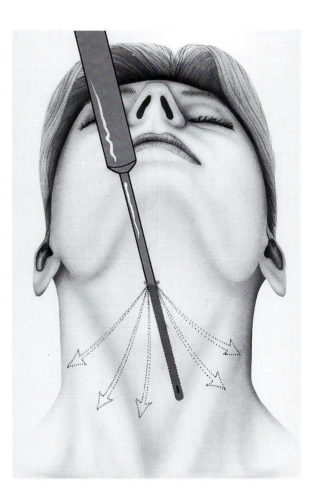

Figure 17-8

In the submental region crisscrossing strokes of the cannula remove localized fat, with an effort being made to "feather" the margins of the treatment area. It is usually necessary to directly scissors-excise fat accumulation just lateral to the incision for more accurate results.

If fat is accumulated beneath the platysmal muscle, we prefer to expose it by direct dissection and excision, with careful attention to exacting hemostasis.

If the borders of the platysma muscle are lax and "stringy," SL may unveil this unrecognized deformity and require concomitant suture-plication of the bands for maximum improvement.

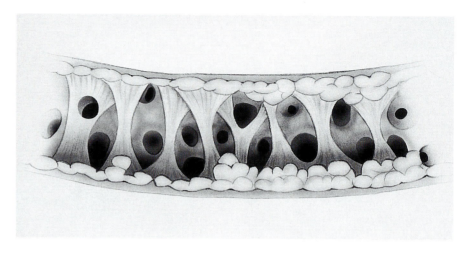

Figure 17-9
Cross-sectional intended condition of subcutaneous fat after SL has been completed. A uniform layer of fat remains on the overlying skin. Multiple crisscrossed tunnels in the central fat accumulations are separated by fibrous septi containing fine vascular structures. The fatty tissue layer assumes the essential characteristics of a sponge—collapsing and thus contracting during the healing process to produce a new, more favorable contour.

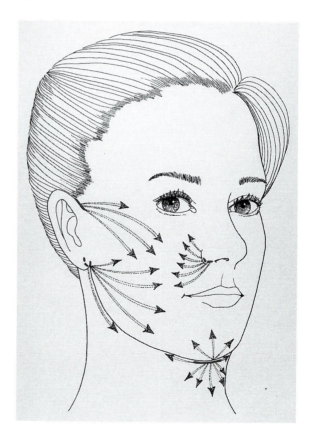

Figure 17-10
Sites of cannula entry for SL with *arrows* portraying the radial direction of SL maneuvers.

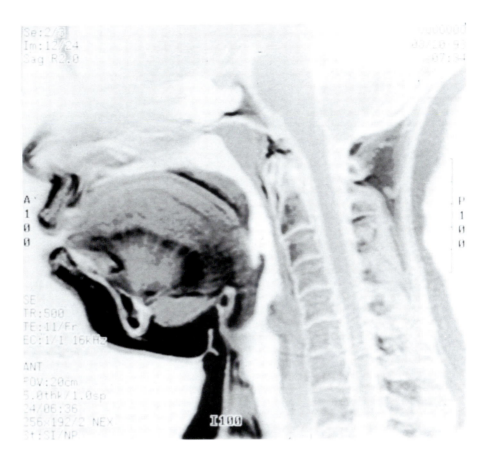

Figure 17–11
Magnetic resonance imaging (MRI) of fat accumulation in the cervicofacial area.

Anesthesia

Locally infiltrative anesthesia such as 1% lidocaine (Xylocaine) with 1:200,000 epinephrine employed for hemostasis is used as a complement to monitored intravenous anesthesia. When smaller localized areas are treated, infiltration anesthesia alone suffices.

Technique

Isolated Suction Lipectomy

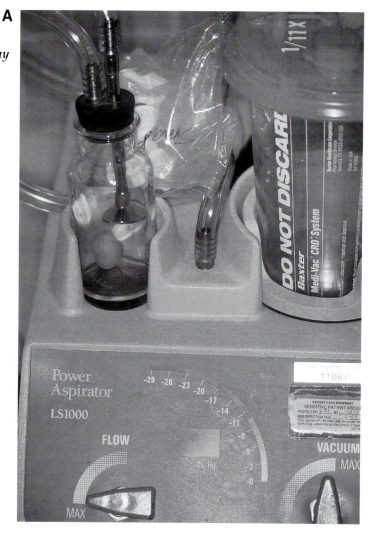

Figure 17–12

A, A variety of vacuums are used for SL. The key criterion for the vacuum is that it should generate approximately 0.75 to 1 atm of negative pressure. The horsepower rating of the pump does not determine the strength of its vacuum but rather the speed at which the maximum vacuum is produced. The maximum vacuum that can be produced by any pump is atmospheric pressure minus water vapor pressure at body temperature. A practical consideration is the pump's ability to reach the desired negative pressure quickly so that there is little delay created during the actual procedure of liposuction. The dimensions of the suction tubing that connect the vacuum apparatus to the suction cannula do not affect the vacuum present at the cannula tip. It is important, however, that the dimensions of the connecting tubing exceed the internal dimensions of the suction cannula in order to prevent obstruction of the vacuum tubing itself.

CHAPTER 17 Lipectomy of the Face and Neck

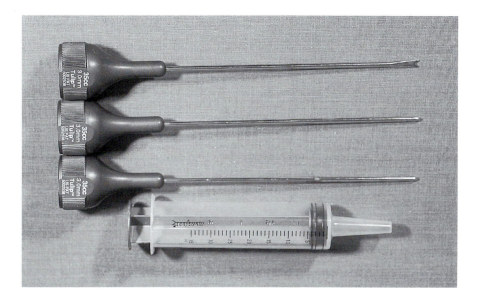

Figure 17-12 (cont.)
B, Suction lipectomy of localized regions of adipose tissue excess may be favorably accomplished with a hand-held syringe affixed to small (Tulip) suction cannulae. This method of lipectomy is highly atraumatic and silent, an added advantage.

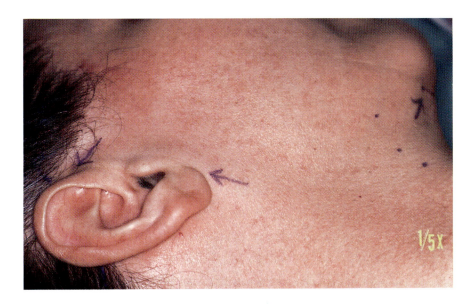

Figure 17-13
The incision should be small (6 to 12 mm) and slightly distant from the localized area of excess fat. Ideally, the incision is placed in a hidden area in or posterior to the submental crease, postauricular area, and preauricular hairline junction. The length of the incision should be sufficient (6 to 12 mm) to allow the curette to be redirected and reangled without causing trauma to the skin insertion site. The proper depth of undermining is in the subcutaneous plane, with a calculated uniform amount of cushioning fat left upon the dermis.

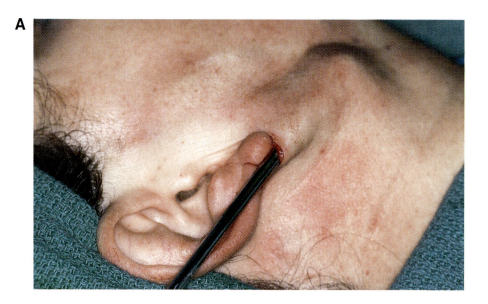

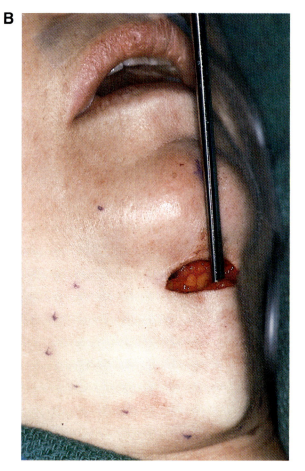

Figure 17–14

A and **B**, the suction curette is best inserted without suction to avoid damage at the incision site. Once situated, full suction is generated, and the cannula is moved back and forth in a radial or fan-shaped direction with the cannula opening facing away from the skin surface at all times. While small tunnel cavities may be created, an intentional side-to-side motion to divide septa that may contain nerves and vessels is not recommended.

CHAPTER 17 Lipectomy of the Face and Neck

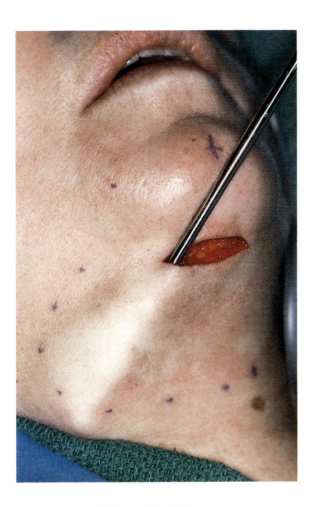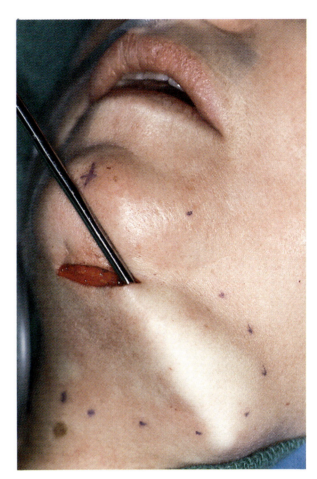

Figure 17–15
The region undergoing SL is "crisscrossed" for more uniform aspiration. An additional zone beyond the area of localized excess fat may be partially treated in a tapering manner (usually tunneled without suction) to create a feathering effect and avoid abrupt changes in contour. Following curettage in one area the suction should be turned off before the suction cannula is removed. Assessing the correct amount of fat to remove is based on direct observation and experience; one should attempt to maintain symmetry and intentionally *undercorrect*. Palpation of the rolled skin pinched between the thumb and forefinger provides an indication of the amount of fat removed and is a talent enhanced by experience.

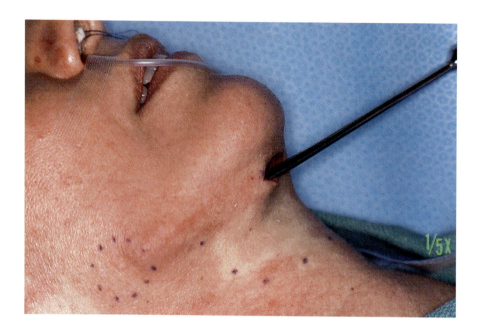

Figure 17-16
Through the same incision, the cannula can be angulated laterally and passed superiorly and superficially into the jowl area. As noted above, the area should be marked with the patient in the upright position prior to liposuction. Care should be taken to remain in the subcutaneous plane and avoid pressure against the mandible or nearby neurovascular structures.

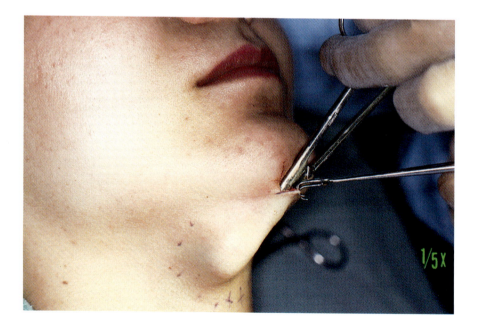

Figure 17-17
In all areas it is helpful to make the initial tunnels with the dissecting Metzenbaum scissors or with small-diameter cannulas passed without suction. A uniformly thick flap in the submental area is quickly defined with scissors dissection followed by SL.

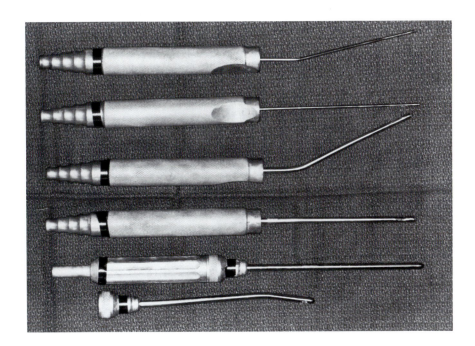

Figure 17–18
Larger cannulas may then be passed for more rapid aspiration if desired. The initial tunnels are typically made with 2-mm cannulas, followed by 4-mm cannulas, and finally with a 6-mm suction cannula. When more subtle refinements are preferred, 2- to 2.5-mm cannulas serve well.

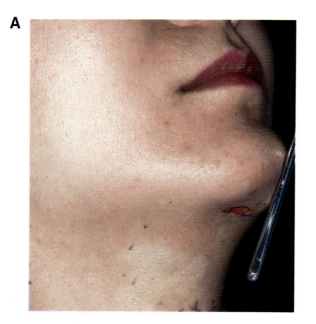
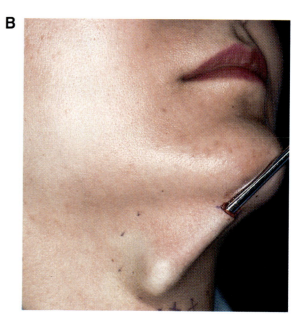
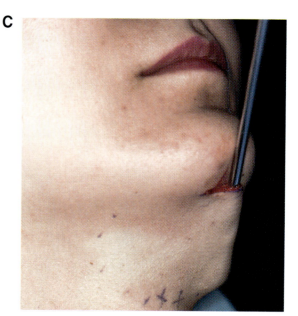

Figure 17–19

A–C, the cannula with the suction activated is passed back and forth in a radial fashion with a "push-pull" motion. The opposite free thumb and forefinger are used to manipulate or "milk" adipose tissue into the cannula tip while it is being controlled by the opposite hand of the surgeon. The opening in the cannula faces away from the dermis and toward deeper tissues. Following completion of one tunnel the suction is turned off and the cannula placed into the next area prior to beginning the suction again, each of the zones within the submental neck area being treated in radial fashion. Once an appropriate amount of liposuctioning has been accomplished, the cannula may be passed beyond the treatment area margins with the suction off to give a "feathering" effect. This allows a smooth transition with surrounding tissues. The cardinal principle of undercorrecting fat removal is again emphasized.

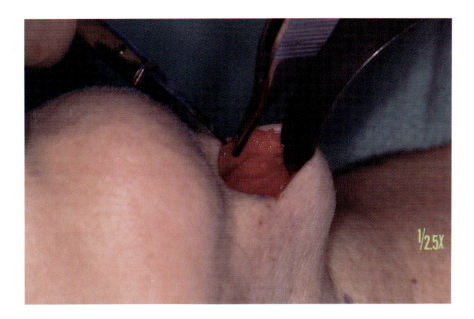

Figure 17–20
An area difficult to sculpt with SL alone lies just lateral to the submental crease on either side. Direct fat excision in this region considerably enhances the SL outcome and avoids leaving a small but unsightly bulge on either side.

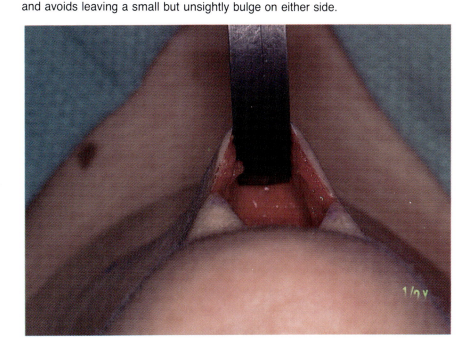

Figure 17–21
Always, the suctioned bed is inspected for uniformity of treatment, and final touches are applied with direct scissors lipectomy. On occasion, spreading the tissues with the scissor blades opened vertical (rather than parallel) to the cervical tissues will open fat spaces previously unaspirated and allow further defining SL at the margins of the treated areas. Minimal bleeding occurs with SL. Hemostasis of any bleeding area is accomplished with bipolar cautery, facilitated by using the narrow S-shaped Cummings retractor (Richards Co., Memphis, Tenn) for exposure. Absolute fastidiousness in bleeding control is mandatory since even minimal postoperative bleeding in the submental and cervical areas produces marked ecchymosis and a delayed favorable outcome.

If sagging of the medial platysmal borders is unveiled after fat removal, suture-plication of the muscle edges is carried out.

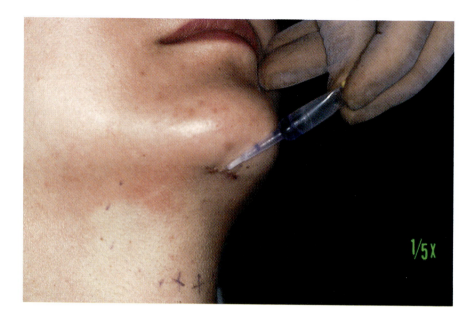

Figure 17-22
The wound is closed with one or two dermal absorbable sutures and 6-0 Prolene skin sutures. Recent experience in skin closure with 5-0 fast-absorbing catgut reinforced with Histoacryl glue has produced superior healing.

Taping the area has been advocated by some; we prefer only a gently compressive dressing. This is changed and inspected 24 hours postoperatively, followed by another 24 to 48 hours of compressive dressing. For 1 to 2 weeks postoperatively an elastic chin support is recommended.

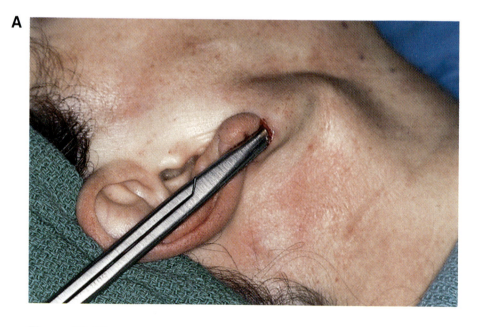

Figure 17-23
A, scissors development of tunnels in the lateral aspect of the neck.

CHAPTER 17 Lipectomy of the Face and Neck

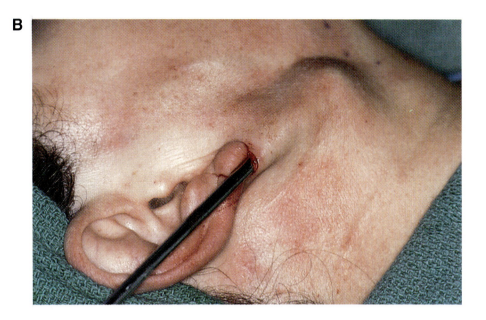

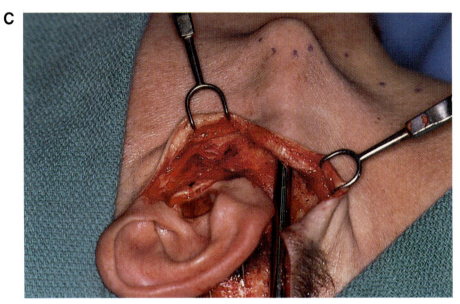

Figure 17-23 (cont.)
B, SL cannula defatting the lateral aspect of the neck. **C,** facial and cervical SL assists in facial flap elevation prior to completion of flap elevation by sharp dissection.

Suction Lipectomy Combined With Lifting Procedures

If liposuction is being utilized in conjunction with a rhytidectomy or facelift procedure, the same submental approach is used as described above. The submental incision may be enlarged following liposuction if the surgeon needs access to other submental structures such as the platysma.

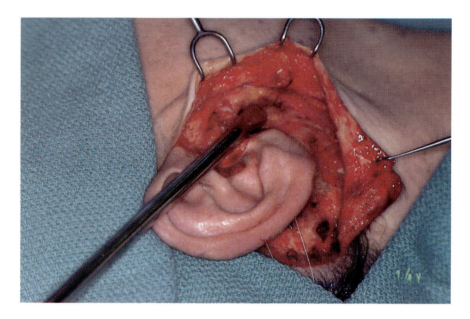

Figure 17–24
Once flap elevation by sharp dissection is completed, open cannula SL with larger-bore cannulas safely removes any excessive localized fat encountered.

CHAPTER 17 Lipectomy of the Face and Neck

Results and Outcomes

SL in the submental region is generally an adjunct to facelifting. Skillful use of SL allows appearance improvements in the jowl and submental region that would be difficult to achieve by other techniques.

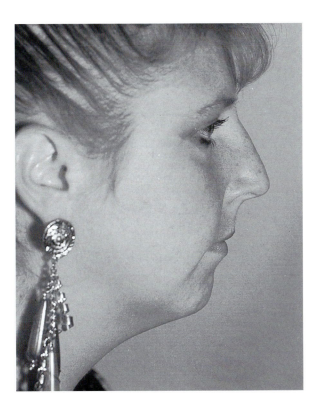
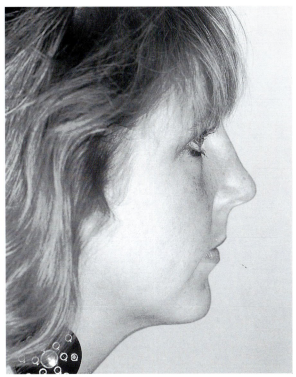

Figure 17–25
Favorable result obtained 1 year following SL of the submental neck with chin augmentation. Despite a lower-than-ideal hyoid position, the cervicomental angle is considerably improved by combining procedures. Elastic skin in this younger (31 years old) patient is essential for the best outcome.

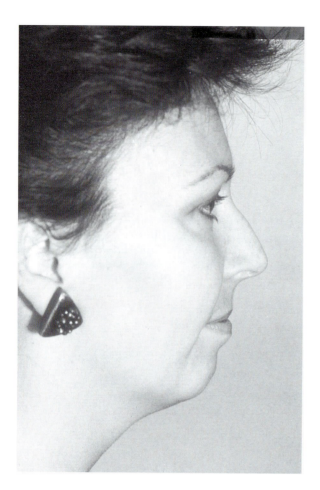 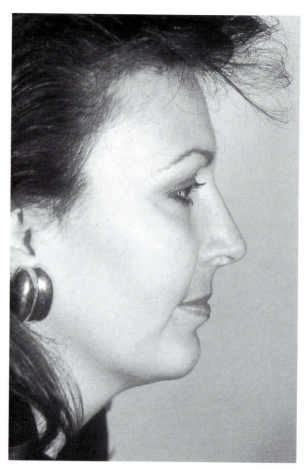

Figure 17–26
Favorable outcome of submental SL combined with further direct excision of cervical fat at 1 year. Chin augmentation adds additional refinement. In her early forties, the patient still retains favorable skin elasticity.

CHAPTER 17 Lipectomy of the Face and Neck

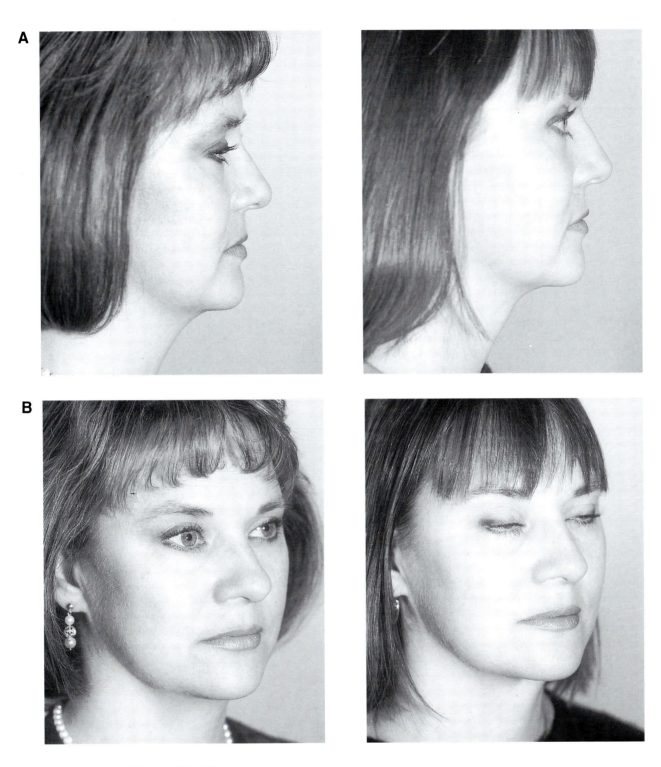

Figure 17–27
A and **B**, submental and lateral cervical SL produces refinement in the cervicomental angle as well as added neck definition at 1 year.

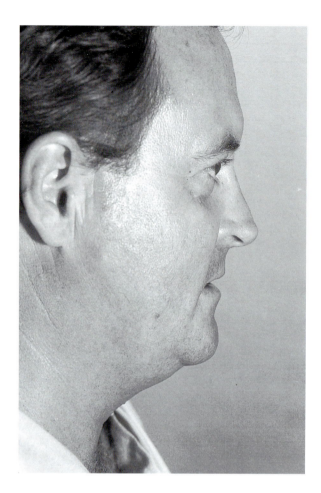 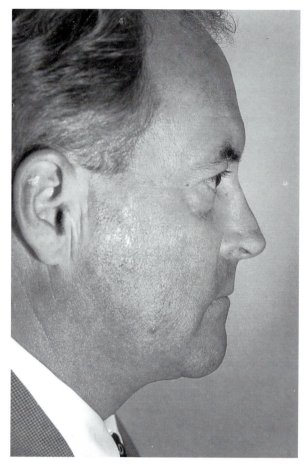

Figure 17–28
Four years following SL of submental and lateral cervical fat excess, this patient's improved configuration has been favorably maintained. One centimeter of excess submental skin was excised during the SL procedure.

CHAPTER 17 Lipectomy of the Face and Neck

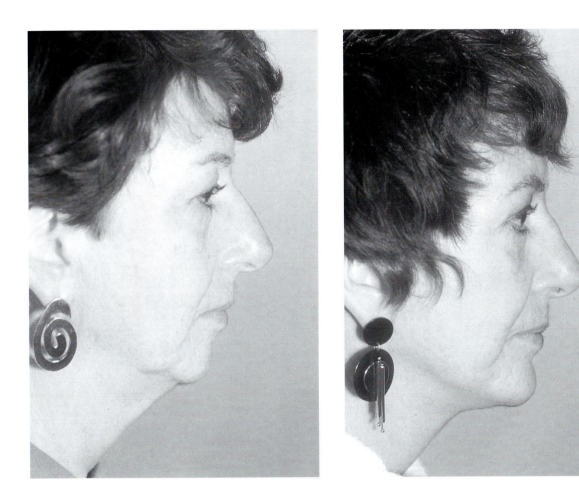

Figure 17–29
Improvement following submental and cervical SL combined with facelifting.

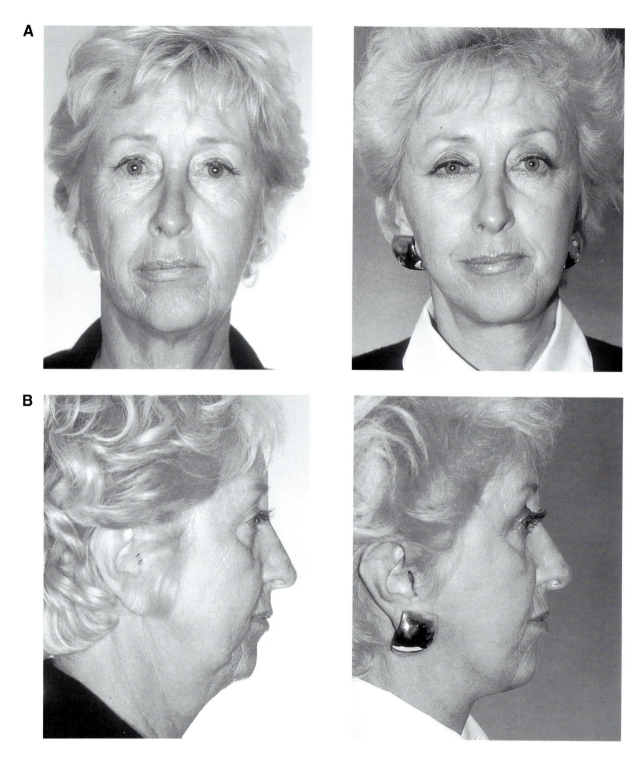

Figure 17-30
A and B, patient demonstrating obtuse cervicomental fat excess contributing to a moderately severe aging appearance. Following submental and cervical SL combined with an SMAS facelift, appearance is improved. Central banding of the anterior part of the neck is eliminated.

CHAPTER 17   Lipectomy of the Face and Neck

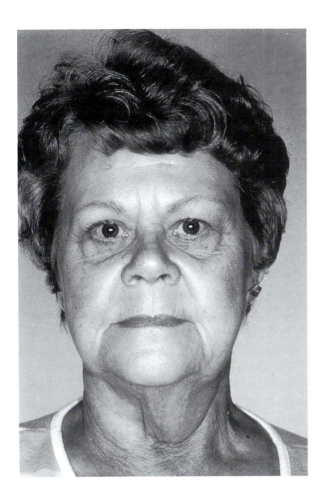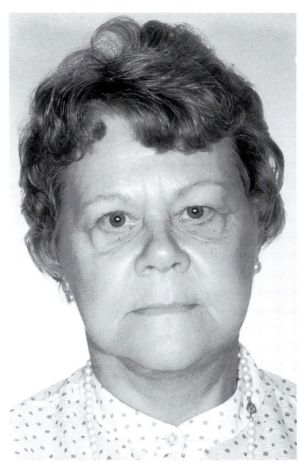

Figure 17-31
Isolated large lipoma of the left submental-cervical region creating marked asymmetry. SL of the lipoma accompanied by unilateral rhytidectomy improves the overall appearance and restores near symmetry.

Complications and Sequelae

Because lipectomy creates potential dead spaces, seromas and/or hematomas are possible unless preventive measures are undertaken. Meticulous hemostasis under direct vision and external compression helps to obliterate potential dead space. If a facelift is combined with cervical SL, the submental area is treated initially and once again inspected and refined *after* completion of the facial lifting and SMAS repositioning procedures. Constant maintenance of firm manual compression of the submental area by the assistant during the facelift procedure significantly reduces intraoperative swelling and edema.

Seroma formation appears to be relatively more common than hematoma formation. Because of the hypoesthesia in the undermined area, drainage is often possible with minimal supplemental local anesthesia should a seroma occur. While seromas are being treated with repeated aspirations, compressive dressings should be continued. Infection in these patients, who are relatively healthy and undergoing clean operative procedures, has been rare. Some authors do not use antibiotic coverage, whereas others advocate prophylactic antibiotics. Patients should avoid aspirin preoperatively and continue to avoid it for 1 to 2 weeks postoperatively.

The postoperative appearance undergoes an evolution over a several-month period. Bruising may be present for 2 or 3 weeks before resolution. In the submental region, elevating the flap with sharp dissection prior to SL significantly reduces the amount and duration of bruising. Rarely, a residual pigmentary change because of hemosiderin deposits may occur. Patients should therefore be advised that their immediate postoperative appearance does not reflect their ultimate outcome and that the appearance evolves favorably over time.

Significant complications with SL have not been encountered. Of major concern is a final contour irregularity, with indentation and grooves being apparent on the skin surface (Fig 17–32). In some instances the deformity may simply represent a failure to remove sufficient fat at the initial operation. Here secondary surgery will remedy the situation. Marked depressions resulting from excessive suction removal with insufficient feathering are much more difficult to treat.

Cardiovascular complications may follow this operation if performed on regions other than the head and neck because of the large fluid shifts that can occur in procedures where large amounts of fat are removed. Estimates that red blood cells make up 10% to 25% of the material aspirated have appeared in the literature. This would not typically be a major consideration in liposuction of the face or neck because of the relatively small amounts of fat removed. Although postoperative drainage will be serosanguineous, significant blood loss has never been encountered. With this procedure free fat has appeared in the urine postoperatively, thus indicating the potential for free fat also being in the blood. While fatty pulmonary embolism is a theoretical possibility, it has not been noted. The results in patients with truly localized fatty collection are far better than those in patients with generalized fatty collections or skin inelasticity. Improvement, as measured by patient satisfaction, can occur with less-than-ideal candidates.

We have experienced no instances of facial nerve paresis following SL.

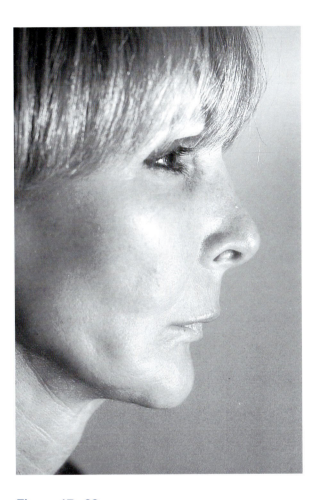

Figure 17–32
Patient operated elsewhere demonstrating contour deformities in the face as a consequence of aggressive facial SL producing non–uniform layering of subcutaneous fat.

Suggested Reading

- Ehlert TK, Thomas JR, Becker FF: *Submental W-plasty for correction of turkey gobbler deformities.* Arch Otolaryngol 1990; 116:714–717.
- Grazer FM: *Atlas of Suction Assisted Lipectomy in Body Contouring.*
- Lambros V: *Fat contouring in the face and neck. Clin Plast Surg* 1992; 19:401–414.
- Thomas JR: Facial plastic surgery applications for liposuction, in Cummings C, et al (eds): *Otolaryngology—Head and Neck Surgery, Update I.* St Louis, Mosby–Year Book, 1990, pp 160–165.

PART VI

ADJUNCTIVE REJUVENATION PROCEDURES

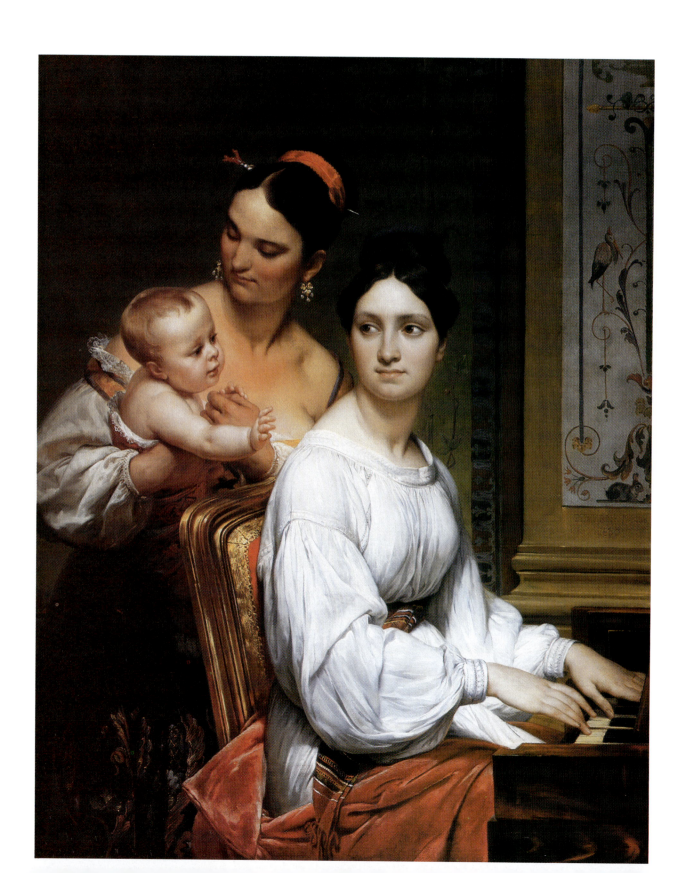

CHAPTER 18

 Dermabrasion

> *Not only does beauty fade*
> *but it leaves a record upon the face*
> *as to what became of it.*
>
> **Elbert Hubbard**

Diagnosis and Candidate Selection

The upper and lower lip wrinkle lines radiating out from the mouth are a source of deep concern to all women who possess them. Although the ideal surgical solution to this unsightly lip deterioration does not yet exist, improvements are possible with either *dermabrasion* or *chemical peeling* (chemexfoliation). Each method possesses advantages and liabilities.

Lip rhytids often make their appearance in relatively young women who have abused their skin with heavy, frequent sun exposure (Fig 18-1). Heredity and ethnic background contribute to early occurrence (Scotch-Irish and English skin appears prone to early rhytid development), and heavy smoking definitely accelerates and worsens the condition. Shrinkage of the skull and perioral jaw structures along with loss of facial fat as a consequence of aging sets the stage for deep rhytid development. Curiously, males are less prone to lip rhytid formation unless constantly exposed to the sun.

Lip dermabrasion with fine wire brushes or diamond fraises is a safe and effective treatment option for lip rhytids and is frequently combined with other facial rejuvenation procedures. Complete surgical control over the depth of the abrasion is possible, healing is uniform and predictable, and the essential histologic makeup of the skin remains unaltered. Dermabrasion, then, may be repeated as required with consistent improvement. When fully healed, skin color is generally unaltered, and the improved texture blends well with surrounding skin. Dermabrasion has been reported to be less longer lasting than the results obtained after chemexfoliation. Properly performed, however, dermabrasion is a safe and effective treatment for perioral rhytids with a substantial duration of improvement. Moreover, if the treated area is kept moist with ointments or occlusive dressings, postoperative pain is negligible, discomfort is essentially nonexistent, and healing is more rapid than when scabbing occurs.

CHAPTER 18   Dermabrasion

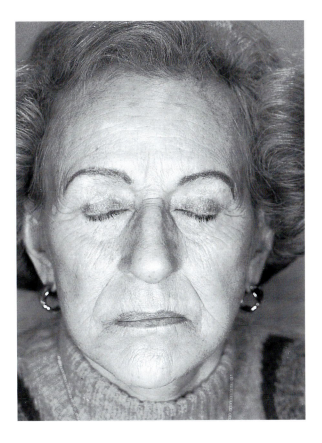

Figure 18-1
Typical lip rhytids in aging patient, compounded by increased vertical length of upper lip.

Surgical Techniques

Anatomy

The anatomy of the skin plays a vital role in dermabrasion since *depth* and *uniformity* of the dermabrasion injury determine the eventual appearance outcome. Fortunately, both are under the control of the surgeon. The dermis, immediately deep to the epidermis, consists of two basic layers: (1) the superficial *papillary* layer and (2) a deeper *reticular* layer. Injuries to the reticular layer produce permanent scar formation, while trauma to the epidermis and papillary dermis almost always heal without visible scarring.

Thus dermabrasion should be limited to these latter two layers and deeper injury to the reticular layer avoided. Histologically, healed skin following dermabrasion is essentially indistinguishable from normal skin, but the collagen of the papillary dermis is restructured, and a smoother-textured, less wrinkled epidermis results. Melasma and senile lentigines are commonly corrected by dermabrasion since these conditions reflect excess or irregular pigmentation in the basal layer of the epidermis.

It has been reported that pretreatment of the region to be dermabraded for several weeks with topical 0.5% tretinoin accelerates healing. Our experience with this pretreatment modality is too short at the present time to completely confirm this reported treatment advantage, but clinically it appears to be valid.

Perioral chemical peels permanently alter the histologic composition of the lip tissues and generally result in a smoother and lighter-appearing skin. Since they are not surgical procedures per se and the result is directly related to the depth of peel and the strength and composition of the peel solution, the surgeon has less control over the ultimate result. For this reason many aesthetic surgeons find chemical peeling unappealing.

Surgical Technique

Lip dermabrasion may be carried out as a single outpatient procedure but more commonly is the final encore to other more major rejuvenative procedures. Commonly associated with blepharoplasty, facelift, and related rejuvenation procedures, lip dermabrasion is deferred until all procedures are accomplished and bandages are in place.

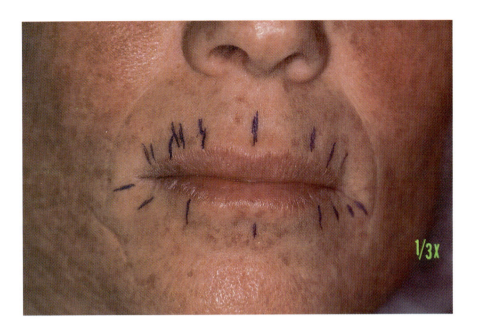

Figure 18–2
The depth and extent of each perioral rhytid are outlined with a surgical marking pen for direction and depth reference. Infiltration anesthesia with minimal amounts of 1% lidocaine (Xylocaine) with 1:200,000 epinephrine provides patient comfort without significant lip distortion; infraorbital and submental nerve blocks, if preferred, provide excellent regional anesthesia. Refrigeration and chilling of the operated site with Frigiderm further help to produce local anesthesia while providing a firmer surface for abrasion.

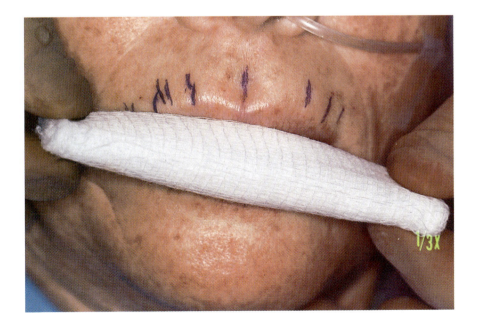

Figure 18–3
A moist, rolled 4 × 4-in. gauze pad inserted into the sublabial sulcus effectively "plumps" the entire lip and aids in stabilizing and leveling it for more effective dermabrasion.

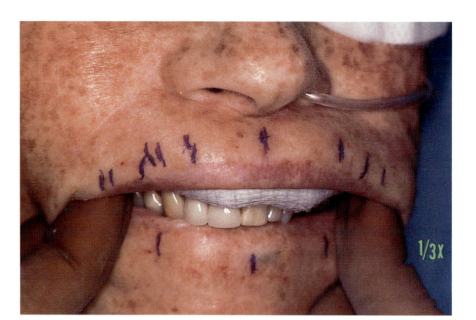

Figure 18-4
Vital to the safety of lip dermabrasion, *constant four-point traction* by the assistant and surgeon on the soft, mobile lip tissues stabilizes and stretches the tissues for more consistent, uniform abrasion. The soft mobile lip is at risk throughout dermabrasion of being "grabbed" by the fraise, with unwanted deeper injury and scarring.

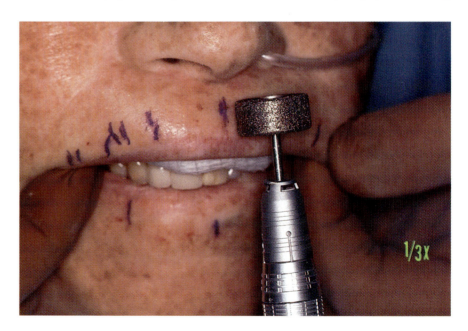

Figure 18-5
Either the diamond fraise or a small wire brush on a high-torque dermabrasion unit is employed to feather-dermabrade the oral rhytids, which are abraded both at right angles to and obliquely across the radiating creases. Eyeglasses and mask protection for all surgeons and nurses at the operating room table are essential. Since blood and tissue products are aerosolized during dermabrasion, a potential risk of transmission of human immunodeficiency virus (HIV) exists.

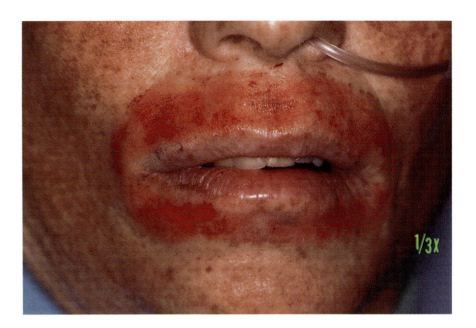

Figure 18–6
Dermabrasion continues deeper until all ink markings in the depths of the creases are eliminated and brisk bleeding from multiple fine points occurs, which indicates that the depth of injury has encountered the small capillary loops of the papillary dermis. Deeper in this plane, faintly visible parallel strands of collagen are exposed and indicate that the proper depth has been reached. Abrasion is carried just beyond the vermillion border into the red lip, and the peripheral edges of the abraded lip areas are "feathered" into surrounding skin at a more shallow depth for ideal skin color blending. Moist compresses control bleeding rather quickly.

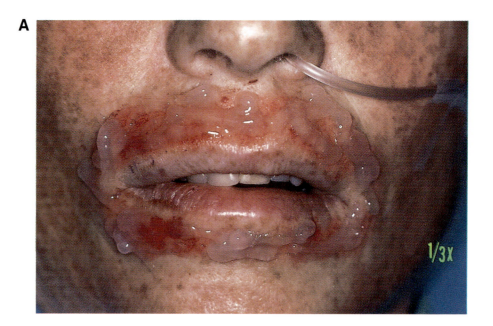

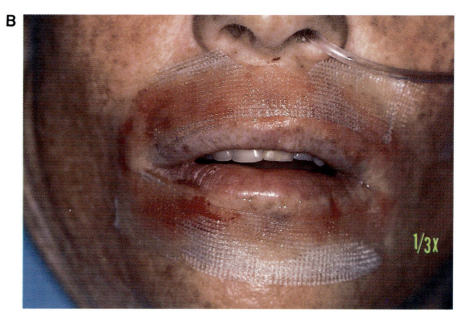

Figure 18-7
A and B, comfort is ensured, and healing proceeds more rapidly if dermabraded areas are kept constantly moist following surgery to avoid desiccation with resultant skin cracking. A dressing of Adaptic Vaseline gauze impregnated with NeoDecadron ophthalmic ointment and secured with Microfoam tape is put in place for 24 hours. Thereafter the gauze is removed and the ointment applied twice daily by the patient for 10 days. Occlusive dressings such as Vigilon or Omiderm may be used instead and left intact until they peel off spontaneously. The latter are more expensive and have not appeared to result in more rapid healing than the regimen recommended. Most important to rapid healing and the avoidance of discomfort is keeping the dermabraded region moist with ointment, thereby avoiding scab formation.

CHAPTER 18   Dermabrasion

Results and Outcomes

Reepithelialization occurs in 6 to 10 days, depending essentially upon the depth of dermabrasion. Erythema usually persists for 3 to 4 weeks but may be camouflaged with makeup after early reepithelialization has begun. Sun avoidance is recommended for at least 3 months.

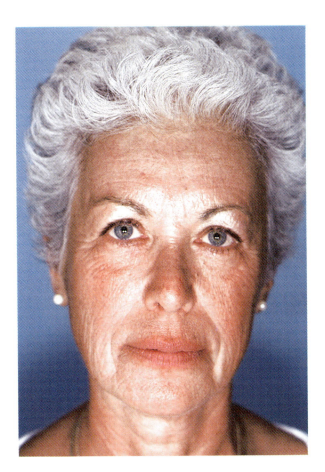
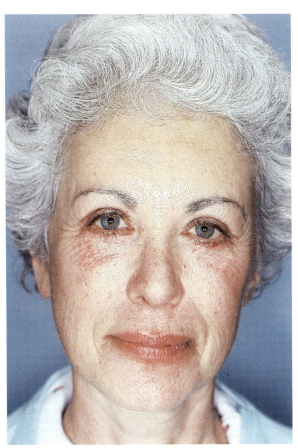

Figure 18–8
Improvement in perioral rhytidosis following lip dermabrasion.

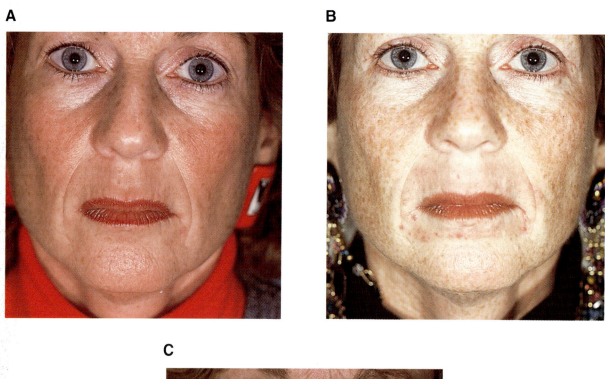
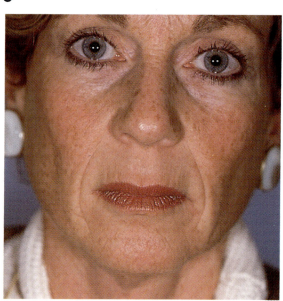

Figure 18–9
Rejuvenation of perioral rhytidosis following labial dermabrasion.
A, preoperative. **B,** 6 weeks. **C,** two years.

Complications

Significant complications associated with dermabrasion are rare in experienced hands and may be divided into early and late complications.

Early complications involve infection, including superficial *Staphylococcus aureus* involvement and, more seriously, herpes simplex virus (HSV) activation around the lips, mouth, and even nose. Both infections are manifested early postoperatively with abrupt, severe pain and erythema. The risk of reactivating dormant herpetic eruptions exists with either dermabrasion or chemexfoliation (Fig 18–10). An exacting history of previous eruptions will diminish this vexing complication—if the history is positive, we prefer to avoid treatment. Unanticipated eruptions are treated aggressively with acyclovir (Zovirax) orally and 0.5% topical idoxuridine (Stoxil) with generally good success for early resolution. Any pain noted after dermabrasion should immediately raise the surgeon's index of suspicion for this potential viral eruption. Some surgeons recommend pretreatment of *all* patients for dermabrasion with Zovirax, 400 mg three times daily for 5 to 6 days beginning 24 hours pretreatment.

Dermabrasion in Oriental and Latin skin colors carries a higher risk of permanent hypopigmentation or hyperpigmentation upon healing. For the same reasons, sun exposure must be avoided for 3 months after abrasion. Hyperpigmentation following lip dermabrasion is usually improved with daily topical tretinoin applications.

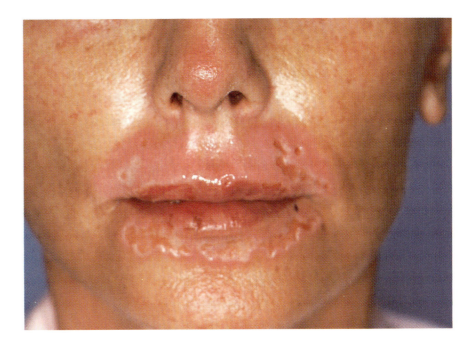

Figure 18–10
Herpetic eruption triggered by perioral dermabrasion in a patient with no previous known history of labial herpes.

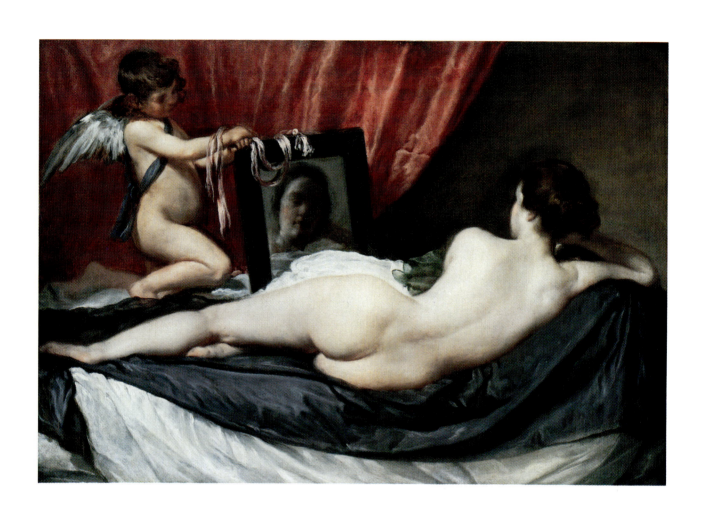

CHAPTER

19

      Chemical Peel

> *What is the worst of woes*
> *that wait on Age?*
> *What stamps the wrinkle*
> *deeper on the brow?*
>
> **Lord Byron**

Diagnosis and Candidate Selection

The chemical face peel, still a controversial form of rejuvenation therapy, has evolved over many years and is carried out with different agents by surgeons with specific preferences. The most frequent agent for significant deep rhytids is the phenol peel solution developed by Baker and Gordon, which has been shown to provide the longest-lasting favorable histologic skin changes.

The indications for appropriate use of the phenol chemical peel have broadened in recent years. The ideal candidate is a fair-skinned female with a complex of fine rhytids. With progressively darker complexions there is a risk of a more visible demarcation of the treated region of the face contrasted to the unpeeled areas. Red haired, fair-skinned patients with freckles will tend to lose the freckles with the peel and therefore are at risk for a distinct line of demarcation at the junction of peeled and unpeeled skin since phenol has been shown to be highly toxic to melanocytes. These patients, however, are often good candidates on the basis of skin texture, color, and the nature of their fine rhytids. Many patients are anxious to diminish freckling and prefer the more uniform skin color change.

Male patients are not ideal candidates for aesthetic peels because of generally thicker, oily skin, which impedes uniform penetration of the peeling solution. Further, the paler, smooth skin that results from the peel may not be as desirable an aesthetic goal in men as it is in women.

Other skin problems related to actinic damage are often improved following a phenol peel. Many patients who have facial rhytids from excessive ultraviolet (UV) light exposure will also benefit from treatment of actinic keratosis and superficial actinic hyperpigmentation with the phenol peel. Blotchy pigmentation from chloasma and melasma may be improved. Finally, superficial acne scarring may show some improvement following a facial phenol peel from the changes in the skin surface and skin tightening that occur; dermabrasion tends to be a better alternative, however, for acne-scarred skin.

CHAPTER 19   Chemical Peel

The preoperative evaluation for a phenol peel should include strict evaluation of the patient's cardiac and renal status. Cardiac arrhythmias have been attributed to phenol, a distinctly cardiotoxic agent. A history of arrhythmias or significant cardiac problems makes the patient less acceptable for treatment. Phenol is excreted approximately 80% unchanged in the urine, and a potential increase in cardiotoxicity could occur in the presence of compromised renal function.

Patients with a history of oral herpetic infections must be warned that significant eruption is possible following the peel, with a potential for permanent facial scarring as a consequence of the viral infestation. Patients with a positive history of herpetic eruptions at any time in the past should begin a course of acyclovir during the week prior to the peel. The medication is continued until the patient's skin is epithelialized over the next 7 to 10 days. If an outbreak of herpetic lesions occurs during the healing phase, the dosage is increased and continued until improvement is accomplished. The onset of unusual pain at any time in the healing process may herald herpetic eruptions.

Active sun exposure must be avoided during the first few months after the peel. Patients may be more susceptible to sunburn because of the hypopigmentation and are admonished to wear a high-number sunscreen (15 sun protection factor [SPF] or greater) during outdoor activities.

Postpeel pigmentation alterations and blotchiness may develop in occasional patients. This cannot be readily predicted, and patients should be aware that they may need to use a concealing makeup to camouflage these areas. Likewise, employing makeup techniques to blend and camouflage the usual line of demarcation between the peeled and unpeeled regions is essential. Blotchy pigmentation seems to occur particularly if there has been significant UV light exposure or sunburn in the first 3 to 4 months after the peel. Also reported are pigmentation changes after using estrogen medications and birth control pills.

Our patients are told that they may return to their normal outdoor activities, *except sunbathing,* as long as they take the UV light exposure precautions (i.e., sunscreen, hats, etc.), which should be a planned routine in those who wish to forestall inevitable aging skin changes.

Thus, comprehensive and detailed informed consent plays a primary role in the discussion with individuals contemplating chemical peeling. The surgeon must select candidates *carefully* in order that the most ideal result can be obtained with the *least* risk of complication.

Of great significance is the fact that it is the depth of injury and not the technique used that determines the epithelial response and ultimate appearance. The histologic skin changes are directly proportional to the depth of injury.

Surgical Goals and Planned Outcome

The face peel is intended to improve facial skin texture and smooth superficial rhytids. The treatment should be regarded as a complement and not a substitute for a facelift and therefore is not intended to correct sagging skin or loose facial tissue. The two complementary procedures become components of a staged facial rejuvenation plan. Regional peels of the perioral area may be used to enhance the common radiating oral rhytids that are not improved by facelift surgery.

Skin chronically exposed to the sun develops an epidermis that is thickened and composed of disorderly cells and irregular cellular architecture. Clinically this results in blotchiness and leathery, wrinkled skin (Fig 19–1). The phenol skin peel returns cells of the epidermis to a more normal appearance microscopically. New collagen fibers are compacted in parallel bundles combined with an improved network of elastic fibers. This new layer of dermis compacts the older damaged layers and results in postpeel appearance of a resilient, tighter, smoother, and more youthful skin. Microscopically, melanocytes are present but are less capable of synthesizing large amounts of melanin. Studies reveal that both the clinical and histologic effects of phenol peeling should be of long-term duration.

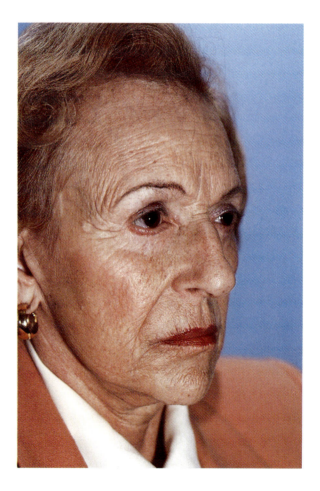

Figure 19–1
Sun-damaged skin has a thickened epidermis composed of disorderly cells and irregular cellular architecture.

CHAPTER 19 Chemical Peel

Surgical Technique

The patient is required to cleanse the face preoperatively with an antiseptic soap. Phenol peeling is best performed in an operative environment that allows cardiac monitoring and sedation since the procedure is uncomfortable and the patient will require sedation and analgesia. An intravenous line is started and the patient hydrated with 500 cc of fluid prior to starting the procedure.

Since phenol is excreted through the kidneys, good hydration is important; intravenous fluids are continued throughout the procedure.

While seated in an upright position, the submandibular area is marked with a sterile marking pen to identify a demarcation line that will be hidden by the mandibular shadow line.

A phenol solution as described by Baker and Gordon is *freshly mixed* prior to initiating the procedure. An individual solution is mixed exactly as described for each patient (Fig 19–2):

Baker's Peel Solution
Phenol, 88% (USP)	3 mL
Croton oil	3 drops
Septisol soap	8 drops
Distilled water	2 mL

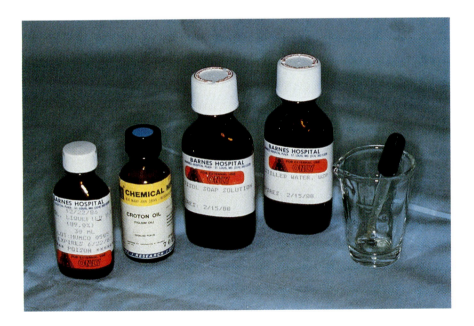

Figure 19–2
The ingredients for Baker's peel formula: phenol, 88% (USP); croton oil; Septisol soap; and distilled water.

Following Septisol facial preparation the patient's face is cleansed with acetone by using a gauze sponge (Fig 19–3). This cleansing is done vigorously for 10 to 15 minutes in order to remove facial oils and skin debris and allow proper and uniform penetration of the peel solution. A failure to cleanse with acetone properly may leave the face with an uneven peel. This initial acetone cleansing is uncomfortable for the patient and should not commence until an appropriate level of sedation is attained.

The solution is applied sequentially to the facial aesthetic units (Fig 19–4). The units are defined as the forehead, cheeks, and perioral and periorbital regions. After treating a unit, at least 10 to 15 minutes is allowed to elapse before treatment of the next unit is initiated. This period of deliberate waiting between peeling anatomic units allows the phenol to be absorbed and metabolized before adding additional phenol, thereby minimizing any likelihood of cardiac arrhythmia.

A predetermined sequence of anatomic unit treatment is preferred in the following order: forehead and perioral areas are purposely treated first

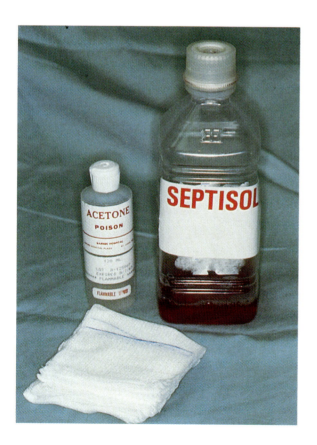

Figure 19–3
The face is prepared with Septisol solution and then cleaned for 10 to 15 minutes with acetone.

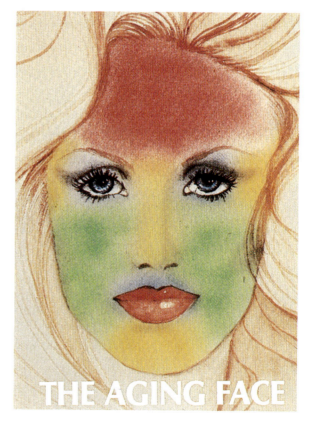

Figure 19–4
The solution is applied to individual facial aesthetic units.

so that if any problem develops that would require stopping the procedure (such as a persistent arrhythmia), the anatomic units already treated would be aesthetically acceptable in appearance. An asymmetrical appearance of a unilaterally treated cheek or periorbital area is thus avoided. The nose is treated as part of the forehead unit, while each cheek is treated as an individual unit. Thus there are five basic regions of the face treated as separate units. With a minimum 10- to 15-minute waiting period between each unit, a typical treatment session lasts a minimum of 1½ to 2 hours. Failure to observe the mandatory time intervals between facial unit treatments invites potential complication and significant additional risk.

All operative personnel are constantly alert to prevent inadvertent contact of the peel solution with the patient's eye. An irrigation syringe with balanced saline solution is available at all times. Should solution contact the eye, immediate copious irrigation is initiated (Fig 19–5). An assistant also keeps a dry cotton-tipped applicator ready throughout the procedure to blot-dry any tears that may form. If tears are allowed to mix with the

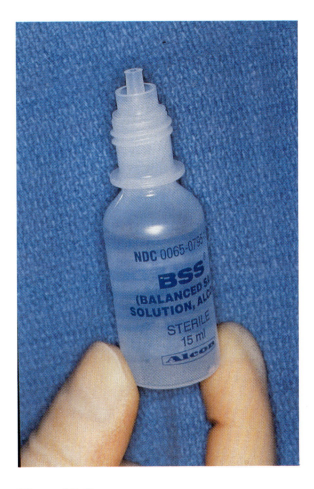

Figure 19–5
A balanced saline solution is available for immediate eye irrigation.

peel solution, the formula becomes diluted, which may cause *deeper penetration* and streaking. Capillary action of the tears could also allow the peel solution to be drawn back into the eye. A second assistant is responsible for continuous stirring and mixing of the peel solution. The solution is actually a suspension that will separate if allowed to stand, thus creating an inconsistent solution for application.

Facial Aesthetic Units

The forehead unit is peeled first by covering the region from the hairline to the brow. It may be extended further to include the nose. Laterally the region extends to the upper temporal area. The solution is carefully feathered with the cotton-tipped applicator into the hairline and eyebrow hair to prevent obvious abrupt demarcation lines. Phenol does not penetrate to the level of the hair follicles, so it does not affect hair growth in these regions. The solution is applied with even strokes on a semidried cotton-tipped applicator that has been dipped into the thoroughly mixed Baker's formula solution (Fig 19–6, A).

Almost immediately a white frost-like appearance will develop on the skin surface because of the active keratocoagulation that develops (Fig 19–6, B). Three to 5 minutes later the white frost begins to fade, and an erythematous appearance will develop. Deeper lines such as those in the glabellar region benefit by having a pointed wooden applicator stick dipped in the solution and used to apply the material within the depths of the individual rhytids (Fig 19–6, C).

Following a 10- to 15-minute wait, the perioral unit is treated. This region includes the base of the nose and upper lip to the vermillion border. Inferiorly it extends from the lower vermillion border past the chin to the previously marked submental extent. Laterally the nasolabial creases form the unit's boundaries. The peel solution should be extended just past the vermillion border to avoid a line of demarcation. By using the wooden applicator stick, the deeper rhytids radiating from the lip, the deep lines of the nasolabial folds, and the lateral commissure rhytids are treated.

Because skin of the upper neck region does not possess appropriate skin appendages for good epithelialization, the peel solution should not be extended to the neck skin.

After a delay, the cheek areas are now treated individually with a 10- to 15-minute wait between sides. The margin of the unit should overlap slightly with the forehead unit in the temple area and the perioral unit at the nasolabial folds. This ensures good coverage and avoids possible "skipped areas." Reactive erythema of 5 to 8 mm can extend beyond the limit of the peeled unit. A failure to properly overlap the margins of treated units can cause unsightly "stripes" if these regions are overlooked and create "skipped" or too lightly peeled areas. The peel may extend on to the earlobes to further camouflage the region.

After further delay, the eyelid skin and periorbital unit are treated. Because of the small surface area involved, both sides may be treated without a waiting period between them.

CHAPTER 19   Chemical Peel

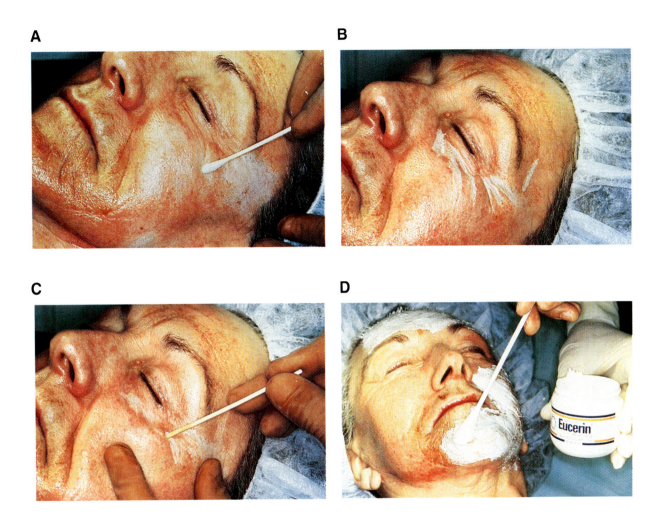

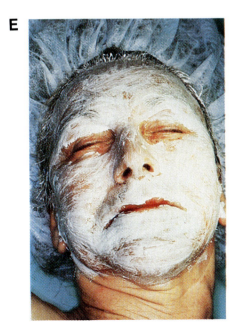

Figure 19–6

A, the solution is applied to individual units with even strokes on a semidried cotton-tipped applicator. **B,** a white frost appears in the treated area, which then transforms to erythema. **C,** deeper rhytids are treated with a pointed wooden stick dipped in the solution. **D,** on completion of treatment for each facial unit Eucerin cream is applied. **E,** the entire face is covered with Eucerin cream. No tape is used.

Because of the proximity of the eye, extreme caution by all personnel is observed. The cotton-tipped applicators are meticulously wrung nearly dry, and the peel is extended to 2 to 3 mm above the superior tarsal plate margin. On the lower lid the peel solution is applied no closer than 3 mm from the subciliary line. Any tearing is carefully but immediately blotted with a clean, dry, cotton-tipped applicator.

The face is now examined to ensure that no areas have been skipped or solution inadequately or unevenly applied. All treated skin is covered generously with Eucerin cream (Fig 19–6, D); no tape is applied. Other moisturizing agents have been described, but Eucerin has worked well for many years, for many surgeons, without frequent problems or reaction. Because it is opaque (Fig 19–6, E), it is easy to apply, and any skipped areas are evident.

Facial taping after the peel is still advocated by some authors. The non-tape method, however, has produced excellent results with less apparent discomfort to the patient. It also avoids the second anesthetic that may be required for removal of the tape. Keeping the face exposed for daily care allows patients and their family to become involved in the postoperative skin care regimen earlier, which is of overall benefit during the recovery period.

Postoperative Care

Intravenous cephalosporin antibiotics are infused during the procedure and continued orally for 1 week. Dexamethasone (Decadron), 8 to 10 mg intravenously, is given at the end of the procedure, and an oral corticosteroid (methylprednisolone) [Medrol dose-pack] is continued on a decreasing dosage in the early postoperative period.

Analgesics will be required for the first 6 to 12 hours. Most patients will require a sleeping medication the first few nights following treatment.

Beginning the first postoperative day the patient showers or gently sprays the face every 4 to 5 hours while awake. The face is gently patted dry and Eucerin cream reapplied. This is a daily routine until reepithelization is completed in 7 to 10 days. Patients are admonished to be gentle with their facial skin. No scrubbing or picking at the eschar is permitted.

At about 10 days the epithelialization has typically reached a point where the residual eschar has separated and sloughed. Now a pink erythema is exposed that will last for several months. At 10 to 14 days the patient is allowed to wear makeup, preferably containing a sunscreen. The patient should use a 15 SPF or higher non–para-aminobenzoic acid (PABA) sunscreen for all outdoor activities. Dry skin is common at this time and requires the use of more frequent nonirritative moisturizers. Oral medications for relief of itching and irritation are provided.

CHAPTER 19   Chemical Peel

Results and Outcomes

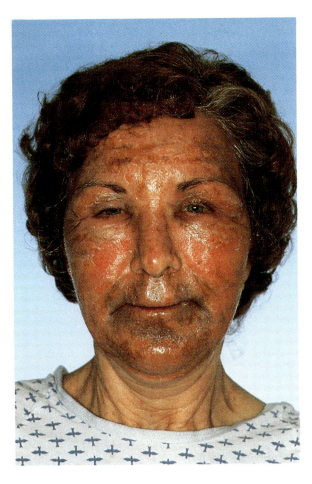

Figure 19-7
The typical patient will progress from facial swelling and eschar formation to reepithelialization and bright erythema in 7 to 10 days.

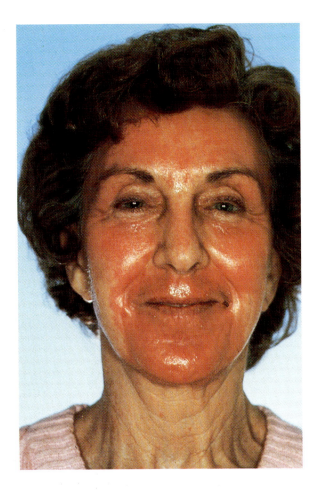

Figure 19-8
Erythema will persist in varying degrees for several months.

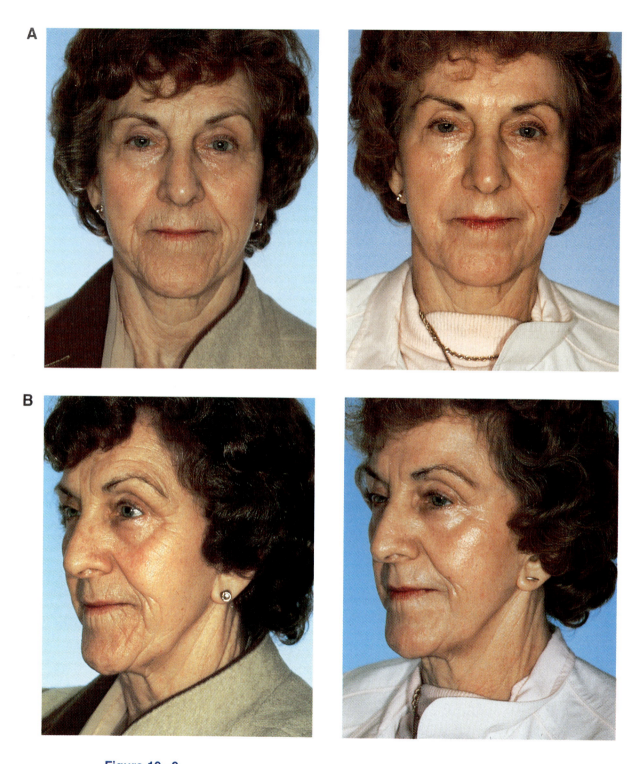

Figure 19-9
A and B, a patient demonstrating improvement in skin texture that minimizes the facial rhytids.

CHAPTER 19 Chemical Peel

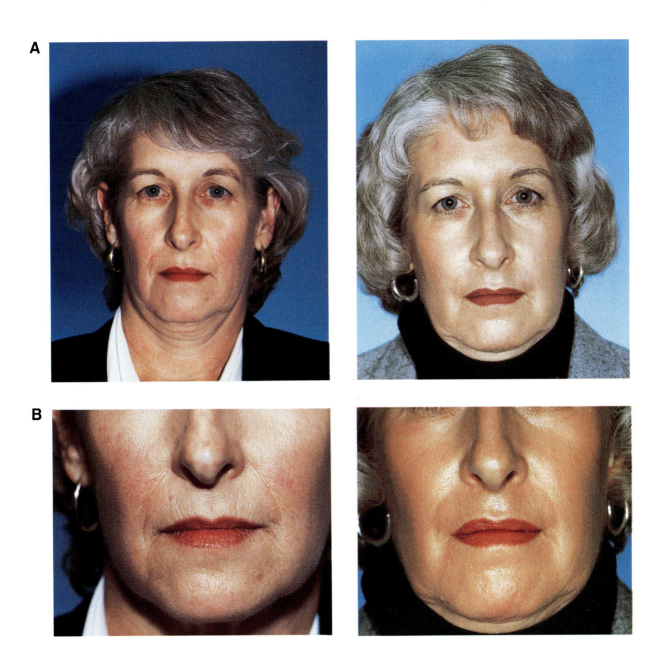

Figure 19-10
A and **B,** a patient with fair skin and fine textural lines and rhytids. The freshening effect of a chemical peel is evident.

Regional Peels

In selected patients a regional peel will provide aesthetic improvement (Fig 19-11, A to L). Appropriate patient selection and rigorous monitoring is required, just as in full face treatment.

If the patient has fair skin and is aware of the risks of possible lines of demarcation, the treatment area may be extended beyond the nasolabial creases to include additional rhytids (Fig 19-12, A to C).

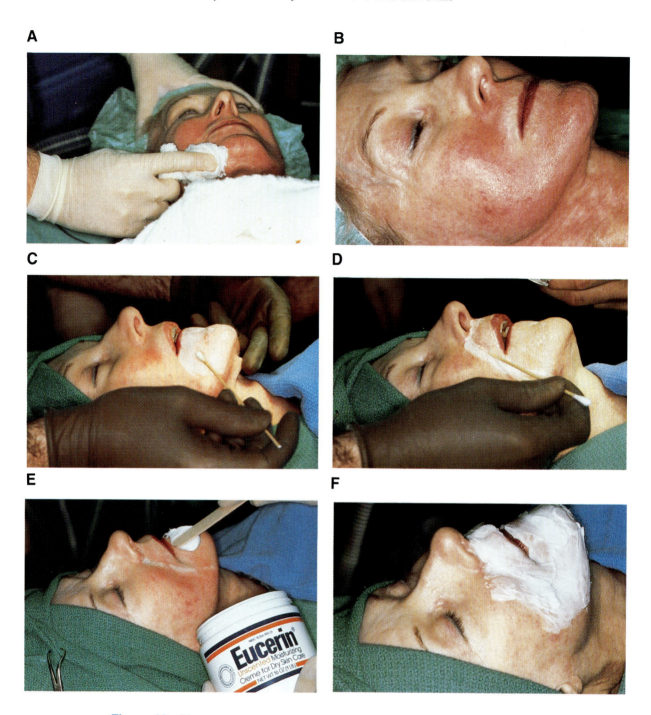

Figure 19–11
A, the perioral area is cleaned with acetone following Septisol preparation. **B**, the perioral area is now free of skin oils and surface debris and ready for the phenol peel. **C**, the peel solution is applied with a cotton-tipped applicator to the perioral unit. **D**, a pointed stick dipped in the peel solution is useful in the deeper nasolabial creases. **E**, Eucerin cream is applied to the treated facial unit. **F**, Eucerin cream is continued until reepithelialization is complete.

CHAPTER 19   Chemical Peel

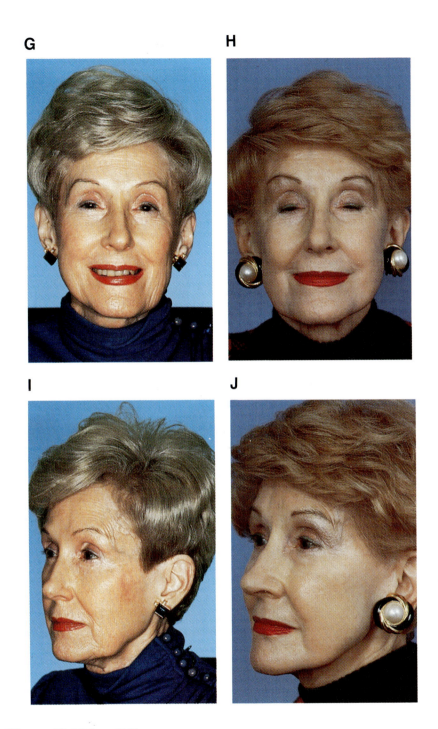

Figure 19-11 (cont'd.).
G, the pretreatment appearance of the patient reveals her to be an excellent candidate with pale skin color and multiple fine texture lines. **H,** the postoperative appearance shows good color match in addition to a smoother skin surface following the perioral peel. **I,** the pretreatment oblique view demonstrates chin, melolabial, and adjacent cheek rhytids. **J,** marked improvement in skin surface smoothing following the peel.

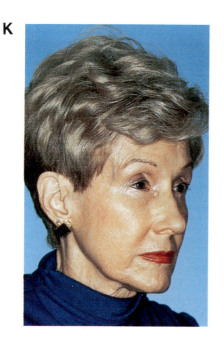
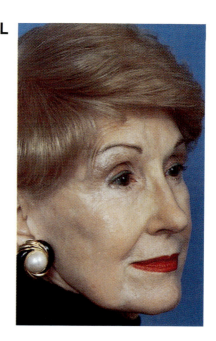

Figure 19-11 (cont'd).
K, the pretreatment opposite oblique view. **L,** the posttreatment appearance with smoother skin and a good color match.

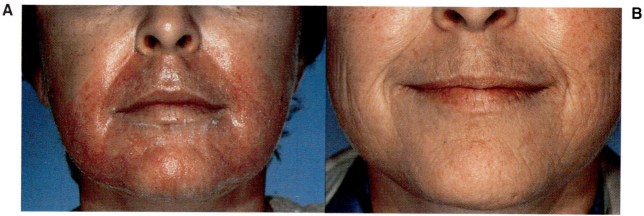
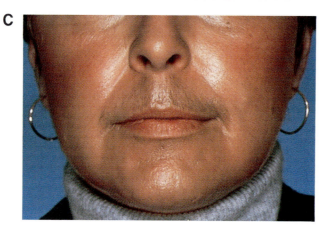

Figure 19-12
A, an "extended" perioral peel; appearance 10 days after treatment. **B,** the patient demonstrates perioral and lateral cheek rhytids prior to the face peel. **C,** the posttreatment appearance with elimination of rhytids and improvement in skin texture.

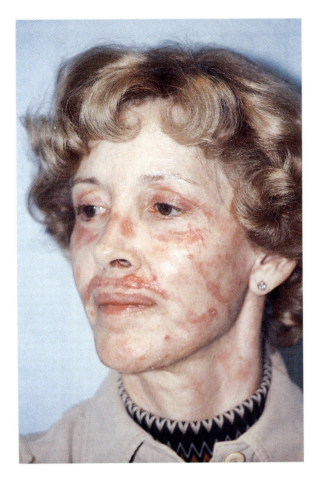

Figure 19–13
Severe facial scarring 4 months following a chemical peel by a highly capable surgeon. Scarring improved considerably over time with serial injections of intralesional corticosteroids.

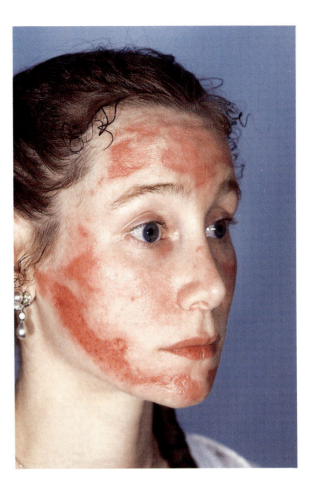

Figure 19–14
Persistent erythema and scarring at 6 months in a young patient treated elsewhere.

Complications and Sequelae

As noted, phenol is significantly cardiotoxic and may result in arrhythmias (although unlikely in the small amounts absorbed during a facial peel performed in the appropriate time frame). Patients with cardiac or renal insufficiency are poor candidates for this reason. Cardiac monitoring throughout the procedure is essential, and patients must be well hydrated throughout the procedure.

Permanent facial scarring has been reported with phenol peels (Figs 19–13 to 19–15). This appears to be more common along the mandibular line. Using the nontape technique may be helpful in avoiding scarring in that the penetration may be slightly less. A pebble-like thickening of the skin will develop in some patients 2 to 3 months after treatment, which seems to be more common in the forehead and malar regions.

Ectropion can occur from the periorbital peel. Patients with a laxity of the lower lid margin or who have undergone previous blepharoplasty should be treated extremely conservatively.

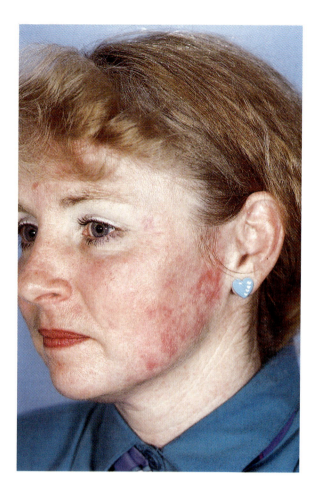

Figure 19–15
Unsightly persistent erythema and scarring 6 months following chemical peeling elsewhere.

Infection is unusual but a distinct possibility. Herpes simplex may be avoided in patients with a positive history by pretreatment with prophylactic acyclovir. *Staphloccus* and *Pseudomonas* infections have been reported and require prompt antibiotic therapy. Prompt skin care and cleansing during healing should help to avoid this. Toxic shock syndrome has been reported after a face peel, but this apparently is rare. Postoperative fever, hypotension, vomiting, and a possible scarlatina-form rash should alert the physician to this possibility.

Other more common problems are more accurately *sequelae* of the treatment and not true complications. All patients should anticipate bright pink erythematous skin for several months. This may be exacerbated by temperature, exercise, or emotional states. The erythema is usually well camouflaged with proper makeup application.

CHAPTER 19   Chemical Peel

Pigmentation changes of varying degrees occur in nearly all patients. The degree of change or hyperpigmentation vs. hypopigmentation is impossible to predict preoperatively. Most patients should expect some hypopigmentation to be present after the erythema stages resolve. Areas of blotchy pigmentation are more likely if the patient fails to use sun protection precautions the first 3 to 4 months posttreatment. As indicated earlier, estrogen medications or pregnancy may also affect pigmentation during this period. When hyperpigmentation does develop, hydroquinone (Eldoquin Forte) and tretinoin (Retin-A) cream have been of help. Another relatively common sequela is the formation of milia, not unlike those commonly seen after dermabrasion. Troublesome milia may be opened with a sterile needle or improved with daily use of a Buf-Puf. More generalized areas may benefit from topical Retin-A.

Patients must be counseled that deeper rhytids may only be improved and not eliminated. Persistent rhytids can be retreated with some success in 3 to 6 months. In the perioral area in particular, persistent individual rhytids may respond to a secondary "spot" dermabrasion.

After reduction of wrinkling following peeling, superficial telangiectasis may become more apparent. Electrocoagulation improves this undesirable sequela.

In summary, candidates for chemical peeling must be selected with all consummate skill to ensure safety and a satisfactory outcome. Because the surgeon cannot *exactly* control the precise depth of the peel and the patient's healing response, less control over the outcome occurs with this procedure than with any of the other facial rejuvenation procedures.

Suggested Reading

- Baker TJ, Gordon HL, Seckinger DL: A second look at chemical face peeling. *Plast Reconstr Surg* 1966; 37:487.
- Cortez EA: Chemical face peeling. *Otolaryngol Clin North Am* 1990; 23:947–962.
- Kligman AM, Baker TJ, Gordon HL: Long-term histologic follow-up of phenol face peels. *Plast Reconstr Surg* 1985; 75:652–659.
- Mandy SH, Landsman L: Dermabrasion and chemical peel, in Papel ID, Nachlas NE (eds): *Facial and Reconstructive Surgery*. St Louis, Mosby–Year Book, 1992, pp 198–207.

*'Tis not a lip or eye
we beauty call
But the joint force
and full result of all.*

Alexander Pope
An Essay on Criticism
1711

Index

A

Aesthetic augmentation procedures, 411–449
Aesthetic blepharoplasty, 223–293
Aesthetic face: proportions of, 129–131
Aesthetic surgery
  of face, 155–409
    ambivalence about, 14–17
    bilateral symmetry in, 4
    complications, 26–27
    education process, 17–20
    follow-up, extended, 25
    nature of, 3–51
    operating environment for, 53–62
    outcome prediction, 20–22
    outcomes, spectrum of, 5
    patient population, 12–14
    photography in (see Photography)
    planned elective, 8–11
    principles, 3–51
    principles, basic, 1–153
    selection of candidates for, 7
    sequelae, 26–27
    setting for, 23–24
    special characteristics, 8–11
    success, 20–22
    treatment plan, overall, 5
    uncertainty about, 14–17
  of neck, aging, 381–409
Aesthetics: analysis and judgment, 126–153
Aging
  brow, ptotic, 162
  changes
    early, in ideal female candidate for rejuvenation surgery, 12
    typical, 11
  characteristics, typical, in male, 13
  face, surgery of, 43–44
  of forehead, 159
  neck, aesthetic surgery of, 381–409
  patients, rhinoplasty in (see Rhinoplasty in aging patients)
  rhytids due to, 159
Alopecia: after forehead lift, 192
Ambivalence: about facial aesthetic surgery, 14–17
Analgesia, IV, 87–90
  monitoring, 90
  pharmacologic agents for, most useful and safe, 93
Analysis: aesthetics and judgment, 126–153
Anesthesia, 85–94
  for blepharoplasty, 241–244
  complications, 91–93
  for facelift, 318
  for forehead lift, 167
  IV, 87–90
    monitoring, 90
  for lipectomy of face and neck, 543
  monitoring, automated, 89
  for plastic surgery, 36
  for rhinoplasty, in midlife and aging patients, 484–486
  side effects, 91–93
Animation: causing rhytids, 159
Aspirin preparations, 16
Augmentation
  aesthetic augmentation procedures, 411–449
  chin (see Chin augmentation)
Auricular deformities: photography in, 122
Authorization, 48
Auto Micro-Nikkor: 105-mm, 109

B

Baker's peel solution, 583
Beautiful faces, 131
Beauty
  concepts of, 127–129
  in Renaissance painting, 128
Blemishes: of face, improving, 42–43
Blepharoplasty, 44, 223–293
  aesthetic, 223–293
  anatomic considerations, specific, 237–240
  anesthesia for, 241–244
  approaches, 244–248
  complications, postoperative, 291
  diagnosis, 227–233
  with forehead lift, coronal, 187
  incisions, 244–248
  instructions after, 51, 283
  outcome, 284–290
    planned, 233–236
  photography in, 122
  postoperative care, 281–283
  preoperative evaluation, 227–233
  results, 284–290
  sequelae, 290
  surgical goals, 233–236
  surgical techniques, 237–280
    alternative procedures, 275–280
    preferred techniques, 249–275
    upper lid, preferred techniques, 249–275
Botticelli's Venus, 128
Brevital, 93
Brow
  female, arching, 161
  lift, 45, 163, 209–221
    direct, 163
    with midforehead lift, 163
    surgical technique, 212–221
  male, normal position, 161
  ptosis, 186
    aging, 162
  sagging, correction, 45
Browplasty, midforehead, 181–185
  in male, 190
  surgical technique, 182–185

C

Camera for photography (see Photography, camera)
Catheter: silicone, 8 F, during intravenous sedation, 59
Chemical peel, 579–597
  Baker's peel solution, 583
  complications, 594–597
    severe, 29
  diagnosis, 580–581
  facial units, 586–588
  outcomes, 589–593
    planned, 581–582
    regional peels, 591–593
  postoperative care, 588
  results, 589–593
    regional peels, 591–593
  selection of candidate, 580–581
  sequelae, 594–597
  surgical goals, 581–582
  surgical technique, 583–588
Chin
  augmentation, 413–433
    complications, 430–432
    diagnosis, 414–417
    outcome, 427–429
    outcome, planned, 418–419
    results, 427–429
    selection of candidate, 414–417

Index

Chin—(cont.)
   sequelae, 430–432
   surgical goals, 418–419
   surgical technique, 419–426
double, correction, 45
implant, outcome, long-term, 15
overdeveloped, correction, 42
postoperative appearance at 5 years, 14
underdeveloped, correction, 42
Collagen augmentation, 46–47
Color slides: projected in operating room, 115
Compulsive-obsessive patient, 75–76
Consent: informed, 48
Consultation: for plastic surgery, 37
Corrugator muscles: in forehead lift, 169
Cost: of plastic surgery, 36–37

D

Depressed patient, 79–80
Depression: after facelift, 360
Dermabrasion, 43, 567–576
  anatomy, 569–570
  complications, 577
  diagnosis, 568–569
  outcomes, 575–576
  results, 575–576
  selection o candidate, 568–569
  surgical techniques, 569–574
Disclaimer form, 19
Discussions: with office personnel, 24
Disengagement: from patient, reasoned, 30–31
Disliking: the patient, 81–82
Droperidol, 93
  complications, 91
  side effects, 91

E

Ear: protruding, correction, 42
Education process: in facial aesthetic surgery, 17–20
Electronic lighting: for photography, 116–120
Equipment: for operating room, 58–60
Eyebrow (*see* Brow)
Eyelid (*see* Lid)
Eyelift: diary, 21–22

F

Face
  aesthetic, proportions of, 129–131
  aesthetic procedures, 155–409
  aging, surgery of, 43–44
  asymmetry, 6
  blemishes, improving, 42–43
  evaluation, 8
  lifting procedures, 155–409
  lipectomy (*see* Lipectomy of face)
  preoperative evaluation, 148–152
  scars, improving, 42–43
  surgery
    aesthetic (*see* Aesthetic surgery, of face)
    plastic (*see* Plastic surgery)
  units in chemical peel, 586–588
Facelift, 45–46, 295–362
  anatomic considerations, specific, 308–317
  anesthesia for, 318
  complications, 355–360
  depression after, 360
  diagnosis, 296–302
  goals of, 303
  hematoma after, 355–357
  infection after, 358
  instructions after, 50
  nerve damage in, 359
  outcome, 347–354
  results, 347–354
  revisional, 365–378
    complications, 378
    diagnosis, 366
    outcome, 374–377
    results, 374–377
    selection of candidate, 366
    sequelae, 378
    surgical goals, 367
    surgical techniques, 367–373
  scars after, poor, 360
  secondary, 46, 365–378
    complications, 378
    diagnosis, 366
    outcome, 374–377
    results, 374–377
    selection of candidate, 366
    sequelae, 378
    surgical goals, 367
    surgical techniques, 367–373
  selection of candidate, 296–302
  sequelae, 355–360
  surgical techniques, 304–354
    alternative techniques, 318–354
    preferred techniques, 318–354
Fat
  herniation of lower lid in 10 year old, 13
  in neck rejuvenation, 383
  submental, of neck (*see* Neck, submental fat)
Fees for plastic surgery (*see* Plastic surgery, fees for)
Fentanyl, 93
  complications, 91–92
  side effects, 91–92
Fiber-optic headlighting: for rejuvenation procedures, 60
Fillers, injectable (*see* Injectable fillers)
Film for photography, 112–116
  Kodachrome 25, 113
Finances: and plastic surgery, 36–37
Flumazenil, 93
Forehead
  aging of, 159
  lift, 157–193
    alopecia after, 192
    alternative techniques, 167–185
    anatomic considerations, 165
    anesthesia for, 167
    complications, 190–191
    coronal, 163
    coronal, forehead paralysis after, 191
    coronal, with blepharoplasty, 187
    corrugator muscles in, 169
    diagnosis, 158–163
    hematoma after, 192
    infection after, 192
    lagophthalmos after, 192
    outcomes, 186–190
    postoperative care principles, 186
    preferred techniques, 167–185
    pretrichal, 163, 173–174, 189
    pretrichal, surgical technique, 174
    procerus muscle in, 170
    results, 186–190
    scalp scar after, 192
    selection of candidate, 158–163
    sequelae, 190–191
    surgical goals, 164–165
    surgical techniques, 165–186
  midforehead (*see* Midforehead)
  paralysis after forehead lift, coronal, 191

Index

ptosis, 186
rhytidosis, improvement of, 188
rhytids, hypertonicity of frontalis muscle producing, 166
Form: disclaimer, 19
Frankfort horizontal plane, 101
Frontalis muscle, hypertonicity of, 150, 162
rhytids produced by, 166

G

Glabella
rhytidosis, improvement in, 188
rhytids in, 160

H

Hair: problems in photography, 104–105
Hand of patient: held during procedure, 58
Head positioning: for photography, 101
Headlighting: fiber-optic, for rejuvenation surgery, 60
Hematoma
after facelift, 355–357
after forehead lift, 192
Herniation: fat, of lower lid in 10 year old, 13
Historian, patient as
careless, 78
poor, 78
Hospital
based operating room, 54–55
operating suite, 55
Hyoid-thyroid complex location: in neck rejuvenation, 384
Hypertonicity of frontalis muscle, 150, 162
rhytids produced by, 166

I

Imagined deformity: patient with, 77–78
Indecisive patient, 76
Infection
after facelift, 358
after forehead lift, 192
Informed consent, 48
Initial encounter: with patient, personal approach, 66–74
Injectable fillers, 435–449
complications, 447–449
diagnosis in, 437
goals of, 437–438
outcome, 440–446
planned, 437–438
results, 440–446
selection of candidate in, 437
sequelae, 447–449
technique, 438–440
test dose injection, 438
treatment injection technique, 438–440
Instructions
after blepharoplasty, 51
after facelift, 50
after nasal plastic surgery, 49

J

Judgment: aesthetics and analysis, 126–153

K

Kodachrome 25, 113

L

Lagophthalmos: after forehead lift, 192
Lenses: for photography, 109–110
Lid
lower, fat herniation, familial, in 10 year old, 13
plastic surgery, 44
surgery, instructions after, 51
upper, blepharoplasty, preferred techniques, 249–275
Lifting procedures: for face, 155–409
Lighting: electronic, for photography, 116–120
Lipectomy of face and neck, 529–563
anatomy, 539–542
anesthesia for, 543
complications, 562–563
diagnosis, 532–533
outcomes, 555–561
planned, 534–538
preoperative evaluation, 538–539
results, 555–561
selection of candidate, 532–533
sequelae, 562–563
suction lipectomy, isolated, 544–554
surgical goals, 534–538
surgical technique, 538–561
technique, 544–554
Litigation: patient involved in, 81

M

Mandibular length: in neck rejuvenation, 384
Mazicon, 93
Mentoplasty, 42
photography in, 122
Methohexital, 93
Midazolam, 93
Midforehead
browplasty, 181–185
in male, 190
surgical technique, 182–185
lift, 163, 175–180
with brow lift, 163
surgical technique, 176–180
Midlife, rhinoplasty in (see Rhinoplasty in midlife)
Minimal deformity: patient with, 77–78
Monitoring
of analgesia, IV, 90
of anesthesia
automated, 89
IV, 90
Motor drive: for photography, 110, 111
Muscle
corrugator, in forehead lift, 169
frontalis, hypertonicity of, 150, 162
rhytids produced by, 166
platysma, in neck rejuvenation, 384
procerus, in forehead lift, 170
Music console: used during surgery, 57

N

Nasal (see Nose)
Nasopharynx: oxygen to, during intravenous sedation, 59
Neck
aging, aesthetic surgery of, 381–409
lipectomy (see Lipectomy of face and neck)
rejuvenation, 383–400
complications, 400
diagnosis, 383–388
fat in, 383
hyoid-thyroid complex location in, 384
mandibular length in, 384
outcome, planned, 388–395
platysma muscle in, 384

Neck (cont.)
  postoperative care, 396–399
  selection of candidate, 383–388
  sequelae, 400
  skin in, 383
  SMAS in, 383
  surgical goals, 388–395
  submental fat and skin resection combined, 400–408
    complications, 408
    diagnosis, 400–401
    outcome, 404–407
    outcome, planned, 401–402
    results, 404–407
    selection of candidate, 400–401
    sequelae, 408
    surgical goals, 401–402
    surgical technique, 402–403
Nerve damage: in facelift, 359
Nose
  plastic surgery, instructions after, 49, 508
  postoperative appearance at 5 years, 14
  rhinoplasty (see Rhinoplasty)
  root, rhytids in, 160
Nurse: surgical, relationship with patient, 68

O

Obsessive-compulsive patient, 75–76
Office
  based operating facility, 54–55
  personnel, discussions with, 24
  photography, 100
    ideal, space required for, 123
    suite, 122–123
Operating
  environment for facial aesthetic surgery, 53–62
  room
    color slides projected in, 115
    equipment, 58–60
    hospital-based vs. office-based, 54–55
    imaged projected on wall of, greater-than-life-size, 61
    personnel, medical, 60–62
    physical surroundings, 56–58
  suite, hospital, 55
Orbit: aesthetic unit, 131
Otoplasty, 42
  photography in, 122
Overflattering patient, 77
Overly familiar patient, 77

Oximeter: pulse, 58
Oxygen: to nasopharynx during intravenous sedation, 59

P

Paralysis: forehead, after forehead lift, coronal, 191
Perfectionist patient, 75–76
Personnel
  medical, for operating room, 60–62
  office, discussions with, 24
Photographs: of patient, preoperative analysis, 9
Photography, 95–123
  in auricular deformities, 122
  background for, 105–107
  basal views, 103
  in blepharoplasty, 122
  camera
    Auto Micro-Nikkor, 105-mm, 109
    body, 108
    single lens reflex 35-mm, 108
  data-back, 112
  f-stops for ideal aperture setting, 121
  film, 112–116
    Kodachrome 25, 113
  hair problems in, 104–105
  head positioning for, 101
  head positions for shadow-free photographs, 119
  lenses for, 109–110
  lighting for, electronic, 116–120
  in mentoplasty, 122
  midsagittal plane in, 102
  motor drive, 110, 111
  oblique view, 103
  office, 100
    ideal, space required for, 123
    suite, 122
  in otoplasty, 122
  patient positioning, 100
    swivel stool for, 100
  preoperative, standard and uniform, 97
  in rhinoplasty, 122
  in rhytidoplasty, 122
  in submentoplasty, 122
  uniform, 95–123
Plastic surgeon, 35
Plastic surgery, 33–47
  anesthesia for, 36
  consultation for, 37
  cost of, 36–37
  of face, 33–47
    definition, 34–35
    facts and fiction, 34–37

fees for, 38
  consultation, 38
  surgical, 38
finances, 36–37
guiding principles, 35–36
of nose, instructions after, 49, 508
outpatient, 37–38
postoperative care, 38
realistic attitude toward, 38–39
risks of, 47
"Plastic surgiholic," 80
Platysma muscle: in neck rejuvenation, 384
Polaroid prints, 115, 117
Premedication, 87
Preoperative
  analysis of patient photographs, 9
  facial evaluation, 148–152
Price haggler: patient as, 80–81
Procerus muscle: in forehead lift, 170
Proportions: of aesthetic face, 129–131
Psychological assessment, 65–83
  initial encounter, personal approach, 66–74
Ptosis
  brow, 186
    aging, 162
  forehead, 186
Pulse oximeter, 58

R

Recovery area: "step-down," 62
Rejection of candidate for aesthetic surgery, 74–82
Rejuvenation
  adjunctive procedures, 565–597
  of neck (see Neck rejuvenation)
  surgery
    aging change, early, in ideal female candidate, 12
    headlighting for, fiber-optic, 60
    of lower lid fat herniation, familial, in 10 year old, 13
    scars after, 27
Renaissance painting: beauty in, 128
Rhinoplasty, 39–41
  in aging patients, 451–527
    anatomic considerations, 476–482
    anesthesia for, 484–486
    complications, 525
    diagnosis, 454–462
    operative sequence, 483–484

outcomes, evaluation, 509–524
outcomes, planned, 469–475
postoperative care, 507–508
principles, general and specific, 469–475
results evaluation, 509–524
selection of candidate, 454–462
sequelae, 525
surgical goals, 469–475
surgical techniques, 476–507
surgical techniques, preferred and alternative techniques, 506
in midlife, 451–527
anatomic considerations, 476–482
anesthesia for, 484–486
complications, 525
diagnosis, 454–462
evaluating midlife patients, assessing needs, 463–468
operative sequence, 483–484
outcomes, evaluation, 509–524
outcomes, planned, 469–475
postoperative care, 507–508
principles, general and specific, 469–475
results evaluation, 509–524
selection of candidate, 454–462
sequelae, 525
surgical goals, 469–475
surgical techniques, 476–507
surgical techniques, preferred and alternative techniques, 486–506
photography in, 122
postoperative care, 41
preliminary steps to, 40–41
Rhytidoplasty, 45–46

photography in, 122
Rhytidosis
forehead, improvement in, 188
glabella, improvement in, 188
Rhytids
aging, animation and excessive sun exposure causing, 159
forehead, hypertonicity of frontalis muscle producing, 166
in glabella, 160
in nasal root, 160
Rude patient, 76–77

S

Scalp scar: in forehead lift, 192
Scars, 27
camouflage, 42–43
facial, improving, 42–43
poor, after facelift, 360
scalp, in forehead lift, 192
Sedation: IV, silicone catheter, 8 F, for oxygen to nasopharynx during, 59
Setting: for facial aesthetic surgery, 23–24
Shopper: surgeon shopper, 79
Silicone catheter: 8 F, during intravenous sedation, 59
Skin
in neck rejuvenation, 383
resection with submental fat, of neck (see Neck, submental fat and skin resection combined)
SMAS: in neck rejuvenation, 383
Stool: swivel, for positioning during photography, 100
Submentoplasty, 45
photography in, 122

"Sudden whim" patient, 76
Sun exposure: excessive, causing rhytids, 159
Surgeon
plastic, 35
shopper, 79
Symmetry: bilateral, in facial aesthetic surgery, 4

T

Talkative patient: overly talkative, 79
Temporal lift, 163, 195–206
outcomes, 202–206
results, 202–206
surgical technique, 198–202
Thyroid-hyoid complex location: in neck rejuvenation, 384

U

Uncertainty: about facial aesthetic surgery, 14–17
Uncooperative patient, 78–79
Unkempt patient, 77
Unrealistic expectations: patient with, 75

V

Versed, 93
"VIP" patient, 78

W

Waiting room, 23

Z

Zyderm augmentation, 46–47